MEDICINE AND HEALING PRACTICES IN ANCIENT EGYPT

MEDICINE AND HEALING PRACTICES IN ANCIENT EGYPT

ROSALIE DAVID

AND

ROGER FORSHAW

LIVERPOOL UNIVERSITY PRESS

First published 2023 by
Liverpool University Press
4 Cambridge Street
Liverpool
L69 7ZU

This paperback edition published 2025

British Library Cataloguing-in-Publication data
A British Library CIP record is available

ISBN 978-1-83764-429-2 (hardback)
ISBN 978-1-83624-524-7 (paperback)

Typeset by Carnegie Book Production, Lancaster
Printed and bound by CPI Group (UK) Ltd, Croydon CR0 4YY

Cover image: Painted wooden coffin of Asru. Late Period. Probably from Thebes, now in the Manchester Museum, The University of Manchester, 1777 (courtesy of the Manchester Museum, The University of Manchester). Images of instruments/implements on the enclosure wall of the Temple of Kom Ombo. Graeco-Roman Period. Redrawn by K. N. White after Nunn (1996: fig. 8.2).

Contents

Illustrations

Figures

Colour plates

Acknowledgements

We would like to thank Dr Campbell Price, Curator of Egypt and Sudan, The Manchester Museum, The University of Manchester, and Dr Anna Garnett, Curator of the Petrie Museum of Egyptian and Sudanese Archaeology, University College London, for providing access to study items in their collections.

We are grateful that it has been possible to illustrate the book with a wide range of images from a variety of sources. We would like to thank Dr Keith White and Mrs Libby Mulqueeny for their skilful production of the line drawings. The photographic credits are included in the individual illustration captions and we particularly wish to thank the following for granting permission to use their images: Dr Campbell Price and The Manchester Museum, The University of Manchester; Dr Anna Garnett and the Petrie Museum of Egyptian and Sudanese Archaeology, University College London; Dr Otto Sosztarits and the Savaria Museum – Iseum Savariense, Szombothely, Hungary; Dr Keith White, The University of Manchester; Dr Anna Loprieno Gnirs, Department of Ancient Civilization, University of Basel; Professor Aidan Dodson, University of Bristol; and the KNH Centre for Biomedical Egyptology, The University of Manchester.

We are grateful to Dr Keith White, Honorary Senior Lecturer, The University of Manchester, and Dr Christopher Gardner-Thorpe, Course Director, The Royal Society of Medicine, London, for their very helpful and insightful comments on the manuscript.

Rosalie David is very grateful to Dr Hedvig Györy of the Vámbéry Ármin Oriental Academy, Budapest, for arranging a personal visit to the Iseum Savariense in Szombothely and facilitating the opportunity to meet the director of the site excavation, Dr Otto Sosztarits.

Multidisciplinary research in Egyptology now encompasses history, archaeology, art, language studies and, more recently, scientific and biomedical investigation. This approach is providing new insights into disease and healing practices, and we have alluded to many of these studies in this book. We would like to acknowledge the contribution that our colleagues on the Manchester

Egyptian Mummy Project (as well as many other researchers) have made in this field over the past fifty years.

Finally, we very much appreciate the advice and support provided by Claire Litt of Liverpool University Press throughout the production process, and the Press's reviewer for helpful suggestions. Also, many thanks to Sarah Davison and her team at Carnegie Book Production for producing the book.

Rosalie David and Roger Forshaw
KNH Centre for Biomedical Egyptology, The University of Manchester

Chronology

Predynastic Period	***c.*** **5300–3000 BC**
Early Dynastic Period	***c.*** **3000–2686 BC**
1st Dynasty	*c.* 3000–2890
2nd Dynasty	2890–2686
Old Kingdom	**2686–2160 BC**
3rd Dynasty	2686–2613
4th Dynasty	2613–2494
5th Dynasty	2494–2345
6th Dynasty	2345–2181
7th & 8th Dynasties	2181–2160
First Intermediate Period	**2160–2055 BC**
9th & 10th Dynasties	2160–2025
11th Dynasty (*Thebes only*)	2125–2055
Middle Kingdom	**2055–1650 BC**
11th Dynasty	2055–1985
12th Dynasty	1985–1773
13th Dynasty	1773–after 1650
14th Dynasty	1773–1650
(*Minor rulers contemporary with 13th or 15th Dynasty*)	
Second Intermediate Period	**1650–1550 BC**
15th Dynasty (*Hyksos*)	1650–1550
16th Dynasty	1650–1580

(Theban rulers contemporary with the 15th Dynasty)	
17th Dynasty	*c.* 1580–1550
New Kingdom	**1550–1069 BC**
18th Dynasty	1550–1295
19th Dynasty	1295–1186
20th Dynasty	1186–1069
Third Intermediate Period	**1069–664 BC**
21st Dynasty	1069–945
22nd Dynasty	945–715
23rd Dynasty	818–715
(Kings in various centres, contemporary with the later 22nd, 24th and early 25th dynasties)	
24th Dynasty	727–715
25th Dynasty	747–656
Late Period	**664–332 BC**
26th Dynasty	664–525
27th Dynasty (*1st Persian Period*)	525–404
28th Dynasty	404–399
29th Dynasty	399–380
30th Dynasty	380–343
2nd Persian Period	343–332
Ptolemaic Period	**332–30 BC**
Roman Period	**30 BC–AD 395**

Chronology based on Shaw 2000.

1

Introduction to Egyptian concepts of disease and medical ethics

(a) Basic concepts of healing

A new perspective on healthcare in ancient Egypt

Medicine was practised from early times in Egypt and Mesopotamia, two great contemporary centres of civilisation. The first extant textual evidence of healing treatments is recorded in cuneiform script on clay tablets towards the end of the 3rd millennium BC (Geller 2010: 27), but there may have been an equally early Egyptian tradition that has not survived because it was recorded on papyrus, a far less robust writing material.

Previous studies on ancient Egyptian medicine have generally categorised and described diseases and medical conditions identified in textual, iconographic, archaeological and palaeopathological sources. These include medical papyri and archaeological evidence from buildings, tomb reliefs, physicians' stelae (inscribed tombstones), votive offerings, surgical instruments and equipment owned by magico-medical practitioners, as well as human skeletal and mummified remains.

This book takes a different, innovative approach, considering the subject afresh from the perspective of both the healing professionals who delivered medical and related treatments and the patients who were the recipients of this care. We provide an overview of the background to healthcare provision, looking at concepts of disease and medical ethics and how these underpinned methods of diagnosis and treatment. We also consider the effects of geographical, environmental and dietary factors upon the general health of the population.

Healers and care providers were essential to the Egyptian medical system and provided a wide range of healing methods. Certain types of healthcare training and practice developed simultaneously in various locations, including temples, palaces, towns and villages, battlefields and building sites. Surgery, pharmaceutical therapy and magico-religious treatments were available that made use of bandages and splints, medical instruments, prostheses and pharmaceutical prescriptions. We consider the training and individual roles of the various groups of healers, and their interaction with each other and with their patients. We assess their contribution, knowledge and expertise, and the extent to which the various treatments were efficacious.

Some questions that explore the patients' perspective are also considered: what was it like to be ill, deformed or disabled? What particular health concerns were encountered by women, infants and children? Were there obvious differences in the medical conditions found in royalty, the elite and the rest of the population, and what treatments did they receive?

This 'people-focused' approach tries to identify and explain the Egyptians' perception of illness and disability and their worthy attitude towards overcoming both physical and mental afflictions. It also addresses particular dangers encountered by certain groups: for example, the trauma, wounds and exposure to epidemics experienced by soldiers, and conditions including blindness, sand pneumoconiosis, trauma and amputations suffered by builders and other workers.

In conclusion, we briefly compare the Egyptian healthcare system and its achievements with medicine practised in contemporary societies in Mesopotamia, Greece and Rome, and summarise the contribution made by Egyptian medicine, via Greek, Roman and Arabic sources, to the principles and practice of modern 'Western' medicine.

Although this book has attempted to address the subject of ancient Egyptian medicine across an extensive timescale (from predynastic times down to the Graeco-Roman era), there is considerable variation in the availability of extant evidence across the whole period. A Chronological Table (pp. xvi–xvii) identifies the various divisions that Egyptologists use as a time-frame when discussing Egyptian history. Generally, the volume of evidence for some of these – such as the Old, Middle and New Kingdoms, and the Graeco-Roman era – is much greater than for, for instance, the predynastic, First, Second and Third Intermediate Periods, and the Late Period.

Current knowledge of ancient Egyptian medicine mirrors this general imbalance of historical evidence, and this is reflected in the extent and depth to which we have been able to describe and discuss various subjects in this book. However, wherever possible, we have drawn on examples from across the millennia, indicating the spread and scope of the medical system and providing some idea of how it was inextricably integrated into the general fabric of society.

Empirico-rational therapies and magico-religious actions

A variety of approaches and treatment strategies was undertaken to cope with infirmities. These combined magico-religious principles with scientific practices that have been the subject of an extensive literature (Grapow *et al.* 1954–1973; Jonckheere 1958; Ghalioungui 1963, 1980, 1983, 1987; Majno 1975; Worth Estes

1993; Bardinet 1995; Filer 1995; Weeks 1995; Nunn 1996; Ebeid 1999; Halioua & Ziskind 2005; Strouhal *et al.* 2014, 2021).

Some previous discussions on healing practices have attempted to distinguish between empirico-rational therapies and magico-religious actions. However, in ancient Egypt these were equally valid parts of a complex cultural system and complementary to each other; healers would have been unlikely to have actively distinguished between them when treating a sick member of the community (Weeks 1995: 1787; Ritner 2001a: 326). A more recent approach, drawing on medical anthropological studies relating to contemporary healing systems in Africa, Asia and Latin America, has discarded terms such as 'rational' and 'irrational' in relation to all healing practices (Wall 1988: 284–336) on the basis that these terms distort our understanding of ancient Egyptian medical practices by viewing them through a 'presentist' lens.

An alternative approach is to consider any medical system from the different starting principles upon which its therapeutics are based. Once a particular set of principles is accepted, any magical practices included in that system cannot be regarded as 'irrational' because they flow naturally and logically from the underlying assumptions. The treatments are not meaningless rites but derive from an individual society's beliefs concerning the causation of disease. From the viewpoint of modern Western medicine, this attribution of disease causation is sometimes erroneous, but the ancient healing methods relating to diagnosis and treatment were nevertheless logically derived from those basic assumptions, and therefore were not 'irrational' in those societies.

This raises questions about complex issues: for example, were magical treatments effective (see section below) and how this can be measured? And, if they were viable, why did they work (pers. comm. L. L. Wall)? Detailed consideration of such issues lies outside the scope of this book, but nevertheless it can be acknowledged that the Egyptians perceived two types of medical condition broadly distinguished by a causative agent, and generally treated their patients accordingly. No terminology is wholly acceptable, but, to discuss diseases and treatments without using the outdated terms of 'rational' and 'irrational', we have chosen to describe the conditions and therapies as either 'empirico-rational'/'pragmatic' or 'magico-religious', while realising that these categories worked in tandem.

Magical rites and the placebo effect

The basic concept that underpinned all magico-religious procedures in ancient Egypt is aptly described in the definition of magic given in *The Oxford Learner's Dictionary*: 'The secret power of appearing to make impossible things happen by saying special words or doing special things.'

The ability to perform magic and control events was vested in the gods, who conveyed these supernatural powers to the king, who in turn delegated them to the healing practitioners. They believed that their principal aim, to expel evil spirits from the patient, could be achieved by adding certain substances to their prescriptions: either disagreeable ingredients such as urine and excrement, that would repel the disease-causing spirits, or pulverised precious stones or special metals that would attract benign spirits and thus enhance patients' well-being.

The magical procedure usually incorporated three elements: the incantation, the magician who would recite this spell and the ritual, which sometimes accompanied the procedure and either took place in the presence of the patient or was enacted on a figurine or representation/depiction of the patient. It was believed that with this performance the healer could influence patients' mental state and change their physical condition.

Sometimes the treatment was accompanied by music and dancing, or the magician would incorporate auxiliary agents (water, wine, oil, perfumes and incense) into the rites to achieve the desired effect. Amulets and *cippi* were also thought to have magical potency and played an important part in rituals. The *cippus* was a statue–stelae usually inscribed with anti-venom spells. Its purpose was to guard its possessor against supernatural creatures in animal or reptile form, and it could either repel attacks by vile creatures such as snakes, scorpions or crocodiles, or heal someone who had been bitten (Pinch 2006: 100). Amulets were special items of jewellery attributed with the ability to confer magical protection on the wearer (Pinch 2006: 105) (see Plate 2). It was believed that their shapes, forms and materials were imbued with the power to protect and preserve the owner in this world and in the afterlife. Sometimes they took the form of animals, whose strengths and qualities of survival could be absorbed by the owner; or they represented individual symbols, including the *wedjat*-eye (wholeness) or the *ankh*-sign (eternal life), which would attract benign influences; or they were images of protective deities such as Sekhmet, Bes or Beset.

It is unlikely that magico-religious remedies recorded in the medical papyri would have contributed any direct or practical therapeutic benefit to the patient. However, they continued to be a significant feature of a healthcare system that was highly regarded over the millennia both in Egypt and in neighbouring lands. It is unlikely that these remedies would have continued to be used if they were ineffectual and it is possible that they produced a favourable placebo effect in at least some patients, perhaps explaining why they continued to be regarded as successful treatments for some conditions.

(b) Disease: concepts of causation and methods of treatment

The healing practitioners: complementary therapies and patient choices

Medical papyri and other documentation indicate that a close association existed between pragmatic and magical therapies. Spells, amulets, healing statues, sanctified water, dream revelation and pragmatic measures were all regarded as acceptable, valid and efficacious healing methods.

The main categories of healing practitioners were the *swnw* (physicians), priests of Sekhmet, priests of Serket, lectors (lector priests), *s3w* (magicians) and 'wise women' (Ghalioungui 1983: 1–15; Worth Estes 1993: 13–27; Nunn 1996: 113; Halioua & Ziskind 2005: 1). Textual and archaeological sources confirm that links existed between these various groups (see Chapter 2c).

Although there is no detailed record of how community practitioners interacted with temple priests, there is ample evidence that both were involved with healing. For example, the Tebtunis Papyri demonstrate that temple personnel were closely associated with medicine and healing (see Chapter 3a). There is no evidence of rivalry between the groups, and a passage in one of the medical papyri, P. Ebers (854a), confirms that different treatments might be attempted to achieve a cure. The sources do not confirm whether a patient had freedom to choose a particular pathway of treatment with one type of healer or if the practitioners would have advised on the best route, perhaps based on their joint diagnosis of the cause of the problem.

Political events towards the end of the Old Kingdom appear to have started the processes of devolution and decentralisation of power from the capital city, Mennefer (Memphis) to the provincial districts, but it is unclear whether this had any impact on the pattern of medical provision across the country. Some evidence suggests that the Priests of Sekhmet increased their presence and influence in the provincial districts during the Middle Kingdom (see Chapter 2b). However, although this may have meant that the priests' expertise in medicine and healing became more widely available to provincial rulers and the elite in these districts, it probably did not benefit lower-status patients and does not necessarily imply that any real democratisation of medical care occurred at this time.

A few instances in the medical papyri identify that particular categories of healer administered certain medicaments. In P. Berlin 3038 three prescriptions mention a lector as such an individual (see Chapter 2c). Inscriptions on various stelae and tombs indicate that some healers possessed a number of these titles. For example, some Priests of Sekhmet also carried a physician's title, suggesting a transfer of knowledge among the named professional groups. The healer could have the knowledge and experience to act as a *swnw* or a *s3w* and so there is perhaps no real need to separate the kinds of treatment each would provide. Irenakhty from the Old Kingdom/First Intermediate Period and Psamtekseneb from the Saite

Period were *swnw* who also carried the title of priest or controller of Serket (*ḫrp srkt*) (Nunn 1996: 120). The funerary stela of Nefer (Clandeboye collection), who practised medicine during the reign of Tuthmosis I (1504–1492 BC; 18th Dynasty), described him as a Priest of Sekhmet and a *swnw* (Halioua & Ziskind 2005: 11).

In addition, the medical title was often not an individual's exclusive occupation or specialisation, as many of the healers carried additional titles. Some were scribes and, particularly in the Old Kingdom, individuals carried numerous titles encompassing a wide range of responsibilities. It is difficult to determine how much of their careers was spent in the performance of healing practices.

Causation of disease and symptomatic diagnosis

One key problem in attempting to examine the role of healers and healing is the extent and quality of the evidence available and the manner in which this evidence has been interpreted. Analysing the past in terms of modern concepts can be misleading and interpretations need to be based on understandings known to be prevalent at that particular period of history. Consequently, to explore the perception and concepts of healing in ancient Egypt it is first necessary to examine beliefs about the causation of illness.

Like other ancient societies, the Egyptians interpreted the experienced world according to patterns of knowledge that differ from those of the modern Western world. Supernatural powers were regarded as major controlling influences in the course of daily life. These included phenomena such as changing weather patterns and the annual flooding of the river Nile, as well as the causation of disease. Illness could be instigated by a variety of agents – malevolent spirits or powers that included not only the deities but also living and dead persons and animals.

The Egyptians' concept of healing was closely allied to their understanding of the causes of ill-health. It was assumed that everyone was born healthy, and every affliction was usually assessed and treated according to its perceived cause. In cases where the physical cause was evident, as with fractured bones, practical measures including bone setting were used. Where the cause was not apparent – for example, with fevers – the condition was attributed to supernatural forces – vengeance of the dead, divine punishment or human malevolence. Magico-religious therapies were usually chosen to treat these afflictions.

However, magic was also sometimes used for minor burns and snake and scorpion bites even when the cause was evident and the condition would have responded to pragmatic treatment. Physicians, probably aware that the venom or toxic material from a sting or bite could cause severe symptoms and even death, treated the patient with local treatments, usually involving a bandage to retain a specified local medication, pharmaceutical remedies and magical incantations (Nunn 1996: 188–89).

In the case of a traumatic injury, a wound or a bite, the agent was the actual perpetrator of the injury, but for a disease the agent was personified as a so-called 'disease-demon' (as termed by Nunn 1996: 96). Sometimes these demons were transmitted by malignant spirits who travelled on the wind and entered the victim through external orifices such as the mouth, nose or a break in the skin (Walker 1990). Once they had penetrated, the body would release excretory products that acted as 'illness inducing substances', which then damaged the tissues and caused symptoms. They also took the form of insects, especially flies, or pests that lurked in food, bedding and household articles. A set of miscellaneous spells added later to P. Edwin Smith includes three incantations intended to exorcise an annual plague or pestilence (Breasted 1930: 469–85; Allen 2005: 107). This one provided protection against the pest-laden atmosphere:

> Another (incantation) for exorcising the plague-bearing wind, the demons of disease, the malignant spirits, messengers of Sekhmet. Withdraw, ye disease demons. The wind shall not reach me, that those who pass by may pass by to make disaster against me … . (P. Edwin Smith verso, incantation 2, XVIII: 11–13; translated Breasted 1930: 502)

Such an understanding is not too far removed from modern interpretations of the transmission of certain diseases. However, lacking any conception of modern theories of disease processes, the Egyptians considered the agents who were responsible to be demons rather than bacteria or viruses. They accredited their spells with the magical potency to exorcise and destroy such disease-causing agents.

In today's world we tend to group a range of linked symptoms together and categorise them as a condition – diabetes, the common cold, gout, cancer. The ancient Egyptians lacked a specific concept of individual diseases or any all-encompassing categorising term, and the medical papyri (which sometimes pose translational difficulties: see below) refer only to selected symptoms (Pommerening 2020: 382). Nevertheless, although healers customarily treated individual symptoms, P. Edwin Smith provides examples where they were sometimes considered together in groups (syndromes) rather than in isolation. This demonstrates that the Egyptian physicians were aware of this significant advance in medical thought long before the Greeks, to whom it is usually attributed.

Physiological concepts: the *metu* and *wekhedu*

The *metu* (*mtw*, singular *mt*) were a key feature of Egyptian physiology. Regarded as essential to life and well-being, they dominated many aspects of medicine, and they and their connections are discussed in some of the medical papyri (Nunn

1996: 44–46; Lang 2013: 112–14). The word *metu* appears to have different meanings in various contexts in the medical papyri, but they were essentially bodily conduits that met at the heart (regarded as the seat of thought and emotions) and the anus. Egypt's geography, with its network of subsidiary canals centred on the Nile, possibly provided the model for this strange concept of human physiology. They included blood vessels, various ducts and nerves, and occasionally tendons and muscles, or 'string-like cords'. Depending on function and origin, references in the papyri specify what is transported via these vessels: blood, air, mucus, urine, faeces, tears and semen. The *metu* could become blocked or overwhelmed by too much transported substance, such that obstructions could result in 'floods' and 'droughts' within the body, which caused illness. P. Ebers 854L describes a condition in which the *metu* supplying the liver caused pain and symptoms: 'There are four vessels to the liver. They are the ones that give it [the liver] water and air and they are those in the last analysis that cause all pains to appear in it through overflooding with blood' (translated Ghalioungui 1987: 230). More intangible bodies – the breath of life, disease-bearing entities and spirits – also passed through the *metu*. The heart is described in more than one text as 'speaking' through each *metu*, which may be a reference to the pulse (see Chapter 2).

The Egyptians also recognised the harm that a substance referred to as *wekhedu* (*wḫdw*) could cause to the bodily structures. The nature of *wekhedu*, a word not defined in the ancient medical texts, is uncertain, but the ancient Egyptians considered that it could arise in open wounds or originate from the faeces and then spread throughout the body via the *metu*. Many scholars have attempted to define or explain exactly what the term referred to, but have not reached any general agreement on this. Expressions including 'purulency', 'pain', 'morbid principle' and 'putrefaction' have been used, but the word is often left untranslated (Nunn 1996: 61).

Medical ethics

The sources demonstrate an ethical awareness and concern for all patients. For example, P. Edwin Smith provides a prognosis of recovery, probable recovery or uncertain outcome for each case. Even when the patient was unlikely to survive, careful examination and assessment were still carried out, and the physician recommended a suitable programme of palliative care.

The Egyptians' perception and treatment of deformity and disability differed markedly from attitudes prevalent in most contemporary societies (see Chapters 5d, 6e; David 2017a). In some early communities, infant deformity was regarded as a disease or a sign of divine retribution, and the babies were exposed to the elements to die. There is no evidence that the Egyptians ever felt this way: tests in the medical papyri to assess the viability of neonates do not include criteria for deciding the fate of deformed infants, and the first known mention of infant exposure in ancient Egypt occurs in a letter dating to the Graeco-Roman Period that relates to the resident Greek population (West 1998).

Remuneration

Extant evidence regarding the remuneration of healing practitioners is scarce, but suggests that the *swnw* received their salaries from the state, particularly those who were attached to the palace, the king or the necropolis, as well as those assigned to teams of quarry workmen, ship crews or military expeditions (Ghalioungui 1983: 96). Diodorus Siculus, a Greek historian writing about ancient Egypt in the 1st century BC, describes physicians as public employees: 'On their military campaigns and their journeys in the country they all receive treatment without the payment of any private fee; for the physicians draw their support from public funds and administer their treatments in accordance with a written law which was composed in ancient times by many famous physicians' (Siculus 1. 82).

The *swnw* could also treat patients other than those identified by the state and in such circumstances received additional private payments, as attested, for example, in *ostraca* (sing. *ostracon* – a limestone flake or pottery sherd used as a writing/drawing surface) found at Deir el-Medina, near Thebes (Austin 2014: 92). There is some evidence that relative values were placed on professional services: in one example that records the payments made by a workman in respect of his wife's confinement, the goods the wet-nurse was to receive were of a higher value than those received by the physician. This may imply that the services of the wet-nurse were considered more important than the physician's contribution, or perhaps her higher payment may reflect a longer involvement with the family (Janssen & Janssen 2007: 15). This document seems to indicate that physicians (whose work included treating gynaecological conditions) were involved in the birthing process, although some researchers disagree with this conclusion (see Chapter 2d, p. 42).

Employment conditions are also discussed in legal contracts of the Graeco-Roman Period drawn up between wet-nurses and their employers. These set out the wet-nurse's duties and obligations, length of service and salary details (Joshel 1986; Heilport & Worp 2007). Similarly, a professional arrangement that benefited both groups may have existed between physicians and embalmers (see Chapter 2e).

(c) Summary of evidence and source material

An analysis of mummified and skeletal remains provides the most direct source of evidence for disease, disability and medicine in ancient Egypt. Iconographic, inscriptional and other miscellaneous resources add further important information, although care has to be taken in their interpretation, particularly in the case of artistic depictions, as they are often subject to bias.

Palaeopathological sources

Palaeopathological evidence is a key source in the study of disease processes, trauma and congenital conditions, particularly in view of the significant numbers and excellent preservation of the skeletal and mummified remains from ancient Egypt. These remains have survived from the entire Dynastic Period, permitting both pathological and epidemiological studies. Originally macroscopic examination was the main approach in this field, but today palaeopathology is very much an interdisciplinary science employing advanced computed tomography and sophisticated DNA and proteomic studies. These and additional scientific methods and approaches have greatly improved our understanding of disease in ancient Egypt (see Chapter 1e).

Early work in this field was pioneered in Manchester in 1908 by Margaret Murray when she undertook the unwrapping, autopsy and scientific study of 'The Two Brothers' (Murray 1910). Investigations continued in Manchester under Rosalie David, with The Manchester Museum Project and the scientific autopsy of Mummy 1770 in 1975 (David 1979). In 2021 the mummy of Takabuti was extensively investigated at Manchester and Belfast, using the latest non-/minimally invasive techniques combined with modern analytical approaches (David & Murphy 2021) (see Plate 3).

Investigations in Manchester and other institutions have revealed the presence of a variety of parasites, such as *Schistosoma* (trematode worm), *Ascaris* (roundworm), *Dracunculus* (guinea worm) and *Taenia* (tapeworm). Malaria, tuberculosis and smallpox have been detected, as well as other abnormalities and disease processes. Extensive examinations of dental remains have revealed a detailed picture of the dental health of these ancient people, perhaps more so than for any other civilisation in antiquity (see Chapter 2f, ii).

In addition to skeletal and human remains, canopic jars containing the viscera of ancient Egyptian mummies are also a useful but underestimated source for histological, radiological, proteomic and ancient DNA examinations (Senti *et al.* 2018).

Iconographic evidence

Important in any study of medicine in ancient Egypt are the iconographic sources such as wall paintings, reliefs and sculptures. However, caution has to be exercised in their interpretation as, although they can provide evidence about disease processes, their representations are often influenced by stylistic and cultural factors.

A well-known example is Akhenaten (1352–1336 BC, 18th Dynasty), with his gynaecomastia and androgynous appearance. Whether the androgynous images were symbolic representations, perhaps meant to represent him as the father and mother of all mankind, or realistic representations indicative of some deforming genetic disorder or disease is the subject of continuing debate. Several genetic disorders have been proposed to explain Akhenaten's condition, including Marfan syndrome, Fröhlich syndrome (adiposogenital dystrophy), Klinefelter syndrome and androgen insensitivity syndrome, although each of these conditions has some features inconsistent with what is known about Akhenaten (Aldred & Sandison 1962; Burridge 1993). The theories are reviewed by Reeves (2001: 149–52). More recently the physical abnormalities of other members of the 18th Dynasty have been brought into this debate, and other syndromes, such a variant of the Antley–Bixler syndrome, have been offered as explanations for his depiction (Braverman *et al.* 2009; Eshraghian & Loeys 2012).

Another often quoted example is the wall scene showing Ati, the Queen of Punt, in the second portico of Hatshepsut's mortuary temple at Deir el-Bahri (Fig. 1.1). The queen is depicted with adipose folds on her belly, large flaccid breasts and rolls of fat on her arms and breasts. Originally, her condition was suggested to be elephantiasis, a parasitic disease that causes the skin to thicken and fluid to collect at the peripheries, producing what is often referred to as 'elephant skin', a detail that is recognisable in the wall scene (Halioua & Ziskind 2005: 106–07). However, this diagnosis was made solely on the basis of the deformities of the limbs observed. More recently it has been considered that the clinical picture seems to be a single phenotype grouping several dermatologic pathologies (lipomatosis, neurofibromatosis, lipodystrophy, Dercum's disease, achondroplasia, Proteus syndrome, X-linked dominant hypophosphatemic rickets, familial obesity). In the absence of any genetic or bioanthropological evidence from a

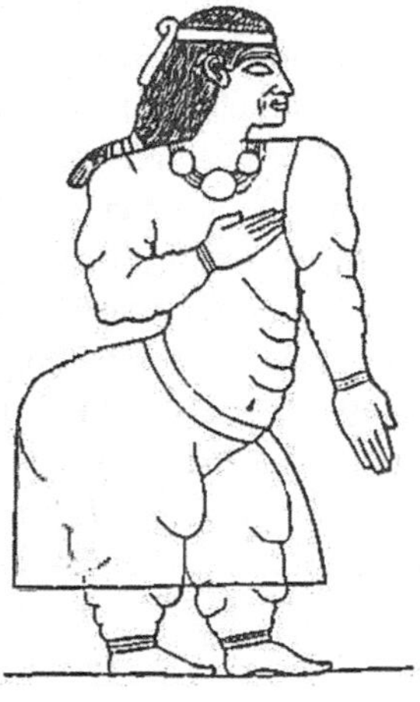

Figure 1.1. Depiction of Ati, the Queen of Punt, from a wall scene in the second portico of Hatshepsut's mortuary temple at Deir el-Bahri. Ati is depicted with adipose folds on her belly, large flaccid breasts and rolls of fat on her arms and breasts. Redrawn by K. N. White after Budge (1902: 407) and Nunn (1996: fig. 4.13).

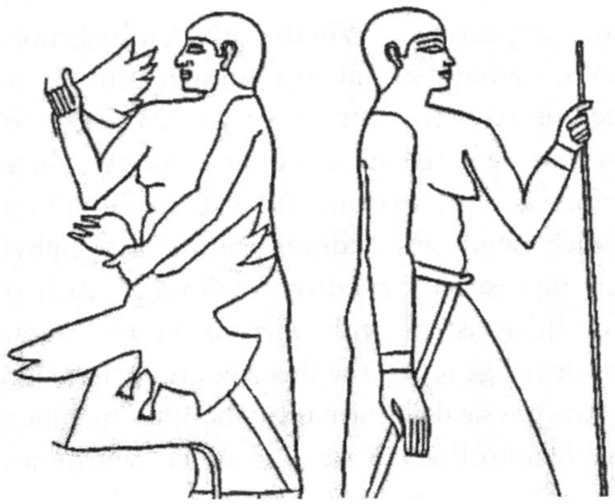

Figure 1.2. Representations of obesity (left figure) and gynaecomastia (enlargement of the male breasts, right figure) in the 6th Dynasty tomb of Ankhmahor at Saqqara. Redrawn by K. N. White after Badawy (1978: figs 27, 28) and Nunn (1996: fig. 4.11).

mummy, the clinical diagnosis that should be ascribed to the Queen of Punt is still far from clear (Christenson 2006; Di Cicco 2008).

The celebrated 6th Dynasty statue of Seneb and his family (found at Giza, now in the Egyptian Museum, Cairo JE 51281), shows him with his wife, Senetites, and their son and daughter (see Plate 4). The statue depicts him as an achondroplastic dwarf, in which the head and trunk are normal but the limbs are short. This is one of more than 200 representations of dwarfs, particularly from the Old Kingdom (Dasen 1993). Today achondroplasia accounts for approximately 1:25,000 births, which would translate to about sixty dwarfs, a fairly low number, in the whole of Old-Kingdom ancient Egypt, in which the population numbered about 1.5 million. In addition, achondroplasia is more frequent in children of elderly fathers and as a result of inbreeding. As the majority of the population of ancient Egypt is reputed not to have lived to an old age, and inbreeding was supposedly restricted to royalty, then achondroplasia may not have been too frequent a genetic disorder. So, the numbers of images of dwarfs give the impression that it was a fairly common condition in ancient Egypt, but the palaeopathological and statistical evidence suggest otherwise. Dwarfs often held privileged positions and were held in high esteem (see Chapter 6e) and this could explain the numbers displayed in the imagery of ancient Egypt.

Many tomb-owners are shown displaying rolls of fat and often signs of gynaecomastia (pendulous breasts) (Fig. 1.2). It is suggested that this may have been a conventional way of depicting an important and prosperous individual, rather than an accurate rendering of their appearance. Similarly, their wives are usually portrayed as tall, slim and attractive individuals, which, as Nunn (1996: 82) has indicated, is often in stark contrast to their mummies. Consequently, the interpretation of such depictions needs to be treated with caution.

Textual evidence

The primary inscriptional sources for our understanding of medicine in ancient Egypt are the medical papyri, which provide information relating to disease, diagnosis and treatment. In many cases the precise provenance of the texts is unknown, as some were purchased on the antiquities market and records of the find-spots of others are lacking. It is likely that only a small proportion of the original papyri have survived, as many will have been lost due to the ravages of time. Others will have been destroyed during tomb robberies, some were utilised to prepare magical remedies and others were even used for fuel in later times. Again, some may yet await discovery, while others may exist in libraries and archives but remain unidentified.

It is often difficult to relate the individual descriptions in the papyri to modern medical understandings of specific disease processes. Translational difficulties with the identification of some of the components of the remedies, notably botanical terms, make it difficult to judge the effectiveness of some of the pharmaceutical preparations, further impeding our ability to understand the treatment of individual infections and ailments.

The content and usefulness of the different papyri vary considerably and there is a degree of duplication among them. Some papyri, such as P. Chester Beatty and P. Ramesseum, have suffered extensive damage. Despite these problems, two of the better-preserved manuscripts, P. Ebers and P. Edwin Smith, are particularly useful in understanding the ancient Egyptian approach to healing, illustrating as they do the skill of the healers in observing and recognising symptoms. The most comprehensive study of the papyri, the *Grundriss der Medizin der Alten Ägypter* ('Outline of the medicine of the ancient Egyptians'), is presented in an extensive series of volumes authored by H. Grapow, H. von Deines and W Westendorf and published in German by Akademie-Verlag, Berlin. The most important papyri are described in the sections below.

Edwin Smith

The provenance of one of the most important medical documents, Papyrus Edwin Smith, is uncertain, but it is thought to have come from a tomb in the Theban Necropolis (Breasted 1930; Grapow *et al.* 1954–1973: IV 1; Allen 2005; Sanchez & Meltzer 2012). The papyrus is named after its original owner, Edwin Smith, an American Egyptologist who purchased it from a merchant in Luxor in 1862. It has been dated on stylistic grounds to about 1650–1550 BC but may be a copy of an older text, although opinions on this suggestion vary (see Plate 5).

The document can be described as a didactic trauma treatise, the oldest known such text in history. In contrast to the other medical papyri, which are mainly lists of recipes or prescriptions, often incorporating a magical incantation within the text, P. Edwin Smith is a systematically organised manuscript in which prognoses are presented and predominately rational therapies recommended (see Chapter 5c).

Ebers

Another notable document is Papyrus Ebers, which, again, was discovered in Luxor at about the same time as P. Edwin Smith and is now housed in the University Library, Leipzig (Ebers & Stern 1875; Joachim 1890; Grapow *et al.* 1954–1973: IV 1; Ghalioungui 1987; Bardinet 1995). On the verso of the document is a reference to the ninth regnal year of Amenhotep I (1525–1504 BC, 18th Dynasty). The manuscript, which is in excellent condition and is written in a clear hand, is the largest of the medical papyri, being a random collection of 877 paragraphs probably from different sources, since parallels can be identified across the range of medical texts, including the Hearst, Berlin and London Papyri.

P. Ebers can be mainly categorised as a treatise on pharmacology and therapeutics, although three paragraphs discuss the function of the heart and its vessels (*metu*), and are important in our understanding of Egyptian concepts of physiology. In addition, clinical cases with their symptoms and treatments are described. These include digestive disorders; urinary problems; intestinal worms; fractures, burns, flesh wounds and bites; diseases of the eyes, ears, nose, throat and skin; gynaecological conditions; stiff and painful limbs; tumours and abscesses; and the care of skin and hair.

London Medical Papyrus

The London Medical Papyrus (EA 10059) is of unknown provenance and has been housed in the British Museum since 1860 (Wreszinski 1912; Grapow *et al.* 1954–1973: IV 1; Bardinet 1995). It is in poor condition and is a palimpsest written over an earlier work. From the original text it is possible to recognise a date close to the reign of Tutankhamun (1336–1327 BC, 18th Dynasty), thus placing the text roughly in the middle of the New Kingdom.

Predominantly a magical papyrus, it is concerned with healing by religious and magical means. Parts of the text are difficult to understand because of their problematic medical and magical terminology. The contents can be grouped into incantations aimed at treating skin complaints, eye complaints, bleeding (especially associated with a miscarriage) and burns. The final incantation is a hymn relating to the image of the sun god Re. Seventeen of the cases have parallels in P. Ebers. One section, mainly relating to skin complaints, incorporates incantations in foreign languages, transcribed into syllabic Egyptian Script (see Chapter 7b).

Several paragraphs list treatments for burns. Trevisanato (2006) has attempted to link these to the volcanic fallout from the eruption of Santorini, which occurred about 1600 BC, noting references in the papyrus to blisters and burns scattered over the body. However, this suggestion is not widely supported.

Berlin Papyrus 3038

The Berlin Papyrus (3038), together with a court record of Ramesses II (1279–1213 BC, 19th Dynasty), was discovered in a clay vase at Saqqara early in the 19th century AD. Otherwise, little else is known of the provenance of this document, but the style and writing are typical of the 19th Dynasty. It was later sold to Friedrich Wilhelm IV of Prussia and is now housed in the Berlin Museum (Wreszinski 1909; Grapow *et al.* 1954–1973: IV 1; Bardinet 1995).

Paragraph 163a states that the original papyrus was 'discovered amongst writings of ancient times in chests of writing materials under the feet of Anubis, in Letopolis, at the time of the Majesty of the King of Upper and Lower Egypt, Den'. Three of the cases in the papyrus (163a, 163h, 190) make a reference to Netjerhotep, who may be the author of the papyrus, although there is no hieroglyphic seated man determinative (the sign placed at the end of the word). Another, perhaps more likely, suggestion is that the word is not a proper name but could be translated as 'one who appeases the god' (Stuhr 2002).

The document comprises nineteen papyrus sheets and 204 paragraphs or prescriptions. Most of the cases are comparable to those found in P. Ebers but cases 193–99 describe the methods of determining a pregnancy, parallels for which can be found in P. Kahun and P. Carlsberg VIII.

Hearst Papyrus

The Hearst Papyrus was acquired in 1901 by the Hearst Egyptian Expedition of the University of California (Leake 1952: 47–75; Grapow *et al.* 1954–1973: IV 1). The expedition members were excavating near Deir el-Ballas when a peasant brought the papyrus roll to the expedition camp. The text is believed to date to the reign of Tuthmosis III (1479–1425 BC, 18th Dynasty) and is now kept in the University of California.

It consists of eighteen pages comprising 260 paragraphs or prescriptions and concentrates on internal disorders, such as those of the alimentary and urinary systems; cutaneous disorders including animal bites; cosmetic matters involving body odour, hair and teeth; and a section on orthopaedic disorders. There is some duplication with other medical papyri, as over a third of the prescriptions can be found in P. Ebers and a number of others in the Berlin Medical Papyri. Prescriptions are given for named diseases, but examination of the patient is not recorded in the same manner as it is in P. Edwin Smith.

Systematic arrangement was apparently not followed by the scribe who compiled the papyrus, as groups of prescriptions are placed without any reference to a logical or orderly sequence. The beginning of the text, which may have provided some clue as to any such structure, is now lost.

Cases 89–92 relate to treatment for skin abrasions and bruising. These prescriptions recommend, among other substances, the application of salt and mouldy breadcrumbs. Advocating mouldy bread may have some rationale; some fungi that grow on mouldy bread, such as *Phycomyces blakesleeanus*, produce the polymers chitin and chitosan, which may accelerate the healing of wounds and shield the wound from infection (Hamlyn & Schmidt 1994).

The papyrus also lists cosmetic prescriptions: prescriptions 144–49 are ointments to encourage hair growth and prevent greyness. Prescriptions 153 and 154 are designed to improve the skin and are similar to P. Ebers 714 and 715 and to those on the verso of P. Edwin Smith. Prescriptions 239–44 are for treating the bites of specific animals such as crocodiles, pigs, hippopotami and lions.

Carlsberg Papyrus VIII

Little is known of the origin of Carlsberg Papyrus VIII, which has been dated to the 19th or 20th Dynasties, but from its style it has been suggested that it could be a copy of an earlier work, perhaps from the 12th Dynasty (Iversen 1939; Grapow *et al.* 1954–1973: IV 1; von Lieven 2007). It takes its name from the Carlsberg Foundation, who own the papyrus, but it is housed at the Egyptological Institute at the University of Copenhagen.

The fragments belonging to the document are in a poor state of preservation. Written in Hieratic, the recto contains part of a treatise on the diseases of the eyes, which is almost identical to chapters in P. Ebers. The verso contains the remains of seven prescriptions dealing with gynaecological subjects, such as the determination of pregnancy, the sex of the newborn child and the ability to conceive. There are parallels with the Berlin and Kahun Papyri.

Kahun Papyrus

The Kahun Papyrus, sometimes known as the Kahun Gynaecological Papyrus, is the earliest known treatise on gynaecology and although badly fragmented is important in our understanding of medical care for women in ancient Egypt (see Chapter 4c).

Ramesseum Papyri

Approximately twenty-four papyri were found inside a wooden box as part of a group of artefacts unearthed in a Middle Kingdom shaft tomb that is often referred to as the Ramesseum collection (see Chapter 5e, i). When the papyri were discovered they were found to be fragmented and in a poor state of preservation, but nevertheless could be separated into various groupings. Three of the Papyri – III, IV and V – include medical prescriptions. P. Ram. III is a magico-medical text for mother and child and in addition includes a section on eye complaints. P. Ram. IV, another magico-medical text, is associated with pregnancy, birth and conditions affecting mothers and children. P. Ram. V contains medical prescriptions mainly dealing with the *metu*, here relating to muscular complaints, rheumatic conditions and stiffness generally. P. Ramesseum has parallels with P. Ebers.

Other papyri

Papyrus Turin 54003 is an early medical text dated to the First Intermediate Period/Middle Kingdom (Fischer-Elfert 2004). Among its remedies are incantations directed against snakes and a formula for removing a fish bone stuck in the throat. P. Berlin 3027, also known as the Erman Papyrus and the Book for Mother and Child, is mostly concerned with childbirth and the health of infants. It contains two prescriptions for unknown childhood diseases as well as magical incantations for childbirth and the protection of infants (Erman 1901; Leake 1952: 14–15; Strouhal *et al.* 2014).

P. Leiden I 343 + 345 date from the Ramesside Period and contain among other things a collection of incantations directed against the ancient Near Eastern disease-demon Sāmānu and his Egyptian equivalent Akhu (Beck 2018). The Brooklyn Papyrus (47.218.48 and 47.218.85) is concerned exclusively with snake bites (see Chapter 2c and 4f). Vindob Papyrus 6257, also known as Papyrus Crocodilopolis, dates to the 2nd century AD and lists ailments and their remedies, some being Egyptian and others originating from the Mediterranean area (Reymond 1976). The Demotic Magical Papyri of London and Leiden (AD 100–300) contain some remedies for treating bites by poisonous animals and others for eye diseases and gout (Griffith & Thompson 1904).

Ostraca

Numerous ostraca record individual remedies, and these range in date from the New Kingdom to the Graeco-Roman Period. Many, dating to the 18th and 19th Dynasties, were discovered at Deir el-Medina and include a mix of magical and more conventional prescriptions used both by workers and by professional healers. Both the Deir el-Medina and the British Museum databases contain information about several of the medical ostraca from Deir el-Medina and include further links (also see Jonckheere 1954).

Miscellaneous

Miscellaneous inscriptions on stelae and tomb wall scenes often record the occupation and career of the owner, some of whom are specified as providers of healthcare. The Old Kingdom tomb of Akhotep and the Old Kingdom/First Intermediate Period tomb of Irenakhty are particularly informative here (Ghalioungui 1983). Some rock carvings, mostly the work of members of expeditions to mines and quarries, allude to the presence of physicians, such as the reference to Heryshefnakht and his colleague Ahanakht found in the alabaster quarries at Hatnub (see pp. 117–18; Anthes 1928). Occasionally, graffiti can provide information relating to healing: for example, certain graffiti inscribed on the walls of temples of the Late Period relate to healing deities and describe treatment provided for individuals with physical or mental ailments.

Cuneiform tablets found at Tell el-Amarna record the diplomatic correspondence between Egypt and either the rulers of the great powers such as Assyria and Babylon or the vassal states in Syria–Palestine. Some of these mention health problems and list the names of individual physicians (see Chapter 7b).

(d) Methodology in the study of human remains

The examination of human remains is a key element in the study of ancient disease, and today the many analytical techniques that are available to investigate bioarchaeological remains are diverse and expanding in number.

Macroscopic inspection

Despite recent progress in the scientific study of human remains, visual recognition of morphological variations continues to be important in the identification of disease processes. Taphonomic changes (physical, chemical and biological processes that cause alterations in organic remains) have to be taken into consideration in order to avoid the misinterpretation of pseudopathological postmortem changes as antemortem disease. Macroscopic inspection is useful for skeletal and unwrapped mummified remains, but for mummified bodies detailed information is now obtained largely by using non-invasive techniques to reconstruct the biological profile of the individual.

Sampling ancient tissue

Prior to modern advances in this field, such as developments in palaeoradiological techniques, invasive methods have been the only means available for the scientific study of mummified tissue. Biopsies were obtained by endoscopic procedures and small gauge needle insertions and the material obtained was examined histologically, palaeomicrobiologically and biochemically, allowing

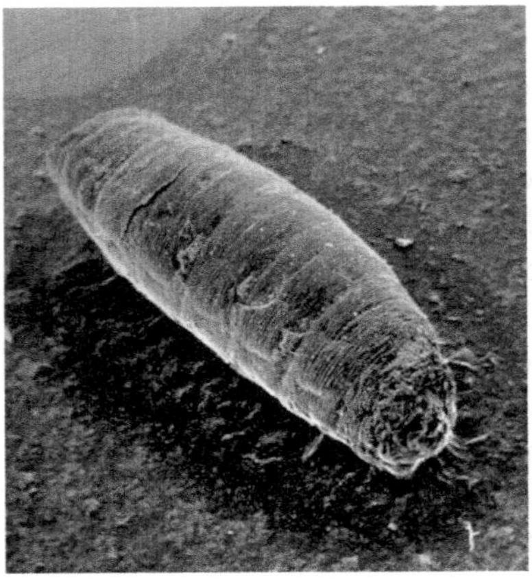

Figure 1.3. Scanning electron microscopy (SEM) can be used to identify insects in mummified remains. This image shows the empty puparium of a dipteran fly, *Piophila casei*, and is shown at twenty-nine-times magnification. This was found in Mummy 1770, Manchester Museum collection. The infestation may have occurred during life or, more probably, after death, contributing to the extreme deterioration of this mummy (courtesy of the KNH Centre, The University of Manchester).

the identification of many diseases and conditions, among them tuberculosis, malaria and parasitic infections (Fig. 1.3). In particular, the histological study of bones and rehydrated mummy tissue has been important in the diagnosis of ancient disease (Grove *et al.* 2015; Denton 2016).

Carbon and nitrogen stable isotope analyses of collagen from bone and teeth help to shed light on ancient diets, an important factor in accessing the health of an individual during life. Developments in gas chromatography/mass spectrometry (GC/MS), isotopic analysis and synchrotron analysis of minimal amounts of mummy hair have enabled significant information to be obtained about the daily lives of ancient populations. These techniques can also detect acute and chronic exposures to heavy metals (Moissidou *et al.* 2015; McCreesh & Gize 2021).

Imaging

Radiography has been in continuous use for the study of mummies since the discovery of x-rays by Wilhelm Roentgen in 1895. Today the use of basic radiographs has largely been superseded by high-resolution computerised

Figure 1.4. Dr Rosalie David and Dr Edmund Tapp discuss the unwrapping and autopsy of the mummy of a young girl (Manchester Museum 1770) at The University of Manchester in 1975. Research has demonstrated that the girl's age-at-death was around fourteen years, and that she suffered from Guinea worm infection (courtesy of The University of Manchester).

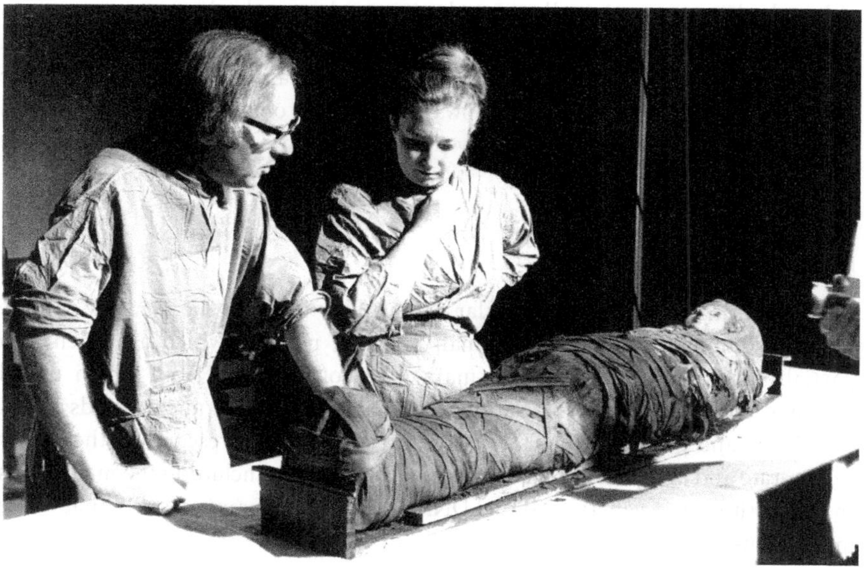

tomography (CT), associated with sophisticated software packaging (see Plate 6). This technology enables not only separate layers in the mummified body to be virtually removed, permitting the observation of bandages, skin, muscles, skeleton and internal organs, but also the viewing of cross sections of the body, achieving a virtual autopsy. Although reliance exclusively upon virtual diagnoses can sometimes lead to inconclusive and misleading interpretations, direct examination of the corpse through autopsy can today create considerable ethical concerns among curators, archaeologists and the wider general public. As a result, the virtual inspection of a corpse has almost completely replaced classical autopsy (Fig. 1.4).

Magnetic Resonance Imaging (MRI)

Although magnetic resonance imaging is the preferred technique for clinical soft-tissue imaging, its application to mummified samples is very limited due to the desiccated nature of the tissue. The presence of hydrogen in water is essential for this method to be successful, as the technique relies on the behaviour of hydrogen atom nuclei when subjected to a magnetic field (Loynes & Bianucci 2021). More recently fast imaging techniques have been able to improve image quality, enabling new approaches to be considered in this field (Giovannetti *et al.* 2016; Baadsvik *et al.* 2021).

Radiocarbon dating

Radiocarbon dating has become a standard dating method in archaeology, although there was originally some hesitancy due to the large error margins associated with the procedure. With continuing technical progress, increased measurement precision and new approaches, radiocarbon dating is now more readily accepted. The procedure allows information obtained from the various scientific investigations to be suitably positioned within a correct historical and social setting (Höflmayer 2016).

Biomolecular archaeology

Research in the field of biomolecular archaeology involves the analysis of large organic compounds present in human remains, most of which are often in a partially degraded state. The two main types of molecule from which useful information can be found in relation to diet and disease are nucleic acids (DNA and RNA) and proteins. The essence of any biomolecular research is the ability to generate and analyse sequences of organic molecules, including the nucleotides that constitute the genetic code in DNA/RNA and the amino acids that make up proteins.

Ancient DNA (aDNA)

Studies of genetic material derived from ancient Egyptian mummified remains can reveal genomic evidence of parasitic and microbiological pathological organisms. Such outcomes point to the presence of acute lethal, chronic or uncleared infection during life.

aDNA analyses have been able to provide molecular evidence of diseases such as tuberculosis (Zink *et al.* 2001; Lalremruata *et al.* 2013), malaria (Nerlich *et al.* 2008), schistosomiasis (Matheson *et al.* 2014) and leishmaniasis (Zink *et al.* 2006). Zink and his co-workers (2000) have detected molecular evidence of bacteraemia, caused by gastrointestinal pathogenic bacteria, in an infant Egyptian mummy. aDNA investigations have also been able to detect disorders caused by gene mutations, including achondroplasia (Pusch *et al.* 2004). It has been possible to analyse past diet by utilising aDNA from dental calculus (e.g., Adler *et al.* 2013), from mummified stomach contents (e.g., Rollo *et al.* 2002) and from coprolites (e.g., Poinar *et al.* 2003).

Proteomics

All the inheritable material possessed by an organism, the genome, is stored as DNA. The proteome is the suite of proteins produced by the genome at any one time. The field of proteomics, the study of the proteome, investigates how different proteins interact with each other, as well as the roles they perform within the organism. Analyses of mummified remains have revealed that diverse ranges of proteins can survive through time. The technique of proteomics utilises mass spectrometry to identify particular proteins and patterns of protein degradation by means of their amino acid sequences (Richards & Britton 2020: 35). Proteins are generally more robust than DNA and RNA, and have been detected in samples that have failed to yield usable DNA.

The proteomic analysis of skin samples from an ancient Egyptian child mummy has provided insights into the preservation and physiological status of the remains, and an indication of the possible cause of death (Ravishankar *et al.* 2020). An investigation of buccal swabs from 500-year-old mummified individuals from the Andes revealed a suite of proteins associated with the immune system, suggesting that an active antibacterial response was present at the time of death (Corthals *et al.* 2012). Analysis of the brain proteome of the Tyrolean Iceman demonstrated an expression of proteins related to wound healing, suggesting a possible head injury (Maixner *et al.* 2013).

Part of the 2018 programme of research into Takabuti (see below) involved a proteomic study of a muscle sample. The results indicated that the ancient muscle sample 'matched' normal muscle of today, making it unlikely that Takabuti had suffered from a muscle disease. In addition, the lack of inflammatory proteins suggest that Takabuti was not suffering from an inflammatory or infectious disease at the time of her death (Freemont & Chasserini 2021).

More recently, a non-invasive sampling technique based on mixed-bed chromatographic media embedded on ethylene vinyl acetate membranes (EVA) has been successfully utilised in extracting ancient proteins from the surface of Egyptian mummies. The method has permitted the recovery of biomolecular markers of disease as well as potential traces of embalming and/or restoration practices, without impacting on the integrity of the body (Demarchi *et al.* 2020).

Proteomics is a fairly recent technique and further scientific advances in this field may well have implications for future ancient protein analysis and the wider field of ancient tissue research.

Multidisciplinary investigations

Today wide-ranging multidisciplinary investigations are becoming the norm in mummy studies. For example, two ancient Egyptian child mummies at the University of Tartu Art Museum in Estonia were submitted for an osteological and archaeothanatological study, radiological investigation, AMS (accelerator mass spectrometry) radiocarbon dating, chemical and textile analyses, 3D modelling, and entomological and aDNA investigations (Oras *et al.* 2020). Takabuti, a 25th Dynasty female mummy, was investigated in Manchester and Belfast using a range of methods including high-resolution computerised tomography, light and electron microscopic studies, and geochemical, radiochemical, aDNA and proteomic analyses, utilising milligram quantities of a needle biopsy sample (David & Murphy 2021).

Collective approaches such as these can generate considerable structural and molecular data that reveal extensive information relating to the lifestyles, disease processes, deaths and mummification practices of ancient peoples.

2

Providers of healthcare: the healer's perspective

This chapter provides an overview of the various groups of professional healers who were responsible for delivering a wide range of healthcare and medical treatments to the Egyptian population.

(a) The prehistoric origins of pharaonic medicine

Advances in medical knowledge and treatment doubtless mirrored the great progress evident in early dynastic times in political and economic development, art and architecture.

The earliest surviving inscriptions regarding medical practitioners and treatment date to the Old Kingdom and indicate that traditions were well-established by that period. A lack of textual evidence for earlier times can only be partly offset by information derived from human remains and some funerary possessions that may have been owned by healing practitioners.

The impact of geography and politics on the development of medical practice

Egypt's unique geographical features and consequent political and religious development provided the context for the origin and emergence of medical practitioners and treatment during prehistoric and early dynastic times. Today, the country is largely desert, with the cultivable land being restricted to the Nile Delta, the Nile Valley and the distant oases in the Western Desert (Fig. 2.1).

The fertility of the Delta and Nile Valley has always been the result of the annual flooding (inundation) of the river Nile. Until the construction of dams at Aswan in the 20th century AD, which facilitated the control of the inundation, this event could be erratic. It sometimes resulted in a 'high Nile', when an excess of floodwater might endanger people's lives and property, or a 'low Nile', which could reduce crop yields and even cause famine.

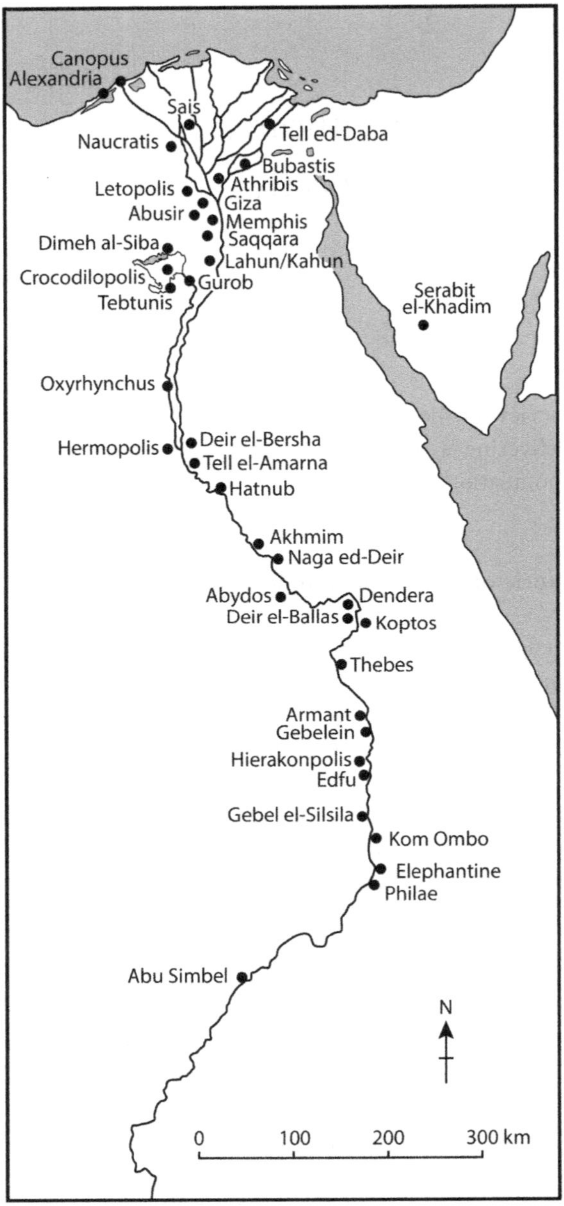

Figure 2.1. Map of Egypt and Nubia showing important locations mentioned in the book. Redrawn by L. Mulqueeny after Partridge (2002: fig. 391) and Baines and Málek (1980: 15, 31, 33, 41, 43).

In the Palaeolithic Period (before *c.* 5000 BC) the Delta and Nile Valley were virtually uninhabitable. The inundation placed the Nile Valley under water for three months each year, and at other times it was covered with dense vegetation that was the habitat of wild animals. Papyrus swamps occupied large tracts of the low-lying Delta. Tools and weapons discovered from this period indicate that people were living on the desert spurs and hunting the prolific game. However, even if any form of medical knowledge or treatment existed in this period, the evidence has not survived.

Once climate change brought about drier conditions and changes in vegetation the Nile Valley became habitable and during the Neolithic Period (*c.* 5000–4000 BC) the inhabitants were able to move down into this area. Gradually, they replaced hunting with a settled existence, living together in communities, cultivating the land, growing crops and domesticating animals.

Social and religious developments in the Predynastic Period

The social structure that emerged during the Predynastic Period consisted of a series of separate communities spread across the cultivable land in the Delta and alongside the river in the Nile Valley. Buildings associated with the living were mainly constructed from organic, perishable materials, and so most information about this period comes from the local cemeteries, which were situated away from the dwellings. Here, the graves and their contents provide some insight into the social organisation and religious beliefs and practices of these communities.

Archaeological evidence suggests that, although geographically scattered, the communities evolved with basically the same political and economic goals. This unity of approach was underpinned and enhanced by the common need to work together to develop an irrigation system that could most effectively utilise the Nile waters for land cultivation. From this baseline, the towns and villages developed similar social, religious and cultural activities.

Sacred places of worship, probably built of perishable materials such as wood, wickerwork, reeds and mud, have not survived, but some are represented on grave goods: shrines are depicted on ivory labels and scenes painted on Decorated Ware pottery show boats carrying gods' shrines and deities.

Evidence indicates that, in each community, statues or symbols of gods were housed in shrines, which were slightly larger versions of people's own homes. Each shrine acted as the dwelling-place of the local god, protecting the divine statue and providing a place where humans could approach the deity. The local chieftain probably brought food and other offerings to the god on a regular basis, in the hope of obtaining divine benefits for the community. These basic features were all continued for thousands of years in the stone-built temples and religious rituals of later periods.

Healers in the earliest communities

The political landscape changed and developed over many centuries, with settlements and areas combining to become larger political and geographical units known later as 'nomes'. Gradually, the most powerful local chieftains gained overall control of the country and became the rulers of two parallel kingdoms, the White Land in the south and the Red Land in the north. In the final stage of this process the southerners conquered the northern kingdom, and in *c.* 3100 BC the two realms were brought together and unified under one king.

Religious developments appear to have mirrored these events. The earliest communities doubtless had quite localised cults, each offering worship to specific deities, but once a settlement had been absorbed or conquered by its neighbours the situation changed: sometimes the victor's god adopted any significant characteristics of the subordinated cult, or perhaps took on the conquered deity as an assistant or follower, although sometimes the latter disappeared altogether from subsequent mythology (Hornung 1996: 101–09).

These political and religious factors doubtless influenced the evolution and course of medicine and healing. In the earliest communities tribal and village chieftains would probably have acted as 'healers', treating their patients through the agency of magical acts and rituals. However, once overarching political power had been seized by one ruler, he alone was credited with this special healing ability (David 2002: 63).

As king, he now in turn delegated his role and responsibilities as a healing practitioner to the temple priests. Acting as his deputies, they acquired an additional role as the most senior physicians in the medical hierarchy. Originally, these priest–doctors were simply religious functionaries who mediated between Sekhmet, the goddess of medicine, and their patients. However, they gradually acquired practical skills through observing their patients and doubtless developing treatments based on trial-and-error procedures. The evolution of the medical practitioner's role, with its increasing focus on practical, rational diagnoses and treatments, was the basis of the Egyptian system of medical science established early in the pharaonic period.

Evidence of disease in prehistoric Egypt

The main evidence for disease in prehistoric times comes from human remains. From earliest times, the limited fertile areas of cultivable land were reserved and utilised for the requirements of the living – food production and housing. Consequently, the dead were interred in burial places (pit-graves, tombs and, during some periods, pyramids for the kings) situated on the edges of the desert or in the nearby cliffs.

At first, both the bodies of the elite and the non-elite were usually covered in a reed or skin mat, and placed in shallow graves dug in porous sand. These conditions, combined with a hot, dry climate, ensured that the bodies were preserved. The sand absorbed the body fluids of the newly buried corpse, thus arresting decomposition and producing a desiccated body that retained its skin and hair. In the correct environmental conditions, these bodies (which exemplify the process known as natural or unintentional mummification) can last indefinitely. A celebrated example is that of Gebelein Man, now on display in the British Museum (EA32751), who was buried in about 3500 BC (possibly earlier) at the site of Gebelein in Upper Egypt.

Simple burial and natural mummification generally continued for the poorer classes throughout the pharaonic period until early Christian times. However, at some point, artificial mummification, which involved evisceration and bodily preservation using a dehydrating agent (natron, a mixture of mainly sodium carbonate and bicarbonate found in natural deposits in Egypt), was introduced for royalty and the elite. The reason for artificial mummification and the date of its introduction are subjects of debate. The procedure was already being practised in the Old Kingdom, and one explanation is that it may have been introduced when more elaborate monumental tombs were introduced for the elite in the early dynasties. These tombs no longer provided the hot, dry conditions conducive to natural mummification, with the result that decomposition of the corpse was accelerated. However, by this period, religious beliefs dictated that the body should be preserved so that the deceased owner could utilise the mummy to derive spiritual sustenance from the food and other offerings placed at the burial site.

Features associated with the artificial process at first involved the extraction of the viscera and the wrapping of specific areas of the body in tight-fitting linen bandages impregnated with resinous substances; examples of these procedures have been found in cemeteries that date from *c.* 4500 BC. Evidence from Hierakonpolis (*c.* 3500 BC) indicates that artificial mummification may have already been introduced in predynastic times, and was used even for non-elite corpses (Davies & Friedman 1998: 206–08; Hierakonpolis Expedition 2012). However, there is debate as to whether such discoveries provide real evidence of early intentional mummification or perhaps simply represent aspects of a funerary ritual (Jones 2007).

Even apart from intentionally mummified remains, naturally preserved corpses provide a considerable resource for disease and injury studies in prehistoric times. The same conditions are often found in later periods: for example, osteoarthritis and ankylosing spondylitis (a form of arthritis that results in fusion of the spine [Aufderheide & Rodríguez-Martin 1998: 102–04]) have been identified in Egyptian human remains from the Predynastic Period through to the Christian era (Zorab 1961; Fritsch *et al.* 2015).

Schistosomiasis has also been identified in predynastic bodies (Miller *et al.* 1993). This disease is caused by a person's physical reaction to the presence of a trematode worm of the genus *Schistosoma* (a schistosome) inside the body. Two of the three main species of this worm are associated with Egypt – *S. haematobium* (Bilharzia), which causes urinary schistosomiasis, and *S. mansoni*, which affects the liver. The schistosome requires two hosts to complete its life-cycle – a freshwater snail of the genus *Bulinus*, found in slow-moving water of a particular temperature, and a human who acquires the infection from immersion in water containing the cercariae (immature forms of the schistosome), which are released into the water by the snail (see Chapter 6a, g).

The fossil snail fauna of the Sahara suggests that schistosomiasis already existed in North Africa in prehistoric times, having originated in East Africa. Early development of irrigation in Egypt provided canals where the snails could flourish and, in fact, the earliest known case of human schistosomiasis dates from around 5000 years ago and occurred in the remains of an Egyptian adolescent (Deelder *et al.* 1990). Early studies on schistosomiasis utilised an enzyme-linked immunosorbent assay (ELISA) to detect schistosome circulating anodic antigen in tissue taken from mummies when other diagnostic methods were unsuitable. More recent aDNA studies have confirmed the presence of schistosomiasis in ancient Egyptian remains (Matheson *et al.* 2014).

In addition to the contribution made by Egyptology to prehistoric disease studies, the region has also provided the earliest-known archaeological and palaeopathological evidence of armed conflict and inflicted wounds, from sixty-one bodies interred in a cemetery at Jebel Sahaba (modern northern Sudan) (see Chapter 4f).

Medical treatments in prehistoric times

Although a lack of textual sources limits our understanding of any medical concepts and treatments that may have existed during the prehistoric era, it is possible, by drawing on evidence from later periods, to offer some tentative suggestions.

Examples of Egyptian rock art have been gathered and collated by a series of desert expeditions, the first of which was led by Hans Winkler (Winkler 1938). Accelerator Mass Spectrometry (AMS) has dated some of the human/animal carvings to *c.* 4400 BC, and some simpler forms to the 8th millennium BC or earlier (Morrow *et al.* 2010: 21). Subsequent studies have focused on the significance and meaning of these images and inscriptions, which may have been predominantly religious (Červiček 1986: 71) or socio-economic and cultural (Morrow *et al.* 2010: 21).

One study investigated whether the rock art provides any evidence of early Shamanism in Egypt (Lewis-Williams 2002). A key element of Shamanism is the shaman, a person whose supernatural powers, acquired while he is in an altered state of consciousness, include the ability to heal the sick. Judd (2009: 61–72) acknowledges that Shamanistic practices are recorded in the rock art of various cultures across several continents, but comments that there is no convincing evidence of its existence in the rock art of Egypt's Eastern Desert. He also mentions that later sources give no indication that it ever occurred in either the predynastic or dynastic eras (Judd 2009: 89–90). However, Morenz (2003: 225) considers that, although the evidence for Shamanism in Egypt is thinly scattered, a similar phenomenon may have played some part in early cultural development.

An indication of contemporary medical treatments can also perhaps be derived from artefacts and materials included in predynastic burials (Petrie 1920). For example, a selection of unguents discovered in some predynastic graves has been analysed as part of the 'Pharmacy in Ancient Egypt Project' at the University of Manchester (see Chapter 5f) (Cockitt & David 2010: 4; Seath-Burrows 2010). The key aims of this study were to characterise and identify the resins and mineral waxes in the unguents and to identify the geographical sources from which, over the millennia, Egyptian physicians obtained their medicinal ingredients. Samples were analysed with minimally invasive techniques: visible light microscopy, environmental scanning electron microscopy, and Fourier transform infrared spectroscopy. The results indicated that some of the compounds found in the samples were also present in much later pharmaceutical treatments listed in the medical papyri, and that the material in some samples originated from outside Egypt, confirming that such commodities were being traded with the Near East from as early as the 4th and 3rd millennia BC. However, we can only speculate as to whether these resins and waxes were already fulfilling a medical purpose in predynastic times and whether they were perhaps included in the burial for this use in the owner's next life.

Slate palettes were another important item found in the burial assemblages of some predynastic and early dynastic graves. Originally, palettes were used for grinding malachite (copper carbonate hydroxide) and galena (lead sulphide) into powdered green and grey pigments that, mixed with oil or fat, were used as eye cosmetics. Larger versions of the slate palettes were produced but had a purely ceremonial function (Petrie 1953; O'Connor 2002).

Later textual sources indicate that these pigments had medicinal as well as cosmetic applications. Galena and malachite were used to treat inflammation and infections of the eye, while copper salts, including malachite, provided a treatment for open wounds. Worth Estes (1993: 66–68) argues that, since it inhibits bacterial growth, malachite probably provided a valid therapeutic treatment for open wound treatment, and references in the medical papyri confirm the medicinal use of such ingredients in dynastic times. For example, malachite was probably the active ingredient in thirty-nine drug mixtures found in the Ebers Papyrus, and was mainly used to treat eye conditions and open wounds (Ebbell 1937: 85; Worth Estes 1993: 65). This is supported by a recent analysis of the minerals used for ocular remedies in ancient Egypt (Argilés *et al.* 2021). The 'green pigment' mentioned in the Edwin Smith Papyrus may be a general term for the copper ores used in wound treatments (Breasted 1930: 365–66; Worth Estes 1993: 65). The Kahun Gynaecological Papyrus recommends the use of green eye paint (probably malachite), boiled in cow's milk, to treat a woman with an infection in the pubic area (Griffith 1898: 5–11; Worth Estes 1993: 68). Given that the pigments were clearly well regarded as treatments in dynastic times, it is possible that the examples from predynastic burials also had a dual function as cosmetic eye-paints and medicinal ingredients.

(b) The transition to priest–physicians: the *wꜥb*-priests of Sekhmet

Imhotep's contribution to medicine

The evolution of medical theory and practice in Egypt mirrored historical and political events: unification as a kingdom in *c.* 3000 BC and subsequent development as a theocracy resulted in the enhancement of the king's spiritual and physical powers. This is reflected in his role as a healer, which he then delegated to the priests who deputised for him in matters of religion (see Chapter 2a).

A well-established system of medical care was apparently already in place by the beginning of the Old Kingdom, when Imhotep held the posts of vizier and chief architect to King Djoser (2667–2648 BC, 3rd Dynasty) (Fig. 2.2). Imhotep is credited with planning and erecting the first pyramid (the Step Pyramid) for Djoser and appears to have been held in high esteem throughout his lifetime. After his death his reputation continued to grow and in the Turin papyri he is described as son of Ptah and became recognised as a patron of scribes.

Imhotep was also regarded as the founder of medical science in Egypt, and in the Ptolemaic Period he was associated with Asclepius, the Greek god of medicine (see Plate 7). A great many statues of him were made and Ptolemy VIII (170–116 BC) built a shrine to him at the Temple of Hatshepsut (1473–1458 BC, 18th Dynasty) at Deir el-Bahri (see Plate 8). Other shrines were put up at the mortuary temple of Ramesses III (1184–1153 BC, 20th Dynasty) at Medinet Habu, at Karnak and at the Temple of Isis at Philae. Pilgrims visited these shrines and in the textual sources there are records of cures that were credited to Imhotep.

A Ptolemaic inscription of Imhotep on the walls of the Temple of Horus at Edfu refers to him as: 'great god, residing at Edfu, at whose order everyone lives, who cures any illness in Egypt'. In the Oxyrhynchus papyri there is an account of how an individual suffering from a fever spent the night in the temple at Memphis and was alleviated of his affliction, a cure that again was credited to Imhotep. The textual sources list tales relating how women appealed to Imhotep to become pregnant. On the funerary stela of Taimhotep (BM EA 147) Taimhotep appeals to Imhotep for a male child, a request that, according to the inscription, was granted. One of the epithets of the last native-born ruler of Egypt, Nectanebo II (360–343 BC, 30th Dynasty), was 'beloved of Imhotep, son of Ptah'. Imhotep continued to be venerated into the Roman Period as a god of medicine and healing.

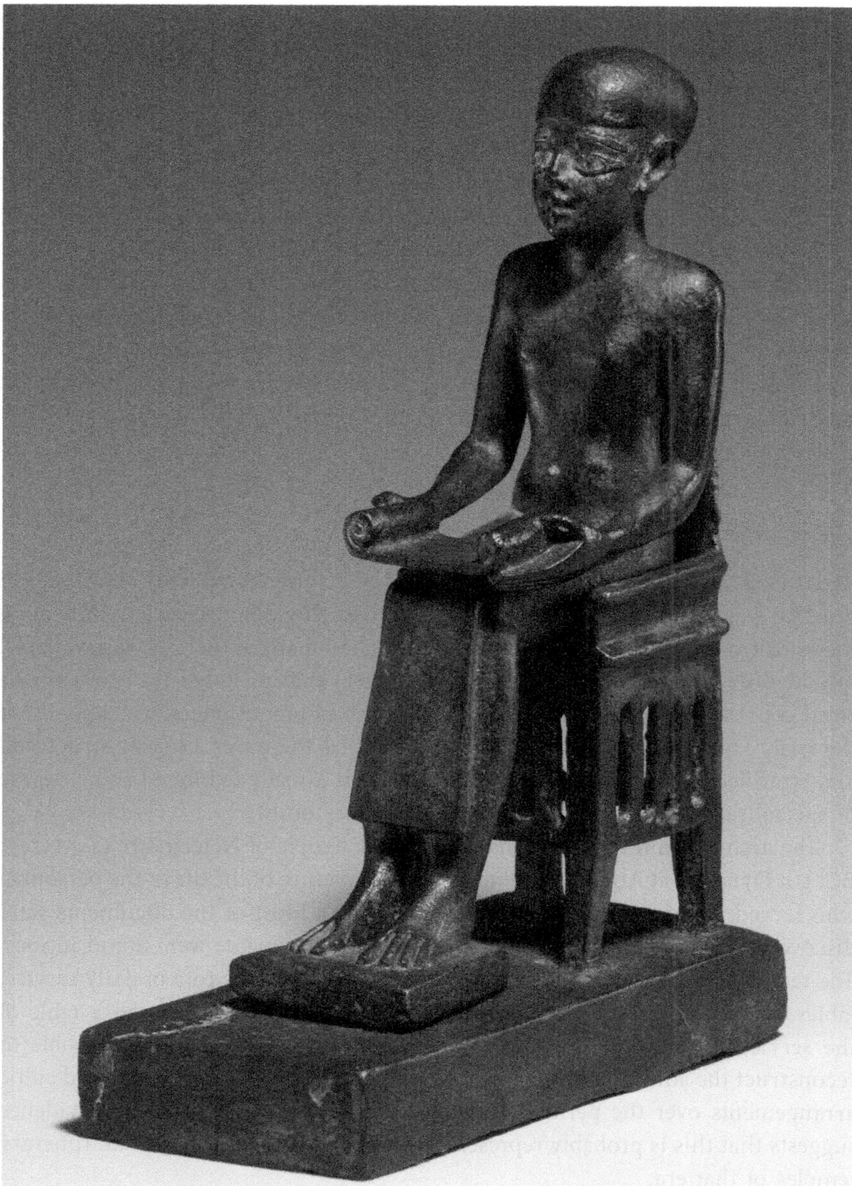

Figure 2.2. Statue of a seated Imhotep. Ptolemaic Period. Thought to have been discovered in the Delta. Cupreous metal, precious metal inlay. Metropolitan Museum of Art, New York. 26.7.852a, b (courtesy of the Metropolitan Museum of Art, New York. Purchase, Edward S. Harkness Gift, 1926).

However, despite his fame in antiquity, direct evidence relating to Imhotep is very limited. He is named on a statue base of King Djoser from the Step Pyramid complex and again in a graffito on the enclosure wall of Djoser's successor, Sekhemkhet (2648–2640 BC, 3rd Dynasty), and is a character in later literary works such as Papyrus Westcar (P. Berlin 3033). After his death a host of myths grew up and many of his accomplishments appear to be built on legend rather than facts. In his *Aegyptiaca* (History of Egypt) Manetho mentioned his medical skills, and he acquired a reputation as a healer, although there is no direct evidence that he ever practised as a physician (see Verbrugghe & Wickersham 2001). Tradition also has him as the author of works of medicine, but again there is no evidence to substantiate these claims. It is not completely certain why Imhotep came to be regarded as a god of medicine, although his reputed success in healing visitors who came to his shrines would have enhanced any such reputation.

The emergence of priest-physicians

Apart from Imhotep's contribution, there is inscriptional evidence that medical practice was already well established by the Old Kingdom. A variety of healing methods from conventional treatments through to magical therapy was available, provided by a professional class of practitioners that included members of the royal court through to community physicians and practitioners of magic. From the Early Dynastic Period, their titles suggest that there was a highly structured and stratified medical organisation in place that already exhibited some degree of specialisation (see Chapters 2a and 2c; Ritner 2001b).

The archive from the 5th Dynasty funerary temple of Neferirkare (2475–2455 BC, 5th Dynasty) at Abusir preserves a detailed picture of the life of the personnel who served in the temples (Posener-Kriéger 1976). Most of the documents were discovered at the site in 1893, and supplementary fragments were found in 1907. The records are organised on a monthly basis and show the rota of daily service, tables of daily revenues, an inventory of religious items in use and a table of the service to celebrate each festival. From this information, it is possible to reconstruct the administrative structure of the temple and its economy and cultic arrangements over the period of a single month; other documentary evidence suggests that this is probably representative of the general routine of all funerary temples of that era.

Records drawn up by highly competent scribes preserve details of this efficient system and provide a unique insight into the lives of the community. Available evidence relating to *wꜥb*-priests – the rank of entry to temple service – covers the long period from the 4th Dynasty to the 3rd century AD. These priests had attained ritual purity through various predetermined measures, and could therefore be admitted to the presence of the god's image. Organised into *phyles* (cohorts) to serve in the temple on a rota basis, their main duty was to act as key celebrants of the rituals (see Chapter 3a). However, the group also included the specialist priests of Sekhmet, listed as one of the various categories of healers (see below).

The priesthood of Sekhmet (also known as the *wꜥb*-priests of Sekhmet)

The priests of Sekhmet had several roles. Inscriptional evidence about their functions, which comes from papyri, tombs reliefs, statues, stelae, sarcophagi (stone coffins), ushabtis (figurines placed in burials to undertake agricultural duties for the owner in the afterlife), graffiti in quarries and Classical writings, covers the millennia from the Old, Middle and New Kingdoms to the Late and Graeco-Roman Periods. The priests of Sekhmet were primarily high-status ritualists and magicians, and had a close association with the House of Life (see Chapter 3b); as such, they made a significant contribution to the spiritual and magical protection of Egypt (Torras 2021: 116). However, P. Edwin Smith and P. Ebers confirm that they were also among those who specialised in diagnosing illness. Inscriptional evidence demonstrates that the roles of these groups were interlinked and all offered a variety of therapies (see Chapter 2c).

The lioness-headed goddess Sekhmet was regarded as a dual-natured deity who could use her breath to destroy mankind, pollute the Nile and bring plague and disease to Egypt. According to a wall inscription in the Temple of Edfu, she brought about these calamities in the month before the inundation, and festival rites had to be performed to placate her (von Känel 1984: 276). Inscriptions in the Temple of Esna state that festival rites performed there to destroy the goddess's power included beating and killing fish (von Känel 1984: 277). However, once assuaged and pacified by her priests, Sekhmet was expected to protect the king and Egypt against common dangers such as enemies and disease. The priests' main duty, therefore, was to propitiate Sekhmet with prayers and rituals, and to emphasise the benevolent aspects of her nature.

Against this background, Sekhmet came to have a wider remit in healing the sick, and although not all the priests who served her functioned as healers (some carried out duties solely as temple administrators or ritualists), most were involved in temple medicine as practitioners and perhaps also provided medical training. Originally, the priests of Sekhmet fulfilled only a religious role, using rituals and magic to mediate between the suppliants and Sekhmet, but over time, as they acquired practical knowledge and experience of the illnesses from which the suppliants suffered, the priests would have gained the expertise to offer medical treatment for many different conditions.

The ritual purity of a priest of Sekhmet allowed him to approach the goddess without fear of incurring personal danger. However, the priests also possessed the dual nature of their deity, and had the ability both to cause and cure disease. The goddess's terrifying attributes could be passed on to the priest during the rituals that he enacted to pacify her (von Känel 1984: 238–39) and, once he possessed these powers, he could act against mankind, spreading disease through his breath or, as in the harem conspiracy against Ramesses III, casting spells to kill the king (Koenig 2001; Torras 2021: 119).

Scholarly studies (Jonckheere 1950; Lefebvre 1952; von Känel 1984; Torras 2021) offer some interesting ideas about the precise roles of the priests of Sekhmet. Jonckheere and Lefebvre proposed that, although these men probably provided guidance and insight relating to medical matters, the *swnw* were the practising physicians. von Känel also suggested that the *wꜥb*-priests of Sekhmet may have had a lower status in medical practice than the *swnw*, a conclusion based on a prescription in P. Ebers (854a) where they are listed before the priests of Sekhmet; however, this order is reversed in P. Edwin Smith.

Ebbell (1937) suggested that the *swnw* and priests of Sekhmet had different functions, the former being responsible for medicinal treatments while the latter specialised in surgery. Nunn (1996: 163), however, regards such a division as unlikely, because surgical techniques do not seem to have had a wide application. Current evidence generally indicates that all groups of practitioners in fact pursued very similar treatment methods and relied on the medical papyri as their main source of information.

Other roles of the *wꜥb*-priests of Sekhmet

Other temple duties undertaken by the priests of Sekhmet may have included the veterinary care of sacrificial bulls and the supervision of ritual procedures in the temple slaughterhouse, where they selected the animals for sacrifice (see Chapter 2d; Lord 2016). The priests of Sekhmet were also credited with a unique ability to identify the distinguishing features of the special black bull that represented the incarnation of the god Apis, an important role since they could ensure that the sacred Apis-bull was never mistakenly chosen for slaughter (Torras 2021: 120).

Beyond their temple duties, the priests of Sekhmet accompanied state-organised mining and trading expeditions to provide medical care for participants (von Känel 1984: 18; Torras 2021). Eventually they also acquired significant roles relating to state and local administration and the economy (see below).

A historical overview of the contribution made by the *wꜥb*-priests of Sekhmet

The role of the *wꜥb*-priests of Sekhmet to a large extent reflects the general political developments that occurred throughout Egypt's history (von Känel 1984). It is possible to chart their course from a limited scope of temple ritual and medical specialism through to undertaking significant administrative roles on behalf of the state.

During the Old Kingdom – a time when there was considerable political and social centralisation – the priests of Sekhmet formed part of the priesthood of the great temples and contributed to the structured medical system then being established. However, following decentralisation of power in the First Intermediate Period, they increasingly occupied additional positions in the provinces throughout the subsequent Middle Kingdom, usually serving in the entourage of a local ruler.

In the New Kingdom their status increased with the burgeoning power of the temples, which were now recipients of massive tribute from the military campaigns sent abroad to establish the Egyptian Empire. From the Late Period onwards the priests' role developed further, with the acquisition of more titles and an increased diversity of functions. Now, they not only undertook duties in the House of Life and engaged in oracular consultations, sacrificial rituals and medical duties in the great temples but also began to take control of many aspects of the country's economy and territorial administration.

The priests of Sekhmet retained their significance and status in the Graeco-Roman Period, continuing to fulfil the many roles they had acquired over the millennia. This importance is exemplified by the Tomb of Petosiris (*c.* 350–330 BC), built in a unique hybrid style combining Egyptian and Greek architecture and decoration. Here, the wall reliefs and inscriptions confirm the high status of its owner, who was director of the priests of Sekhmet at nearby Hermopolis (Sauneron 2000: 9).

(c) *Swnw*, *sau*, priests of Serket and lectors

Introduction

The medical papyri detail different groups of individuals who practised healing in ancient Egypt. For example, there are references to physicians (*swnw*), *wꜥb*-priests of Sekhmet (see above) and magicians (*sꜣw*) in P. Ebers 854a and, with a slightly different wording, in Case 1, gloss A of P. Edwin Smith:

> There are vessels in him for every part of the body. As to these, if any physician (*swnw*), any *wꜥb*-priest of Sekhmet or any magician (*sꜣw*) places his two hands or his fingers on the head, on the back of the head, on the hands, on the place of the heart, on both arms or on both legs, he measures the heart because of its vessels to every one of his body-parts. It (the heart) speaks forth in the vessels of every body-part. (translated Allen 2005: 72)

This extract also indicates that placing the hand upon the patient was part of any physical examination, and that the ancient Egyptians recognised that the peripheral pulse reflected the beating of the heart. The placing of the hand on the patient recurs frequently in the medical texts and appears an important aspect of any physical examination. Another suggestion is that cures were effected by 'the laying on of hands' (Westendorf 1992: 58–59).

Aside from these groups of healing personnel, other professionals that can be identified as being associated with healing include the priests or 'Controllers of Serket' and lectors.

(i) *swnw* – physician

The ancient Egyptian healer who appears to have been the closest equivalent to the modern doctor or physician was the *swnw*, of whom there are over 150 identified examples from all periods of ancient Egyptian history (Jonckheere 1958: 87–94; Ghalioungui 1983: 16–37; Nunn 1996: 211–14). There is a body of evidence that supports the translation of *swnw* as 'physician' or 'doctor' and which also links him with the care of the sick. There are many instances in the medical papyri where the occupation of the *swnw* is apparent; for example, P. Edwin Smith (Case 9, Gloss A) reads: 'As for 'the bandage of cloth belonging to a physician's medical kit,' it is 'a head binding which is under the charge of this bandager (embalmer), which he ought to place over this medication that is on that wound that is in his forehead' (translated Sanchez & Meltzer 2012: 97).

In P. Berlin (164b) there is: 'a remedy against "pain matters", art of the *swnw*' (translated Wreszinski 1909: 96). P. Ebers (188), when offering a remedy for a stomach complaint, has this passage: 'You should prepare a secret herb remedy which the *swnw* makes' (translated Ghalioungui 1987: 54). The non-medical literature of ancient Egypt, such as poems and inscriptions, similarly contains instances that point to the occupation of the *swnw* (Jonckheere 1958: 143–47; Kamal 1967: 235), while a connection has been made between the Coptic word for a physician, *SAEIN*, and the transliteration *swnw*, as derivations of many Egyptian words have survived in Coptic (Nunn 1996: 115–16).

The *swnw* is linked with all the different elements of the medical process, ranging from the initial examination to treatment and aftercare, including treatment protocols such as remedies, recitations and surgery. The principal sources of information relating to the drugs or medicaments that the *swnw* would have utilised are the medical papyri, particularly the Ebers and Hearst, which list hundreds of drugs and remedies. However, the components of some of these remedies are unknown to us and there are translational uncertainties in the identification of others. The glossary in J. Worth Estes's 1993 publication *The Medical Skills of Ancient Egypt* (pp. 139–57) provides an extensive *materia medica* of pharaonic Egypt. However, an important source for some of the information contained therein is Ebbell's 1937 translation of the Ebers Papyrus, which is sometimes considered unreliable because there is no firm linguistic basis for the translation and interpretation of many obscure Egyptian words (Nunn 1996: 30).

Hierarchy and specialisation

Although the majority of the physicians carry the *swnw* title, a number held additional administrative or hierarchical designations such as 'Administrator of Physicians' (*ẖrp swnw*), 'One with Authority over Physicians' (*ḥry swnw*), 'Overseer of Physicians' (*imr-r swnw*), 'Chief of Physicians' (*wr swnw*) and 'Physician of the Palace' (*swnw pr ꜥꜣ*). Although these titles would appear to offer varying degrees of administrative authority, it is uncertain if they represent a recognised hierarchical structure. As with many ancient Egyptian titles it is difficult to define the range and scope of a particular office, and these titles may have evolved over time, though, as with most titles, we see a general reduction in their usage by the New Kingdom.

The question of possible specialisation among the *swnw*, as potentially represented by titles such as 'Physician of the Abdomen' (*swnw ẖt*) and 'Oculist of the Palace' (*swnw irty pr ꜥꜣ*), has often been debated in the literature relating to healing practices in ancient Egypt. This subject was first addressed by Herodotus, the 5th-century BC Greek historian, in his *Histories* (II, 84): 'The practice of medicine they split into separate parts, each physician being responsible for the treatment of only one disease. There are in consequence, innumerable doctors, some specialising in diseases of the eye, others of the head, others of the teeth, others of the stomach … ' (Fig. 2.3).

In considering specialisation it is possible to view the topic from two different perspectives. If we define specialisation as perhaps we would today, then the implication is that medical knowledge was extensive and highly developed, and that, due to the extent of the knowledge, an individual had to specialise, much as occurs in the modern world. However, it is possible that ancient Egyptian specialisation represented merely a division of the known medical knowledge, with every practitioner treating a particular part of the body. This may have been related to the ancient Egyptian perception that the body did not function as a complex single organism, as we now understand it, but more a loose association of separate anatomical entities. Each individual body part was considered to have a divine nature and was associated with a deity, whose particular divinity was related to a set of divine attributes. This suggestion is borne out by alternative translations of the extract from Herodotus reproduced above. Here, instead of de Sélincourt's translation 'some specialising in diseases of the … ', Rawlinson (1956: 108) provides 'some undertaking to cure diseases of the … '.

Another possibility is that the various titles simply indicate aspects of medicine in which the *swnw* had developed a reputation, due to his expertise

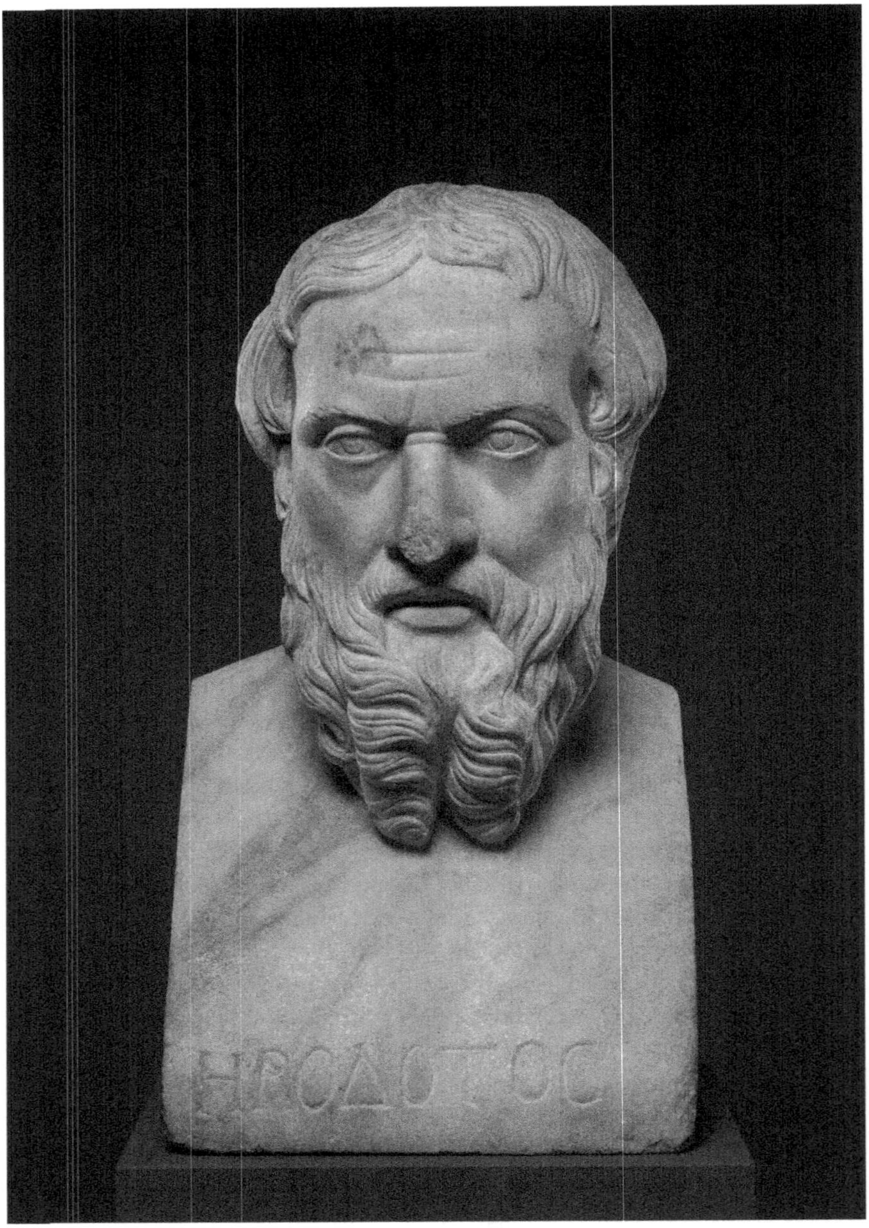

Figure 2.3. Bust of Herodotus. Herodotus lived *c.* 484–424 BC and achieved fame in his own lifetime as a Greek traveller and historian. Copy of a Greek bronze statue, 2nd century AD, Roman. Marble. Metropolitan Museum of Art, New York 91.8 (courtesy of the Metropolitan Museum of Art, New York. Gift of George F. Baker, 1891).

in that particular field. When considering physicians who treated eye complaints (*swnw irty*), there are, for example, Nefertjes and Wa from the Old Kingdom, and Irenakhty from the Old Kingdom/First Intermediate Period. Later, during the Saite Period, Cyrus II, ruler of the Achaemenid Empire, requested that Ahmose II (Amasis, 570–526 BC, 26th Dynasty) send an Egyptian eye specialist to his court to cure him of an ocular complaint (see section 5a).

There is limited evidence of female physicians in ancient Egypt and only two known examples, Peseshet and Tawe (Ghalioungui 1983: 92; see below).

(ii) *s3w* – magician

The word *s3w* is translated as 'magician' in ancient Egyptian and shares the same hieroglyphic ideogram as *s3*, meaning amulet and protection. This perhaps points to this role as being a maker of protective amulets, an advisor on their use and a composer of spells or incantations to be used with them. He may also have acted as a divine intermediary, and his services would have been sought in preventative medicine. Case 1 of the Ebers Papyrus includes the *s3w* among the healers who took the pulse, perhaps indicating that their role was more widespread than just their association with amulets and suggesting their involvement with healing practices.

Evidence for the *s3w* is limited, but in the Sed-festival scenes from the 22nd Dynasty temple of Osorkon II (874–850 BC, 22nd Dynasty) at Bubastis there is a procession of so-called wise men. Within their ranks there are depictions of

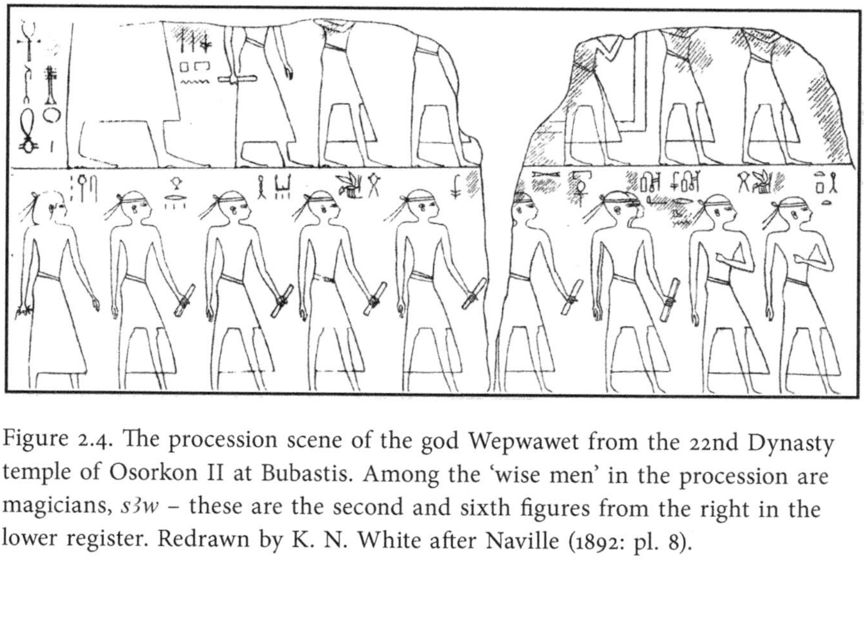

Figure 2.4. The procession scene of the god Wepwawet from the 22nd Dynasty temple of Osorkon II at Bubastis. Among the 'wise men' in the procession are magicians, *s3w* – these are the second and sixth figures from the right in the lower register. Redrawn by K. N. White after Naville (1892: pl. 8).

a *s3w* of Upper Egypt and another individual, probably a *s3w* of Lower Egypt (Naville 1892: pl. 8) (Fig. 2.4). The title is sometimes linked with Serket, the scorpion goddess in the title 'Amulet Man of Serket' (*s3w-šrḳt*), seemingly otherwise known as 'Controller of Serket' (Ritner 1993: 53). This individual is found accompanying mining expeditions and two of the three *swnw* listed on stelae in the temple at Serabit el-Khadim in a quarry in Sinai, Akmu (stela 117) and an anonymous *swnw* (stela 121), probably held this title. Both date to the reign of Amenemhat III (1831–1786 BC, 12th Dynasty) (Gardiner *et al.* 1952: pl. 40, 48; Nunn 1996: 99).

(iii) *ḫrp srḳt* – priest or controller of Serkẹt

Serket was a scorpion goddess normally portrayed as a woman with a scorpion on her head, but also depicted on occasions as a scorpion with the head of a woman, or merely as a scorpion (a key text is von Känel 1984). Her appearance was generally attractive, her influence usually benign, and she was attested for her protective role since at least the Old Kingdom. In the mythological tale of the birth of Horus Serket aids Isis in protecting her infant son Horus from venomous scorpions and snakes. She is also mentioned in the Pyramid Texts and is one of the four protective goddesses who guarded coffins and canopic jars, with the specific responsibility of protecting the god Qebesenuef. An example of this is Utterance 555, PT 1375 (Faulkner 1969: 215).

The cult of Serket is known to have existed since at least the 1st Dynasty, as attested by a reference to a scorpion on the funerary stela of the high official Merka (Tomb 3505) at Saqqara and by her appearance in the Pyramid Texts (Emery 1958: pl. 39; von Känel 1984). There were priests of Serket, but they were not considered to be the servants of the temple; rather, having the title *ḫrp srḳt*, 'One who had Control over Serket', they were believed to have a special role in the treatment of venomous bites from scorpions and snakes. They were later employed by the state to accompany mining expeditions, where such creatures posed a constant threat. Records from Deir el-Medina indicate that additional payments were made to them on an ad hoc basis (Austin 2014: 95).

A major source relating to the role of the priests or 'Controllers of Serket' is the Brooklyn Papyrus, a medical work in two parts that dates to the 30th Dynasty, but is thought to be a copy of an earlier work (Sauneron 1989). This first part (47.218.48) describes the type of snake, its habitat and the symptoms of a bite from the snake, as well as the god or goddess of whom the snake is a manifestation. From a description of the snake, its habitat and the prognosis following a bite it has been possible to identify and distinguish many of the snakes that existed in ancient times from those found today in Egypt. The second part (47.218.85) is mainly concerned with treatment (Chapter 4f).

Again, care has to be taken with a precise categorisation of this role, as several of these figures bear other healing titles, such as Irenakhty and Psamtekseneb, mentioned previously, who were also designated *swnw*.

(iv) *ẖry-ḥbt* – the lector

The term lector (*ẖry-ḥbt*) is translated as 'one who is in control of the papyrus rolls'. This figure was a regular officiant at ritual performances in ancient Egypt. He is recognised as being closely associated with magic, was an important ritualist at funerary ceremonies and was active within the temple sphere (for a fuller discussion of the role of the lector see Forshaw 2014) (Fig. 2.5).

There is also a body of evidence to indicate the lector was involved in healing activities. There is a reference to a lector in P. London (15, l. 8–13):

> Another [conjuration] for [repelling] *nsy*-disease and *tmyt*-disease, which [Isis] did for her father … . This amuletic protection was found at night, descended into the broad court of the Temple of Koptos as a secret of this goddess, by the hand of this lector of this temple, while this land was in darkness. It is the Moon-God who shone on this book on all its way. It was brought as a marvel to the king of Upper and Lower Egypt … . (translated Leitz 1999: 81)

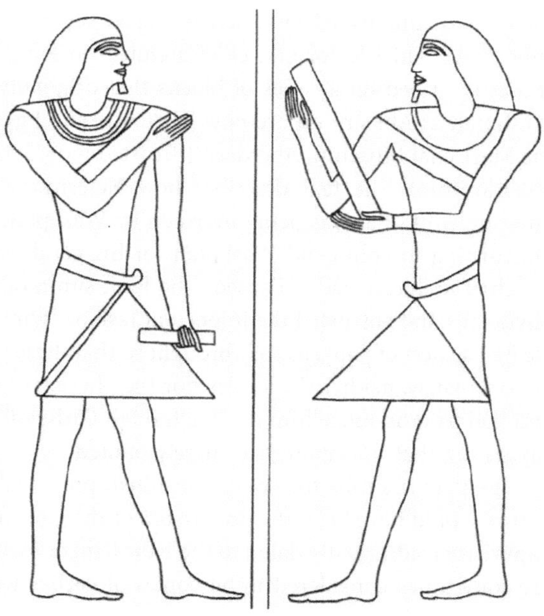

Figure 2.5. Depiction of two lectors from the 6th Dynasty tomb of Qar (G7101). The lector is predominately portrayed wearing a broad sash from his shoulder across his chest and carrying a rolled or unrolled papyrus scroll in his hand. Literacy and ritualistic knowledge were his principal qualifications. Redrawn by K. N. White after Simpson (1976: fig. 28).

The translation of *nsy*-disease and *tmyt*-disease is uncertain, but it has been suggested that the terms refer to unknown illnesses thought to be caused by disease demons (Nunn 1996: 225; Leitz 1999: 80). In this text, although the lector is noted as the agent who discovered the amuletic protection, it does not directly confirm his involvement in the treatment of the particular disease.

As well as reading set incantations from the papyrus scrolls, some of a healing nature, there are references to the lector having more of a direct involvement in healing activities. In P. Berlin 3038 (10, l. 10–11) there is: 'Another ointment to dress a wound: Pork grease. To be coated by an excellent lector, who knows this ointment' (translated Wreszinski 1909: 19, no. 100). In P. Chester Beatty (P. BM. ESA 10695: 15, 1.5–8) there is evidence of a lector knowing about a particular remedy: 'Remedy for the driving out of thirst [illness?] from the mouth [...] a [book?] relating to [the activities] of a lector. Acacia leaves; leaves of the arou tree; panther skin ... ' (Grapow *et al.* 1954–1973: IV 1, 170; Bardinet 1995: 478).

The three prescriptions above are some of the few references to a lector having knowledge of a particular compound or protection aimed at treating a medical condition. In addition, they are rare instances in which a particular professional is named as being the person to administer a medicament; the overwhelming majority of the remedies listed in the medical papyri are not connected with a specific category of healer or individual.

Documentary evidence of the lector's role in healing is found in a number of textual and inscriptional sources. One of these is an inscription in the Old Kingdom mastaba tomb of Washptah. (The mastaba tomb was a special type of tomb for the elite, distinguished by a bench-shaped superstructure.) Washptah was vizier, chief judge, chief lector and chief architect to King Neferirkare. The fragmented text is inscribed on a series of blocks that originally formed part of the tomb of Washptah at Abusir and are now located in the Egyptian Museum, Cairo and in the Marischal Museum, Aberdeen (Breasted 1906: I, 111–13; Strudwick 2005: 318–20; Picardo 2010). The text describes how Neferirkare was inspecting progress on building work that was being overseen by Washptah in his role as chief architect. On turning to commend Washptah for his good work, Neferirkare realised that his chief architect had collapsed. The king summoned both his lectors and chief physicians and entrusted the important task of trying to revive Washptah to them. He had a chest of papyrus rolls brought so that these specialists could consult them. Unfortunately, neither the lectors nor the physicians were able to revive Washptah and had to pronounce him dead, although Grdseloff (1938) interpreted the text by suggesting that Washptah had merely fainted.

The papyrus rolls that were consulted, presumably of a medical and magical nature, could have been the precursors of the later medical papyri. Most medical papyri are traditionally dated to the New Kingdom, but on palaeographic grounds are sometimes considered to be copies of earlier works. The king's summoning of both these groups of individuals again emphasises the multifaceted nature of ancient Egyptian healing practices, with lines of demarcation between the activities of such personnel being blurred.

The participation of both a lector and a physician can be seen again in an event that occurred during the reign of Ramesses II. Hattusili III, the ruler of the Hittites, wrote to Ramesses requesting that Egyptian physicians prepare drugs to help his married sister, Matanzi, to have children. Ramesses replied in a rather undiplomatic manner:

> Now see [here], as for Matanzi, my brother's sister, the king your brother knows her. Fifty, is she? Never! She's sixty for sure! ... No-one can produce medicine for her to have children. But of course, if the Sun-God and the Storm-God should will it ... . But I will send a good lector and an able physician, and they can prepare some birth drugs for her [anyway]. (translated Edel 1976: 69; Kitchen 1982: 91–92)

Again, the treatment involves both magical incantations by the lector and the preparation of drugs by the physician. This passage and similar communications between the Egyptians and the Hittites illustrate the reputation that Egyptian medicine had in the ancient world.

The above examples provide some insight into the lector's association with healing practices. The references to the lector in the medical papyri indicate that he was directly involved with dispensing some of the remedies, suggesting that he had a 'hands on' approach to healing practices as well as a more traditionally perceived role as a narrator of healing incantations and a ritualist.

(d) Paramedical staff

Introduction

The titles, roles and working practices of medical personnel are relatively well attested, although the interactions between different categories of practitioner are less evident. In contrast, textual, iconographic, archaeological and palaeopathological sources provide only limited information about the working lives of paramedical personnel and their relationship with each other and with the physicians. Nevertheless, some tentative conclusions can be drawn regarding the treatment provided to patients by midwives, dry- and wet-nurses and other paramedical personnel, and also the possible interactions between priest–physicians and veterinary practitioners.

The extent and limitations of source material

Archaeological, iconographic, textual and palaeopathological evidence indicates that the care of patients was largely undertaken by midwives, dry-nurses and wet-nurses, who functioned at various levels throughout society. Obstetric and nursing assistance was clearly available, but the limitations of the source material leave many questions unanswered (Cole 1986).

For example, the exact status of midwifery and nursing remains unclear. To what extent did 'professionals', perhaps with some level of formal training, undertake these duties? How much did their roles complement or replace the age-old obstetrical and nursing traditions of the early communities, when patient care would have been undertaken by family, friends or perhaps local magico-medical healers?

Again, little is known about individual practitioners' roles and functions. Although midwifery and wet-nursing were undertaken exclusively by women, both women and men seem to have fulfilled other 'nurturing' roles – for example, as nannies and tutors in elite households. A well-known male example of this role is that of Senenmut, who was tutor to Princess Neferure, daughter of Tuthmosis II (1492–1479 BC, 18th Dynasty) and Queen Hatshepsut (Roehrig 2005). Some evidence suggests that both men and women carried out dry-nursing duties, although it is unclear how this was organised. Male nurses doubtless tended to sick or injured colleagues at work sites, but it is not known whether both men and women provided nursing care in the home, or whether nurses assisted the physicians in treating the sick.

There is also speculation about the social status of midwives and nurses. In the absence of firm evidence, it seems likely that an individual's standing reflected the position of the family they served.

Names and titles of midwives and nurses

There is no evidence that female medical doctors, entitled *swnwt* ('lady physicians'), played any role in obstetrics. However, little is actually known about these women: for example, no information survives about the medical duties of Peseshet, the earliest known holder of the title *'Imyr swnwt* ('Chief Woman Physician' or 'Lady Director of Female Physicians'), who lived during the 5th and 6th Dynasties (Elhabashy & Abdelgawad 2019).

Most names and titles for paramedical practitioners (midwives and wet- or dry-nurses) are associated with wet-nursing or childcare. Some are rather confusing and misleading (discussed in Nunn 1996: 132; Janssen & Janssen 2007: 104–05). There are no definitive Egyptian words for gynaecologists, obstetricians or midwives. However, some researchers translate the title *smyt* as 'midwife'. It accompanies the representation of Hekat (the frog-headed goddess of childbirth) in the Divine Birth scenes in the Temple of Hatshepsut at Deir el-Bahri (see Plate 8). Support for this translation is provided by the description of Hekat's role as a divine midwife in the Westcar Papyrus. The term was also used for the goddess Nekhbet in the Late Period.

The Egyptians had several names and titles for nurses. The most common, *mnꜥt*, is translated as 'wet-nurse' or sometimes 'foster-mother'. The hieroglyphic determinative is either a female breast or a seated woman suckling a child. A variation of this word, *mnꜥy*, was sometimes used for men employed in the royal household as instructors or tutors for the royal children. Although this is a masculine title, a female breast appears as the hieroglyphic determinative, emphasising the title-holder's role as a 'nourisher' and promoter of children's educational development. These men were considered to be very powerful and influential members of the Royal Court.

The term 'dry-nurse' has been suggested as a likely translation for the word *ḫnmtt;* here, the hieroglyphic determinative depicts a woman seated in a chair with a child on her lap. This same image is used as the determinative for the word *rnn*, which means to 'nurse' or 'rear, bring up'.

The roles of nursing and midwifery in society

The training and working practices of midwives

Very little information is available about the training of midwives. According to a late source, they received tuition in the art of obstetrics in the House of Life in Sais, and then transmitted this knowledge to the physicians (Schäfer 1899; Feucht 2001).

Working practices: Textual evidence

The Westcar Papyrus is the only extant textual source that actually provides details of the birthing procedure and confirmation of midwives' active involvement in this process. Also known as 'Tales of Wonder' or 'Tales of the Court of King Khufu', the papyrus describes a series of magical events narrated by Khufu's sons to entertain the king (Blackman & Davies 1988; Parkinson 2001). The fourth tale includes a description of the labour and delivery of triplets to Rededet, the wife of a priest of Re. These infants, the sons of the sun god Re, are destined to become kings of Egypt.

Re directs four goddesses – Isis, Nephthys, Hekat and Meskhenet – to assist Rededet's delivery. Disguised as dancing girls and accompanied by the god Khnum, they seek out Rededet, who is in great pain. Reassuring her distressed husband that they have knowledge of midwifery, they are invited inside to supervise the births.

The first birth is described in detail: Isis and Nephthys stand in front of and behind Rededet, while Hekat hastens the birth. As soon as the child is born, Isis pronounces his name. Then they cut his umbilical cord and wash him, before placing him on a cloth-covered brick. Meskhenet declares that each child will become a king. Then Khnum gives health to the child's body. The text mentions that Rededet isolated herself for a fourteen-day period of purification after the births.

Perhaps surprisingly, the medical papyri provide no direct references to midwifery or obstetrics, although the Kahun Gynaecological Papyrus (Quirke 2002) and the Ebers Papyrus (Ghalioungui 1987; Strouhal *et al.* 2014: 97–203) contain a wide range of treatments for women's diseases and some detailed information about contraception, diagnosis of pregnancy and assessment and treatment of neonates.

However, fumigations, special concoctions for the mother to drink and preparations to be applied to her abdomen are prescribed to ease the pain of childbirth and hasten delivery. One group of remedies in P. Ebers (800–07) and an incantation in P. Ramesseum IV (C 28–30) (Gardiner 1955) were to 'release a child from the belly of a woman'. A prescription in P. Ebers (799) that 'date juice, Lower Egyptian salt, and oil/fat should be taken by mouth' is one of a series (797–99) intended to cause a woman to 'give to the earth' (i.e., to hasten the birth). Another remedy, P. Ebers 823 (with unidentified ingredients), was intended to 'pull together' or contract the uterus, perhaps intended to 'hasten the birth' or alternatively to expel the placenta, or help the uterus return to its normal size. Other remedies address conditions encountered after birth. P. Ebers (828) provides a remedy to 'draw out the blood' – that is, to stop bleeding – and for treating a birth injury to the perineum, P. Kahun (4) indicates that a preparation of oil should be soaked into a woman's vagina.

Working practices: Iconographic evidence of Divine Births

Iconographic evidence relating to midwives' working practices is scanty. Temple scenes provide rare examples of divine or royal pregnancy and births, but add little information about birthing procedures. In a couple of examples, the wall reliefs are still in situ: these depict the Divine Births of Hatshepsut in her temple at Deir el-Bahri (Naville 1896), and Amenhotep III in the Temple of Luxor (Gayet 1894). They represent the New Kingdom myth that every future legitimate ruler was the offspring of a divine union between the ruling pharaoh's chief wife and Amun (the dynasty's foremost deity), who approached the queen in the guise of her own husband.

Scenes of Divine Births of gods or rulers continued in temples of the Late and Graeco-Roman Periods. However, they were now placed in a small, free-standing building known as a 'mammisi' or 'birth-house'. The mammisi (as exemplified at Edfu, Denderah and Philae) stood adjacent to the main temple. The scenes mainly continued the themes found in the New Kingdom temples: the moment of birth, when goddess-midwives attend the queen, seated in a delivery chair; Khnum's modelling of the royal child and its double on his potter's wheel; acknowledgement by the chief temple god that the child is his own legitimate offspring; and his confirmation of the child's rights as a future ruler. There is no evidence that the mammisi ever had an obstetrical or birthing purpose,

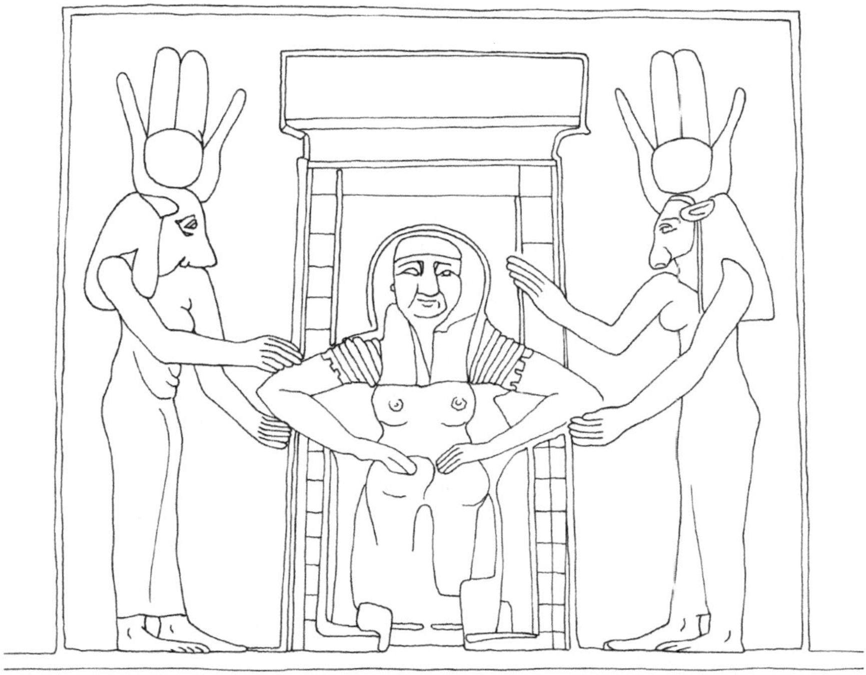

Figure 2.6. Representation of a stone-carved wall-relief showing the mythical birthing scene of Queen Cleopatra (centre) in labour, supported by two Hathor deities. Ptolemaic Period, 1st century BC. Temple of Hathor at Denderah, now located in the Egyptian Museum, Cairo, 40627. Redrawn by L. Mulqueeny after Nunn (1996: 193).

although women may have visited them simply to pray for children or for a safe confinement and delivery.

Additional details of midwifery are preserved in two other iconographic sources. A carved relief from the mammisi of the now-destroyed Temple of Armant survives in a copy made by Napoleon's expedition to Egypt (AD 1798–1801) and published in *Description de l'Égypte* (1809). Dated to the Ptolemaic Period, this relief depicts Cleopatra giving birth. She kneels on the ground, supported from behind by three standing women: Neith and an assistant act as midwives, while an onlooker holds an *ankh*-sign. Two other midwives, and a nurse who suckles the newborn child, kneel in front of the queen. The other relief, which comes originally from the Temple of Denderah, is now in the Egyptian Museum, Cairo (JE 40627). It depicts a squatting woman (shown frontally and in three-dimensional form) resting on her two arms, flanked and attended by two figures of Hathor (Fig. 2.6). These sources indicate that high-status women were attended in labour by at least two or three birth attendants and a wet-nurse. Non-elite women may have been similarly supported, perhaps by older female relatives or professional midwives and wet-nurses.

Working practices: Palaeopathological evidence

No palaeopathological evidence of the methods or treatments employed in midwifery or nursing survives. However, pathological conditions found in human remains can provide information about the problems that midwives and nurses would have encountered. Pregnancy and childbirth were viewed as times of great danger: miscarriages were frequent, as were deaths of the mother and/or her child as a result of complications such as puerperal fever or abnormal pelvic anatomy, as well as a general lack of hygienic conditions. Indeed, studies on mummies have shown that, because women often died in childbirth, their life expectancy was two to four years lower than that of men (for further discussion on life expectancy, see Chapter 6d; Masali & Chiarelli 1972; Chamberlain 2006). Anthropological research into childbirth deaths in ancient Egyptian and Nubian populations is not extensive, however. Studies include several adult females buried with foetuses or neonates in a cemetery at Gabati in central Sudan and research on the remains of two women from Tomb 16 at Thebes, who possibly died from childbirth-related conditions (Onstine *et al.* 2018).

Women with abnormal pelvic skeletal structures faced the possibility of birth obstruction and death in childbirth. This is demonstrated in the body of a 4th Dynasty dwarf excavated at Giza: the woman probably died in childbirth because the head of her normal-sized baby was unable to pass through her birth canal, which was both small and deformed. A similar death was experienced by a Nubian woman whose narrowed birth canal – the result of congenitally absent sacroiliac joints – led to an obstructed delivery (Derry 1909). Royal examples include Princess Hehenit, who lived during the 11th Dynasty. When the anatomist Douglas Derry examined the mummy he noted that an abnormally small pelvis (reported by Williams 1929) had probably caused her death soon after childbirth. A vesicovaginal fistula (a tear from the vagina to the bladder) may indicate that she experienced a protracted delivery.

The mummy of another royal lady, originally identified by Grafton Elliot Smith as Queen Mâkeri and suggested to be the wife of Pinudjem I, was discovered in the Royal Cache at Deir el-Bahri in 1881 and subsequently unwrapped by Grafton Elliot Smith in 1909. He concluded that the queen had probably died during or soon after the birth of her daughter, as indicated by the enormous enlargement of her breasts, the method used to pack the body cavity and the loose and puckered appearance of the abdominal skin (Smith 1912: 98–101; Pls LXXII, LXXIV). This theory was initially supported by the discovery of a small mummy buried alongside the queen in her coffin, although Smith did not unwrap it at the time. This was assumed to be the body of Mâkeri's daughter, but subsequent radiological studies have revealed that the bundle contained a female hamadryas baboon, included in this burial for reasons that remain obscure. Additionally, radiographs revealed that the queen's pregnant appearance was apparently due to over-packing by the embalmers. It has since been established that the mummy was that of Pinudjem's daughter, Maatkare, God's Wife of Amun (Harris & Weeks 1973: 173–75; Dodson & Hilton 2004: 126–27, 329).

The birthing environment

The Egyptian word for 'birth' (*mswt*) is translated as 'to come down to the ground'. The hieroglyphic determinative of this word shows a kneeling woman from whose body the head and arms of a child emerge. The rare iconographic and textual descriptions of childbirth also indicate that the vertex method, in which the woman squats or kneels and rests on her arms, was the normal means of delivery. Turin stela 102 states: 'He left me like a woman on the bricks', and in the Bible (Exodus I: 16) the pharaoh says: 'When you do the office of a midwife to the Hebrew women, and see them upon the stones … '.

From earliest times, women squatted on two bricks separated by a space into which the child was delivered. The birthing bricks became a religious and magical focus: spells were recited over them to drive away evil forces and it was believed that, after birth, the child's destiny was inscribed on them by Thoth, god of writing. The bricks were personified by the goddess of childbirth, Meskhenet, as were the birthing stools or chairs that developed from them: the centre of the seat was removed in these, to facilitate a normal vertex delivery. Similar chairs are still used today in some rural areas of Egypt.

A wall relief in the Temple of Kom Ombo depicts the goddesses Nephthys and Isis crouching on birthing stools, but no examples of birthing furniture have been conclusively identified from ancient Egypt. An item found in the tomb of Khenmose may have been used for this purpose, or as a portable night stool (see Plate 9).

Special accommodation was provided for the lying-in, birth and subsequent period of isolation and purification (Janssen & Janssen 2007: 1–6). Special confinement pavilions, built either in a garden or on a roof-top, consisted of papyrus stalk columns, walls woven from plants, and roofing mats. They are depicted in mural scenes in houses at Deir el-Medina and Amarna; another example occurs in a wall relief in the Royal Tomb at Amarna, which records the death of Princess Meketaten in childbirth.

In some circumstances, a particular room in the home was used as a birthing chamber – for example, the front room in the small, cramped houses at Deir el-Medina. This had a low, inbuilt brick platform, and the mural decoration and contents of the room (such as beds with mattresses, head-rests, cushions and stools) often featured deities associated with fertility and childbirth (such as Bes and Taweret). However, key items associated with birthing – such as apotropaic wands and birthing chairs or stools – have not been found here.

Mural scenes in the houses and statuettes indicate that, throughout the lying-in period and after the birth, the mother wore no clothing except for a collar and girdle, and her hair was dressed in a distinctive manner. During the birth she was attended and supported by several older women, but her husband does not appear to have been present (Janssen & Janssen 2007: 1–6).

After the birth the attendants cut the umbilical cord with an obsidian knife (Herodotus II: 84); according to P. Westcar, this took place once the newborn had been washed and placed to rest on a pillow. The umbilical cord and placenta, mentioned in a few texts, were regarded as important and received special treatment. After delivery, the mother was isolated in the birthing room for fourteen days, where she was assisted and fed by girls whose nudity and hairstyle mirrored her own appearance.

Magical protection during childbirth and pregnancy

To alleviate the considerable uncertainties associated with childbirth, practical measures to protect the mother and child were augmented with magico-religious rites. Amulets were placed on the woman's body and prayers and magical

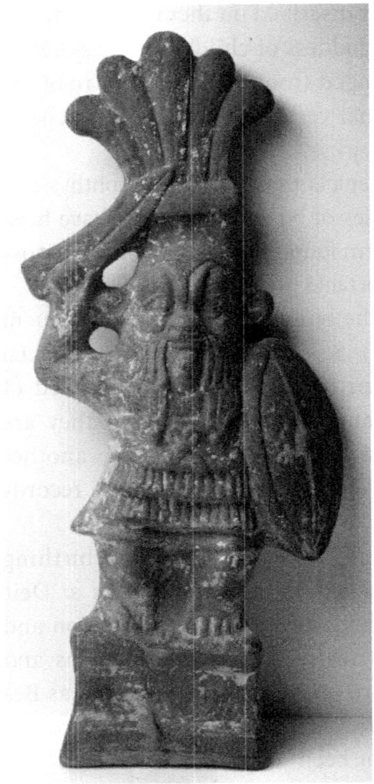

Figure 2.7. Terracotta statuette of the dwarf deity Bes wearing his characteristic feathered headdress. He was believed to protect women and children by using music, singing and dancing to drive away evil. Because of his defensive nature he was sometimes depicted in the garb of a Roman soldier during the Roman Period. Graeco-Roman Period. Unprovenanced. The Manchester Museum, 11244 (courtesy of The Manchester Museum, The University of Manchester).

spells were recited both by attendants supervising the birth and by priests and magicians (Fig. 2.7). For example, P. Ramesseum IV contains spells to assist with procreation, pregnancy and neonates. Two magical birth prognostications are given in the Ebers Papyrus and P. Berlin 3027 provides the 'Magical Spells for Mother and Child', all of which were probably recited by lectors or 'Magicians of the Nursery'.

Some female figurines were associated with childbirth (Pinch 1983), and deities including Bes and Taweret provided divine protection during pregnancy and childbirth. Iconographic images of Bes often show him playing musical instruments to drive away evil forces from the birthing chamber, while Taweret's hybrid form, combining the characteristics of a woman, hippopotamus, crocodile and lion, gave her unique powers to protect women and infants (see Plate 10).

The status of midwives in society

Despite inconclusive evidence, some professionally trained midwives probably did exist in ancient Egypt (Töpfer 2014). However, their social status is unclear. According to the Westcar Papyrus, the goddesses dressed themselves up as dancing girls when they went to deliver Rededet's triplets, and this may imply a relatively lowly status, perhaps because of the 'ritually impure' nature of their work (Janssen & Janssen 2007: 6). However, some of them seem to have achieved privileged positions: as with wet-nurses and nannies, their individual status probably depended on the social standing of the family they served.

Some midwifery would have been undertaken by local healers. A canvas mask (probably representing Bes or his consort Beset) and pair of apotropaic ivory wands were discovered in a house at Kahun (Petrie 1890: 30, pl. VIII). They were probably owned by a local female magician who practised magico-religious rites within the community to promote women's fertility and protect them and their offspring during pregnancy and childbirth (further discussed in Chapter 5e, ii).

Confirmation that such wands were associated with childbirth comes from a wall scene in the tomb of a local governor, Dhutihotep, at Deir el-Bersheh, which shows a woman (probably a wet-nurse or nanny) carrying one of these wands (Janssen & Janssen 2007: 8). Various uses of the wand have been suggested: it may have been placed directly on to a woman's stomach during childbirth; used to outline an area on the ground where the practitioner could perform protective rites around pregnant women; employed as clappers in ritual dances to banish hostile spirits from a sacred space or birthing area; or placed directly on to a child's body to identify the baby with Re and transmit the god's powers and strengths to the infant.

It is impossible to determine whether professionally trained midwives or local practitioners of magic had any direct association with the *rekhet* ('wise woman' or 'knowing one'), whose precise role and duties within communities also remain unclear (see Chapter 4d). These groups may all have been involved in obstetrical procedures. The 'wise women' perhaps offered a combination of magical and rational treatments, but although evidence seems to indicate that they were consulted both as diviners and healers some research has disputed this dual role.

The background and working practices of nurses

Professional nursing care was probably provided by two distinct but interwoven groups of paramedical personnel.

Dry-nurses were probably engaged in tending sick or severely disabled patients, or sometimes assisting the elderly, although this duty generally rested with a person's own children. Palaeopathological and inscriptional evidence attests that the sick, disabled and elderly were supported by a system of social care and some level of medical or paramedical attention. There is palaeopathological evidence of a substantial numbers of healed fractures, and individual cases of recovery and survival have been identified that demonstrate the effectiveness of nursing regimes.

One textual source preserves an order given to Papet (probably a professional nurse or orderly) requiring him to care for his co-workers at a Theban work site (Jonckheere 1945). Another source records that, in a group of men punished with a hundred blows, many died but some survived, including an elderly man who was restored to health after being comatose for four days and receiving nursing care for three months (Worth Estes 1993: 74). There are also cases of paraplegic patients whose survival would have depended on dedicated nursing care; these include an example in the Edwin Smith Papyrus (case 8) and a male burial at Shurafa (Derry 1913).

A radiological and neurological investigation of a body presumed to belong to Geheset, an elite woman at the Royal Court (*c.* 2000 BC), has produced some significant results (Nerlich *et al.* 2010). Radiological studies have shown that the right hand was deformed, with a severe malposition of the hand bones. There was also a strong indication of paralysis of the right side of the face. The researchers concluded that the woman had probably suffered from a severe neurological disorder, probably cerebral palsy, a disease that affects neonates, and may have experienced a range of disabilities throughout her lifetime. Nevertheless, she apparently supervised an important elite household – a role that would have depended on a high level of personal support and nursing assistance.

More information is available about wet-nurses. Mothers usually breast-fed their own children but, particularly in elite households, wet-nurses were often engaged, perhaps for social or medical reasons, to provide breastfeeding services for their children. Many probably stayed on to serve as nannies. According to iconographic and inscriptional sources, children were breast-fed for up to three years, perhaps because it was regarded as a viable method of contraception. The close bond created between child and wet-nurse was underpinned by religious beliefs. Milk, symbolising the divine liquid with which Isis had healed her son Horus, was thought to contain magical, life-giving properties, and mothers' milk, stored in special vessels in the form of a squatting woman holding a child in her lap, was used in a range of medicinal treatments. Wall scenes in religious contexts quite often show the king being suckled by a cow, and a unique ancient scene, preserved only in a 19th century reproduction, shows a cow simultaneously suckling a non-royal child and its own calf. However, there is no confirmatory evidence that animals were used as surrogate wet-nurses.

The status of nurses in society

Source material emphasises the importance attributed to wet-nursing. There are many depictions of a god or the king being suckled and nourished by a goddess, and bronze statuettes representing Isis breast-feeding her son Horus were particularly popular in later periods (Fig. 2.8).

A royal heir was usually attended by a wet-nurse, a royal nurse and a chief royal nurse. Stelae, statues representing nurses with royal children and burial assemblages all confirm the important role of nurses in royal households and their ability to achieve high social status and wealth. Typically, some were wives or mothers of high officials, who used their position at court to advance the career of a husband or son and promote the interests of their own families. Tey, the chief royal nurse and wet-nurse of Queen Nefertiti, is a celebrated example: her husband, Ay, progressed from chariot-commander to vizier, and ultimately to the kingship.

The privileged status of these women sometimes continued after death: they were honoured with the highest standard of mummification and even burial near the royal family. One example is Lady Rai, the wet-nurse of Queen Ahmose-Nefertari and possibly of her husband, King Ahmose I (1550–1525 BC, 18th Dynasty). Although the location of her original tomb is unknown, her well-preserved mummy, with its abundance of false hair, was discovered in the Royal Cache at Deir el-Bahri in 1881. Elliot Smith, who unwrapped and examined the mummy in 1909, described it as: 'the most perfect example of embalming that has come down to us from the time of the early XVIIIth Dynasty, or perhaps even of any period' (Smith 1912: 11).

Other prestigious burials include those of Maia, the 'Great Royal Nurse' of King Tutankhamun, at Saqqara; Sit-re, Hatshepsut's nurse, close to the queen's own Theban tomb; and, also at Thebes, the tomb and burial assemblage of Djesraperet, wet-nurse of the daughter of King Taharqa (690–664 BC, 25th Dynasty) (Guiddotti 2008: 130).

Wet-nurses were also greatly respected members of elite households. Some scenes on stelae and in officials' tombs depict them among members of the

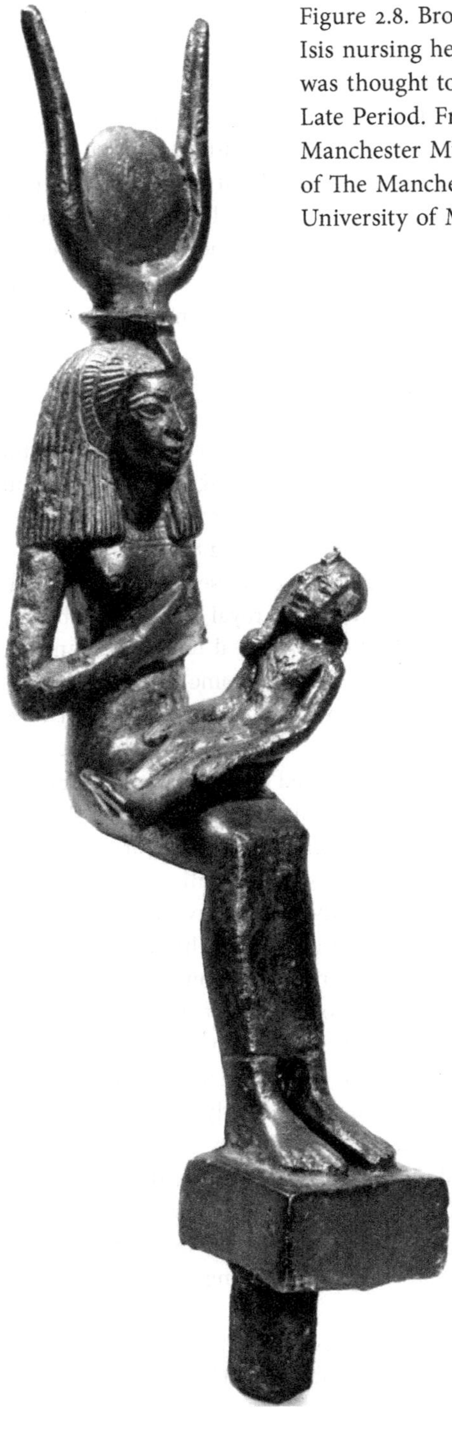

Figure 2.8. Bronze statuette of goddess Isis nursing her son Horus. Her milk was thought to have healing properties. Late Period. From Saqqara, now in The Manchester Museum, 1971.25A (courtesy of The Manchester Museum, The University of Manchester).

family, indicating that bonds continued to exist with their employers' families. Even in non-elite families, wet-nurses were held in high regard. For example, a letter from a scribe of the community at Deir el-Medina requests that his son should make provision not only for a woman and her daughter but also for the nurse (Janssen & Janssen 2007: 15).

Relative values placed on professional services are addressed in a papyrus in the Turin collection that records the payments made by a workman in respect of his wife's confinement (see Chapter 1b). The wet-nurse was to receive goods of a higher value than was the physician. This may imply that the services of the wet-nurse were considered more important than the physician's contribution, or perhaps her higher payment may reflect a longer involvement with the family (Janssen & Janssen 2007: 15). Although this document seems to indicate that physicians (whose work included treating gynaecological conditions) were involved in the birthing process, this conclusion is not universally accepted.

Other paramedical personnel

Evidence from two 6th Dynasty tombs at Saqqara belonging to Ankhmahor and Khentika depicts practitioners who have been variously described either as possibly manicurists/pedicurists, physiotherapists or reflexologists (Fig. 2.9).

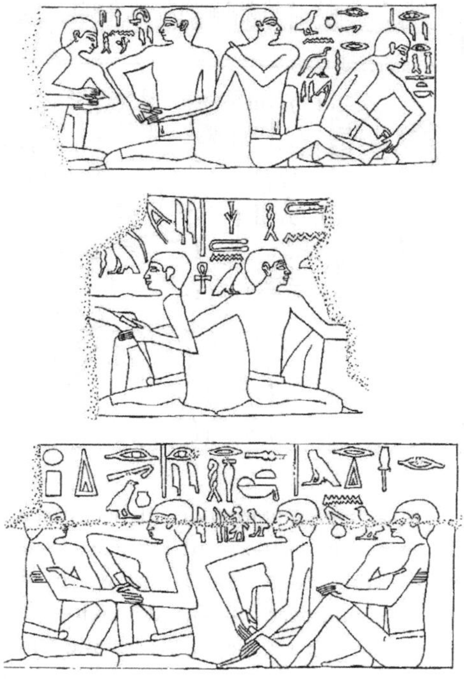

Figure 2.9. Scenes from the 6th Dynasty mastaba tombs of Khentika and Ankhmahor at Saqqara depicting ritual purification, manicurists/pedicurists, physiotherapists or reflexologists. Redrawn by K. N. White after James (1953: pl. 9), Badawy (1978: figs 27, 28) and Nunn (1996: fig. 6.14).

Other inconclusive evidence of paramedical activity occurs in wall scenes and accompanying inscriptions elsewhere (discussed in Chapter 4e).

Veterinary practitioners

Veterinary provision for domesticated and tamed animals

The main iconographic sources of information relating to animals are the wall scenes in tombs and temples from the Pharaonic and Graeco-Roman Periods (Houlihan 1996: 10); Neolithic rock art in the Saharan desert provides other examples.

Tomb and temple art shows herdsmen engaging in a whole range of activities related to animal husbandry and management (Brewer *et al.* 1992; Brewer 2001; Scanlan 2004). They doubtless also provided treatment for sick animals in their care. However, according to the conventions of religious art, only healthy

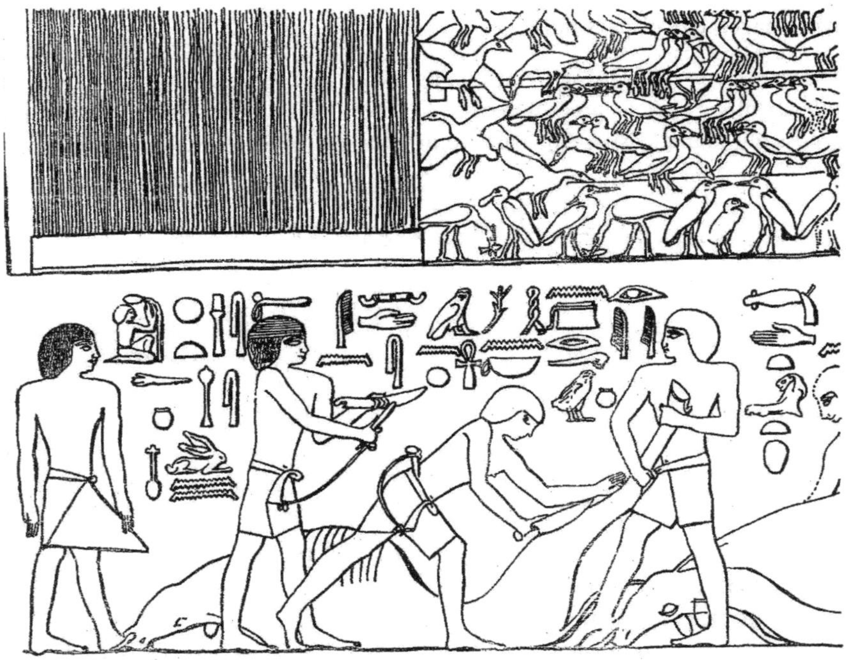

Figure 2.10. Representation of butchers preparing joints of beef to be offered to deities as part of the regular rituals carried out in the temples. 5th Dynasty tomb of Ptahhotep. According to the hieroglyphic text, Wenennefer (extreme left) is presiding over this sacred activity. Designated here as a *wꜥb*-priest and physician, he was a 'Chief of Priests and Chief Physician to the King'. Redrawn by K. N. White after Mariette (1889: 335) and Ghalioungui (1961: fig. 12).

animals were represented, to ensure perfection in the afterlife, and thus there is insufficient iconographic evidence to determine the true nature of the herdsman's veterinary role or to identify the involvement of any other practitioners.

The need for veterinary provision would have arisen with the establishment of settled communities and the parallel developments of animal domestication. Crowded accommodation in farms and villages where humans and animals lived in close proximity led to an increased vulnerability to disease in both groups. Domesticated animals would have been exposed not only to endemic parasitic conditions but increasingly to animal diseases brought back through warfare or trade (Dunlop & Williams 1996: 73; Lord 2016: 143). Parallel therapeutic treatments for humans and animals probably emerged in the earliest communities, perhaps undertaken at first by the same personnel. However, there is no record of how such links may have originated or developed.

In addition to the herdsmen who cared for animals in the food chain, veterinary supervisors were employed by the temples to oversee butchery of sacrificial offerings or to nurture and treat the cult animals (Figs 2.10 and 2.11). However, it is unclear whether the priests supervising the temple sacrifices had any veterinary skills or were more akin to public health inspectors (Lord 2016: 147–48).

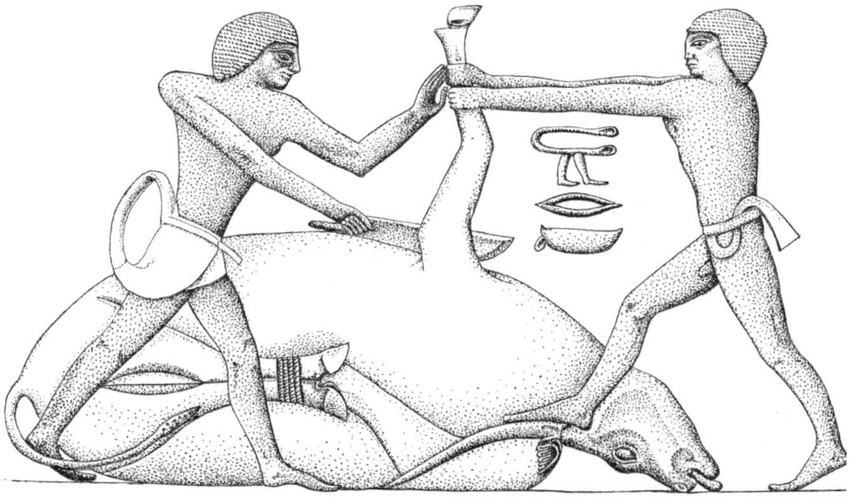

Figure 2.11. Representation of a temple scene depicting the butchering of a sacrificial bull. This meat formed part of the regular meals offered first to the gods and then to the priests as their daily stipend. Drawing based on New Kingdom examples of temple wall-scenes.

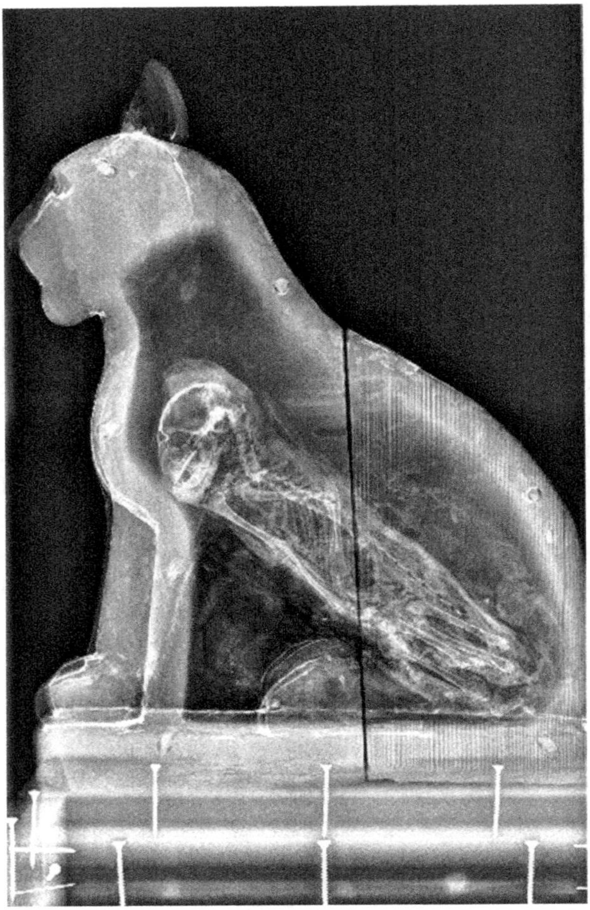

Figure 2.12. Radiograph reveals a mummified cat contained within a cat-shaped painted wooden coffin. A wealthy owner probably provided this elaborate burial for a favoured pet. Late Period. Unprovenanced, acquired 1921. Manchester Museum, 9303 (courtesy of The Manchester Museum, The University of Manchester).

The Egyptians did not simply regard animals as a food source. Throughout the millennia, animals remained an integral and vitally important part of society. Their major role in religious beliefs was characterised by the hybrid human and animal forms of most Egyptian deities, and by the worship of cultic animals in some temples. Animals were also kept as family pets, and some were specially bred to accompany their owners on hunting expeditions (Fig. 2.12). Animals mummified and interred in catacombs and cemeteries (Bleiburg *et al.* 2013) included cultic animals, domestic pets and vast numbers dedicated by pilgrims as votive offerings at sacred sites (Martin 1981; Davies 2006). Many of the latter would probably have been reared at high density, thus increasing the risk of disease. Practitioners with extensive experience and perhaps some specialised training would have been required to supervise the well-being and medical treatment of these animals.

Veterinary treatments: palaeopathological sources

There is a marked discrepancy in the number and range of scientific investigations that have been undertaken on human and animal mummies. This is partly because many animal mummies are badly damaged or poorly preserved and there is considerable variation in the quality of mummification. However, the limited range of surveys already undertaken has revealed injuries, developmental abnormalities and disease in animals. These have included a radiological study of fifty-three mummified cats in the British Museum collection (Armitage & Clutton-Brock 1981); investigation of baboons and Barbary macaques from the baboon catacombs at Saqqara (Goudsmit & Brandon-Jones 1999); and the use of high-magnification macrophotographs to examine mummified dogs from el-Deir (Roman Period) (Huchet *et al.* 2013). In an elite predynastic cemetery (HK6) at Hierakonpolis, where various animal remains have been discovered, the healing process observed in the fractured remains of seven baboons suggests that the animals were given a safe place and human attention during their recovery (Hierakonpolis Online 2014).

The vast numbers of surviving mummified animals provide a potential resource for future palaeopathological studies on animal disease and veterinary medicine (Ikram *et al.* 2014). These include ample resources from excavation sites and museum collections (Ikram 2015). The *Ancient Egyptian Animal Bio-Bank* provides other opportunities: established in 2010 in the KNH Centre at the University of Manchester (McKnight *et al.* 2011), it collates information on mummified animal remains in museum collections outside Egypt and undertakes macroscopic and imaging studies on animal mummies (McKnight & Atherton-Woolham 2015: 65–81).

Veterinary treatments: inscriptional and iconographic sources

Textual evidence relating to disease, treatments and medical practitioners associated with human conditions is very limited, but sources available for veterinary medicine are even rarer. There is only one extant and fragmentary document – the Kahun Veterinary Papyrus (UC 32036, Lot LV.2) (Walker 1964; Collier & Quirke 2004: 55). Found among the papyrological documentation discovered at Kahun, a Middle Kingdom town occupied by the families of royal workmen, this document is now housed in the Petrie Museum at University College London (Petrie 1891; Griffith 1897).

Only the main section survives, providing three treatments probably all relating to bovines. As with treatments indicated for human diseases in the medical papyri, these case studies include a title, symptoms, treatment, prognosis, re-examination, further symptoms and finally, further treatment (Lord 2016: 150–51). Evidence from the smaller fragments indicates that the document originally also addressed conditions in other animals.

Veterinary practitioners: possible links with human healthcare
There is no specific word in hieroglyphs for a veterinary practitioner, but it has been suggested that human and veterinary practitioners may have worked interactively, and that perhaps some *wꜥb*-priests of Sekhmet had an additional role as veterinary specialists (Ghalioungui 1963: 113; Nunn 1996: 119–20; Lord 2016: 147–48) (see Plate 11). However, problems with the translation and interpretation of the inscriptional sources make it difficult to establish these associations.

For example, the meaning of particular titles remains unresolved. The title *rḫ kꜣw* ('One who knows Bulls') has been variously interpreted as 'veterinary surgeon' or as the person responsible for deciding if cattle were fit for sacrifice (Lord 2016: 148). Perhaps it is worth considering whether some priestly titles may have had a wider remit than hitherto recognised. For example, the duties of priests who supervised the food provision for temple animals may also have been responsible for veterinary care.

(e) Mummification and embalmers

Ancient Egyptian embalmers acquired a direct and detailed knowledge of human anatomy through the practice of mummification and the techniques of wrapping and bandaging the body. According to Herodotus (II, 86), they were a distinct profession, but some of their experience and skills may have been transmitted to medical practitioners, since tenuous links probably existed between the two professions (see Chapter 3a).

Source material relating to embalmers is closely associated with evidence about mummification. Current knowledge of this procedure is based on examination of mummified remains and associated palaeopathological studies (Evershed & Clark 2021), archaeological and iconographic evidence from tomb wall scenes, coffins and canopic jars, and literary evidence.

Archaeological and iconographic evidence

Tomb wall scenes
Embalmers are depicted in wall scenes in two Theban tombs, where they are engaged in various stages of the mummification procedure and the production of funerary goods. These 19th Dynasty tombs belonged to Tjay (TT 23), a scribe of the royal dispatchers in the reign of Merenptah (1213–1203 BC, 19th Dynasty) (Ivanov 2018), and Amenemope (Ipy) (TT 41), 'Royal Scribe and Chief Administrator of the Domain of Amun' in the early 19th Dynasty (Assmann 1996).

Another example occurs in the rock-cut tomb (TT 1) belonging to Sennedjem, located in the cemetery near the royal workmen's town of Deir el-Medina

(Bruyère 1959; Porter & Moss 1994). This Ramesside Period tomb has a wall scene showing Anubis, the god of embalming, attending to a mummy lying on an embalming table inside an embalming booth.

A purification ceremony associated with mummification is also found in the 19th Dynasty tomb of Khabekhnet at Deir el-Medina (TT2) (Davis 1999). He was the son of Sennedjem and held the title 'Servant in the Place of Truth'. This wall scene shows a rite taking place inside an embalming tent where a priest, wearing the jackal-headed mask of the god Anubis, undertakes the purification of a large fish lying on the embalming table. The fish is a very unusual replacement for the human mummy usually depicted in such scenes. It represents Osiris, divine king of the underworld, and the rite was believed to play an important part in the tomb-owner's resurrection.

Coffins, canopic jars and other artefacts

Further examples occur in vignettes painted on coffins and canopic jars. These include the Late Period coffin of Djedbastetiufankh (No. 1954) in the Hildesheim Museum, Germany. A scene in the upper register shows a naked corpse lying on an embalming table, attended by three embalmers and the officiating priest who wears the jackal-headed mask of Anubis. A lower register scene depicts a cleansing and purification rite performed by attendants who pour water over a naked corpse lying in a bed of natron.

In the 19th Dynasty Papyrus of Ani, which contains the Book of Going Forth by Day (Book of the Dead), a vignette shows Anubis attending a mummified body inside an embalming booth.

Literary evidence: Egyptian sources

No extant Egyptian sources provide a complete description of the technical processes involved in mummification, but some papyri and stelae contain scattered literary references to mummification and associated religious rituals.

The embalming ritual

Details of the Ritual of Embalming are preserved in P. Boulaq 3 (Egyptian Museum, Cairo), Papyrus 5158 (the Louvre), P. Durham 1983.11 and P. St Petersburg 18128. These documents, which may be derived from a common source, probably all date to the Roman Period (30 BC–AD 395). The papyri provide a major literary source for the mummification technique in ancient Egypt (Smith 2009), and may be more important in this respect than Herodotus or Diodorus Siculus (Töpfer 2017).

The beginning of the text is missing and thus the original title is unknown, but it is known by the name of 'Embalming Ritual', as suggested by Maspero (1875: 16). It includes a detailed set of instructions to guide the embalmer in his performance of rites accompanying the mummification process. Although this probably reflects contemporary embalming practices of the Ptolemaic and Roman Periods, perhaps in use at different locations across Egypt, it does not set out any major innovations or depart in a significant way from methods employed in earlier times (Töpfer 2017: 24).

The texts do not merely provide a simple order of procedure focused on anointing and wrapping. The aim of the ritual was to reproduce in every detail the method which, according to mythology, had been used to mummify Osiris and ensure his resurrection. To this end, these documents include a collection of prayers and incantations with religious symbolism and many mythological allusions; intended to glorify the dead, these were recited after every rite.

The Rhind Papyri

Discoveries made by Alexander Henry Rhind (1833–1863) during the two seasons he spent in Egypt (1855–1856 and 1856–1857) include papyri from an 18th Dynasty Theban tomb which have references to embalming ceremonies.

Literary evidence: the Classical sources

The earliest and nearest to complete extant account of the mummification procedure is provided by Herodotus (II, 86–88). The Greek historian Diodorus Siculus (I, 91) provides some additional information about the mummification process.

The reliability of Herodotus' account

Herodotus' description of three distinct methods of intentional mummification, available according to cost, has formed the basis of our current understanding of this procedure. However, he was writing centuries after the development of mummification had reached its peak, and sometimes his sources may not have been entirely reliable: for example, the Egyptian priests who were often his major informants may not always have wished to fully divulge the secrets of their religious beliefs and practices.

Because of this, scholars have sometimes questioned the veracity and accuracy of his work, and aspects of his account of the mummification process have come under scrutiny. However, scientific studies focused in particular on the timespan he allots for mummification, and whether natron, the dehydrating agent, was used in a dry or liquid state, have tended to support his statements (Lucas & Harris 1962: 270–326; Garner 1979). Nevertheless, palaeopathological studies continue to demonstrate that, although all embalmers appear to have pursued the main well-defined stages of mummification, they did have some flexibility regarding whether, for example, excerebration (brain removal) and evisceration (removal of thoracic and abdominal organs) were performed (Wade & Nelson 2013).

The mummification procedure

By drawing on all these sources, it is possible to reconstruct the main stages of mummification. The best-quality procedure involved the performance of elaborate funerary rites as well as a series of physical interventions intended to preserve the body. The two crucial steps to arrest decomposition were evisceration of the corpse and dehydration of the bodily tissues. The viscera were sometimes left in situ in the body, but more often were removed from the thoracic and abdominal cavities through an abdominal incision in the left flank (or sometimes through the anus). The heart was usually left in place, probably because it was thought to be the locus of the individual's life-force and personality; however, there are examples where it has been removed (Loynes 2015). The kidneys were left in situ: there is no known religious or philosophical reason for this, but they may have been difficult to identify or excise because of their position inside the body.

Although never a universal practice, excerebration was introduced at least as early as the Middle Kingdom and was in widespread use by the New Kingdom. The nasal route, via a perforation in the ethmoid bone, was most commonly used, and demonstrates the embalmers' high level of technical skill. Following excerebration, the brain tissue was discarded. The Egyptians probably recognised the brain's significance in controlling bodily functions, as described in P. Edwin Smith, Case 8 (Breasted 1930: 12–13; 201–16; Sanchez & Meltzer 2012: 86–94). However, since they did not regard the brain as essential for continuing existence in the afterlife, there was no necessity to retain it after death.

The body cavities were then washed out and a temporary filling of dry natron, gum resin and vegetable matter was inserted. In the next stage, the body was covered entirely with a dehydrating agent: research has confirmed that this was usually natron, used in a dry or solid state rather than in solution (Garner 1979). According to Herodotus, this process lasted no longer than seventy days, but studies have indicated that a period of forty days may have been the optimum, with religious rites occupying the remaining time (Garner 1979). This is supported by literary evidence: the Embalming Ritual confirms that mummification occupied the final forty days of the mummification process (Töpfer 2017: 24).

After dehydration, the temporary packing mixture was taken out of the body. Eviscerated organs were dehydrated separately and, wrapped as four individual packages, were reinserted into the cavities or stored in four containers (canopic jars). Less frequently, they were wrapped together in a large package and placed on the legs of the mummy. Although the intention was that each individual organ would always be allocated to a specific jar or package, studies have demonstrated that this distribution was sometimes a random and careless process, with organs not always distributed correctly.

These procedures were essential to prevent putrefaction of the body, but they were followed by steps that were largely cosmetic, including closing the abdominal incision, plugging the nostrils with resin or wax and anointing the body with gum resins and oils.

The embalmers then wrapped the body in a series of linen cloths and bandages, inserting amulets between the layers in order to provide magical protection for the owner on the journey to the next world. Finally, a liquid resinous substance was poured over the mummy and coffin before they were taken from the embalmers' workshop to the family home in readiness for the funeral and burial.

Herodotus mentions two less expensive methods of mummification, neither of which involved complete evisceration. Liquefaction of the viscera was a key feature of the second method: oil of cedar was injected into the anus and the body was treated with natron; once this had taken effect, the oil was drained away, bringing with it the liquefied intestines and stomach. The body, consisting of only the skeleton and surface skin, was now returned to the family. The third method, used for poorer clients, involved purging the body cavities to remove the intestines and then treating the corpse with natron.

Over the millennia, only two major innovations were added to the mummification procedure: excerebration and various techniques introduced by the embalmers in the 21st Dynasty to give the mummy a more rounded and realistic appearance. Subcutaneous packing of the body and face was a key feature: sawdust, butter, linen and mud were introduced through small incisions in the skin and mouth, and the wrapped viscera were re-inserted into the body cavities. The skin was painted with red ochre (for men) and yellow ochre (for women), false plaits and curls were woven into the natural hair, and artificial eyes were sometimes inserted into the orbits. However, these intricate, expensive and time-consuming processes were discontinued after the 23rd Dynasty.

The embalmers' roles and functions

The Classical literary sources indicate that embalming was supervised and undertaken by distinct categories of personnel. The 'cutters' (Greek 'paraschistos') made the abdominal incision in the mummy and removed the viscera. They belonged to the lowest social class, which may have included convicted criminals, and were regarded as ritually impure, perhaps because their work was associated with health hazards and bodily contamination. Religious beliefs centred on respect for the dead may also have influenced the social ostracism of this group, since their work arguably involved some defilement of the corpse. Other menial workers included the men who washed and cleaned the mummy and viscera and prepared the natron, resin and oils.

However, the mummification process also involved elite practitioners: the daily work was overseen by scribes, while a specialist class of embalmers was in overall control. They held various high-status, sometimes priestly, titles that were probably hereditary; they belonged to a special guild, and stood at the forefront of an important industry that generated considerable income and employed many workers, including those who produced coffins and tomb equipment.

According to Herodotus (II, 87), the embalmers played a key entrepreneurial role in advising relatives of the deceased about the available methods of mummification. They used painted wooden models of mummies to illustrate and explain the three procedures, and fixed a price with their clients once they had selected their preferred method of mummification. However, the embalmers' prime function was to supervise all the mummification ceremonies and to perform the associated rituals, for which they wore a jackal-headed mask to impersonate Anubis, the patron deity of embalming and Lord of the Necropolis. According to mythology, Anubis had mummified the body of Osiris, thus ensuring his resurrection as a god, and, by impersonating Anubis and recreating this process in detail, the embalmers were reaffirming that mummification was not merely a physical process. By carrying out appropriate rituals and funerary recitations, they sought to ensure that their clients would also experience the Osirian rebirth.

The Embalming Ritual (see above) provides some very detailed descriptions of the technical and religious procedures undertaken by embalmers to transform the corpse into a mummy and a glorified spirit. Each of the twelve chapters listed in the papyri contains two sections. The first provides practical instructions on how to deal with body parts, referring to the bandages, unguents and plants used in anointing and wrapping the body during the second half of the seventy-day period of mummification. It describes how the process was carried out from the head downwards: this was supervised by the 'Chief of Embalmers' (*ḥry-sštꜣ*), and the 'God's Sealer' (*ẖtmw-nṯr*) anointed the head and face of the mummy.

Different types of cloth and bandage used to wrap the mummy are described, as are the procedures of wrapping and inserting artificial gold and electrum nails between the bandages of the fingers and toes. There are no references to evisceration or dehydration, although these may have been mentioned in columns of text missing from the beginning of the documents. There is also no description of the outer components of the mummy: the linen shroud, funerary mask, and cartonnage chest and foot covers (cartonnage is a composition of papyrus and gum or glue used to manufacture items of funerary equipment). The second section of each chapter focused on the glorification spells: these were recited later, on the final night of the mummification rites, after the technical procedures were finished.

Other groups involved in the liturgical and funerary preparations included priests of Osiris and lectors who recited passages from the sacred texts at specific points in the embalming ritual and led the chants and prayers at the funeral.

The association between embalmers and physicians

There is no evidence from pharaonic times that physicians performed human dissection in Egypt. However, according to Classical sources, the practice occurred briefly in the Ptolemaic Period when Herophilus – a Greek physician working in Alexandria – undertook dissection on human cadavers (see Chapter 7). There is also some evidence that living criminals were supplied for him to practise vivisection (von Staden 1989).

However, the embalmers' work would certainly have enabled the Egyptians to acquire a detailed knowledge of human anatomy and, with the possible exception of the kidneys, to make a correct identification of the viscera. The preparation of a mummy also required a high level of expertise to apply the bandages and wrappings to the body, but it is unclear whether this was carried out by the embalmer himself or a specialist bandager to whom the embalmer supplied the materials.

The embalmers' wealth of experience regarding anatomy would have been invaluable to contemporary physicians, and may have been handed on to them, although the exact nature of professional links between embalmers and physicians, and possible routes of transmission, are unclear. In discussing these issues, Nunn (1996: 42–44) comments on Herodotus' statement that embalmers were regarded as unclean, suggesting that this may have obstructed any formal interaction between the two professions. However, he also quotes an earlier source (P. Edwin Smith: Case 9, Gloss A and Case 19, Gloss A) that implies that some links probably did exist. For example, the embalmer may occasionally have had direct contact with a sick client before death, and this was perhaps an opportunity to have a discussion with the physician attending the patient.

The family context provided another possible route for the transmission of individual knowledge and expertise. Nunn (1996: 44) speculates that, in the case of physicians and embalmers, this was most likely to happen if they belonged to the same family, citing the example of Nebneb, an embalmer, and his grandson, Minemsehenet, a chief physician (van de Walle & de Meulenaere 1973), as a situation where this may have occurred.

(f, i) Professional pharmacists

Inscriptional source material

The medical papyri provide an extensive list of pharmaceutical treatments used for a wide variety of ailments. Although translators of these texts continue to face difficulties in identifying some of the medicinal ingredients, it is now evident that an efficacious and therapeutic pharmaceutical tradition existed from an early period (see Chapter 5f).

Dioscorides' *Pharmacopoeia* is another major source for the study of ancient Egyptian medicinal plants and the treatments derived from them. Coptic medical texts from the latter part of the 1st millennium AD also make a contribution, since the medical practices of early Christians in Egypt, although largely derived from Greek and Arab traditions, also retained some remedies from pharaonic times (Manniche 1989: 59).

Dioscorides Pedanius, a Greek born in Anazarbus, in Cilicia in southern Anatolia, in the 1st century AD, compiled his *De materia medica* around AD 68/69. As a physician in the Roman army, he had the opportunity to gather information about the medicinal remedies found in various countries through which he passed, although the places he visited are not recorded. This knowledge became the basis of his *Pharmacopoeia*, which was written on five scrolls. It lists pharmaceutical ingredients and their properties, derived from a wide range of animal products, minerals and 500 listed plants, and also discusses methods of application (Scarborough 2018: 520).

It has been claimed that this is the oldest extant pharmacopeia, but an earlier Mesopotamian example has been identified. Nevertheless, Dioscorides' work remains an important pharmacological source for the early Roman Empire (Gunther 1934; Scarborough 2018) and, copied and translated into several languages and transmitted through Arab and European medicine, it ultimately became the basis of a tradition that lasted for over 1500 years (see Chapter 7c).

Dispensing drugs

The ancient records provide few details about the people who actually prepared the medicines. There is no Egyptian word for 'pharmacist', although a distinct profession of dispensing chemists may have existed (Jonckheere 1955). Instructions and remedies carefully inscribed on a group of potsherds may be attributable to such a group; alternatively, they may be notes jotted down by physicians or even pupils' exercises (Ghalioungui 1963: 146–47).

The medical papyri appear to indicate that specific individuals were responsible for dispensing medicines: the phrase usually included at the beginning of each prescription states: 'Thou shalt prepare for him' or sometimes: 'Then you shall cause one to prepare for him'. Nunn (1996: 132) suggests that these instructions were written for the *swnw*, implying that they or their assistants were responsible for preparing their own medicines. This arrangement may have existed in communities where the role of a local physician was perhaps synonymous with that of apothecary, and preparation of drugs may have been carried out in his own dispensary. However, some recipes that involved complicated procedures and access to special equipment and materials were possibly carried out in special laboratories or on apothecaries' premises (Ghalioungui 1963: 147).

It is also unclear what role, if any, was played by temple personnel in preparing pharmaceutical drugs. Prescriptions for aromatic oils and ointments (and references to technicians involved in their production) are carved on the walls of some special chambers in temples of the Ptolemaic era. These rooms may have served as temple laboratories for producing medicaments, although the inscribed prescriptions – which relate to religious rather than medicinal purposes – do not confirm this. Alternatively, the space could have been used to store the aromatic substances regularly employed in temple rituals (Ghalioungui 1963: 147–48).

Very occasionally, names and titles provide additional information about those involved in the preparation of medicines. One example comes from a foreman's journal preserved on an ostracon (BM 5634) from Deir el-Medina. Dated to the fortieth year of Ramesses II, this records how a royal workman, Paherypedjet, absented himself from work to attend to the needs of two fellow workers who had fallen sick. His duties included the 'preparation of medicines' (Černý & Gardiner 1957: pls 83–84; Janssen 1980), suggesting that ordinary members of this community were responsible for producing some of their own remedies.

Some of the titles held by important politico-religious dignitaries indicate that they provided medical care in the palaces and temples (Ghalioungui 1963: 147), although it is most unlikely that they made their own pharmaceutical remedies. Although Chui the Venerable, a high priest at Heliopolis, held no special titles, P. Ebers (419) credits him as the maker of a medicinal ointment (Ghalioungui 1987: 121).

Archaeological, iconographic and botanical source material

Inscriptional evidence about the pharmaceutical tradition is limited. However, archaeological, iconographic and archaeo-botanical sources provide some additional information about the medicinal ingredients derived from animal, mineral and plant sources.

Tomb and temple scenes depict gardens, while mineral and plant remains (including floral wreaths and adornments from mummies) are found in museum collections. Many of the plants present in ancient Egypt still exist in the country today, and these, together with the archaeo-botanical material, provide an important resource for comparative studies on the flora of ancient and modern Egypt.

Acquiring raw materials for medicines

It is likely that both temple and domestic gardens played a key role in supplying plants for medicinal preparations. A famous New Kingdom garden, created by Queen Hatshepsut in the precinct of her temple at Deir el-Bahri, featured incense trees brought back from Punt, while a set of reliefs carved on the walls of a small chamber in the Temple of Amun at Karnak provides a lasting pictorial record of the plants Tuthmosis III acquired during his military campaigns in Western Asia. Unfortunately, there are no accompanying inscriptions here or elsewhere to confirm if the main or exclusive purpose of herbal gardens was to produce plants for use in medicinal preparations.

Additionally, medicinal plants would have been acquired from agricultural or horticultural sources, and some may have been gathered in the wild, perhaps by the healers themselves or by professional foragers (Nunn 1996: 138).

There is no record of the ways and means by which the healers obtained their supplies of mineral and animal ingredients, although most minerals (with the exception of lapis lazuli, which came from the region known today as Afghanistan) would have been available locally, and animal ingredients would have been collected from wild and domestic fauna.

Preparation of drugs

The medical papyri give instructions on how the drug-dispenser should produce his remedies and deliver them to his patients. They describe in some detail how the ingredients should be prepared, and the appropriate vehicle (water, honey, milk oil, wine or beer) to be used for each medicine. They also include the route by which the treatment should be administered to the patient: these were, specifically, oral (the commonest), rectal, vaginal, external application or fumigation (Nunn 1996: 139–42; Campbell 2008: 222–24).

The papyri also provide the appropriate dosage in volume measurements for these preparations (Nunn 1996: 140–43; Campbell 2008: 223–24). Precise measurements for each ingredient in a preparation start to appear at the beginning of the New Kingdom (*c.* 1550 BC); this has prompted and facilitated research on the exact units of measurement used in the recipes (Pommerening 2010: 132–37). The aim of such studies is to produce further evidence about dosage requirements and the therapeutic efficacy of Egyptian medicines generally (Pommerening 2017a; 2017b).

The role of pharmacists in ancient Egypt

At present, there is insufficient evidence to demonstrate how the overall structure and hierarchy of the pharmaceutical tradition functioned in Egypt, and to what extent the various groups interacted with each other. The scattering of high-level priestly/political titles perhaps suggests that some individuals carried out their duties in the contexts of royal palaces or temples, supervising specialist 'pharmacies' or 'laboratories' that may have existed there. They may have provided a special service for the royal family and some of the elite.

However, other healers doubtless worked in the community, combining the roles of physician and pharmacist/apothecary, and possibly working from premises that combined a surgery with a basic dispensary. According to Ghalioungui (1963: 146), 'It is more than probable that the physician himself often prepared his remedies, as our country doctors did before the introduction of patent drugs'.

Even in 2007, researchers from the University of Manchester were able to observe the traditional approach of Beduin medicine still continuing alongside conventional clinics and pharmacies. As part of the Pharmacy in Ancient Egypt Project they visited the South Sinai Environmental Agency (Conservation and Sustainable Use of Medicinal Plants in Arid and Semi-Arid Ecosystems in Egypt) at St Katherine's (see Chapter 5f), and were introduced to a practitioner of traditional Beduin medicine who combined the roles of physician and apothecary. He regularly collected his own plant ingredients in the locality and processed them in his surgery/dispensary to provide treatments for patients suffering from a variety of medical conditions.

(f, ii) Dental health, disease and dental care

Dental health, dental disease and dental care are important factors in the health and well-being of any population group. What does the evidence reveal about the dental condition of the ancient Egyptians? Did the populace suffer from toothache, and was there a dedicated dental profession that tended to the needs of the inhabitants of the Nile Valley?

Dental health and disease

Teeth are composed of the hardest and most chemically stable tissues in the body, are well preserved in archaeological remains, being resistant to decomposition in the soil, and usually survive long after their supporting structures have deteriorated. In ancient Egypt the dry climate and the burial customs have resulted in the survival of large numbers of well-preserved skeletal and mummified remains. Extensive examinations of these remains have demonstrated the many pathological and non-pathological conditions seen in the dentitions of these ancient people. This, together with the surviving documentary, archaeological and ethnographic evidence has enabled a detailed picture of the dental health and dental care of the ancient Egyptians to be revealed, perhaps more so than for any other civilisation in antiquity (Forshaw 2009a: 421).

These analyses indicate that the ancient Egyptians suffered from extremely worn teeth, periodontal problems and numerous dental abscesses. Significantly, these disorders were experienced not only by the peasants, the overwhelming majority of the population, but also by the pharaohs and the elite of society.

Many of them would have experienced symptoms ranging from minor discomfort to severe throbbing pain. The dental abscesses would have resulted in infection that may have caused local and systemic problems, and in severe cases could have resulted in death.

The most significant dental pathology was tooth wear, a condition so widespread that it has been found in the teeth of many of the surviving ancient Egyptian skulls throughout the dynastic period (Ruffer 1920: 348–56; Leek 1967a: 51–52; Hillson 1979; Forshaw 2009a: 421). Leek (1966), in a study of over 4000 ancient Egyptian teeth, found that nearly 90 per cent of them showed some evidence of tooth wear. This wear was brought about by the chewing of a coarse fibrous diet, made even more abrasive by the presence of inorganic particles in bread, their staple food. These inclusions were derived from several sources, but primarily they were granules of sand blown in from the desert. Contamination would also have been caused by the fracturing of small splinters from their flint-tooth sickle harvesting tools as well as the ingress of particles from the soil where the grain was growing, and which were later not sieved out. Additionally, grinding the grain with soft sandstone implements and baking the bread on the outside of stone ovens would have contributed further to this process. Evidence of these practices is well illustrated in the various colourful scenes of daily life that are painted on the walls of many of the ancient Egyptian tombs, such as the ploughing, reaping and sowing scenes depicted in the tomb of Sennedjem (TT 1), and the winnowing scene in the tomb of Nakht (TT 52) at Thebes. Similarly, models retrieved from such tombs also provide indications of these activities.

The consequence of this tooth wear was a rapid reduction in the outer protective layer of the tooth, the enamel, and subsequently the underlying dentine. Not only does this cause the tooth to become sensitive to temperature and pressure, but the pulp chamber, the centre of the tooth, becomes exposed to the oral cavity, which permits the ingress of bacterial contamination from the mouth. This would cause the living tissue inside the tooth to necrose and the chamber to then fill up with bacteria and pus. This infective material can then leak out of the root canal into the surrounding bone, become a source of infection, and result in abscess formation at the root tip.

Another dental disease affecting the ancient Egyptians was periodontal or gum disease. This is primarily due to bacterial irritation caused by the accumulation of plaque and calculus deposits on the teeth and gum margins, mainly due to inadequate oral hygiene. These deposits can cause inflammation of the gums, leading to tissue destruction, and in severe cases can result in abscess formation and loss of teeth.

Caries, or tooth decay, a common dental pathology in the modern world, was also evident in ancient Egypt. Caries is caused by bacteria found in plaque breaking down fermentable carbohydrates in the diet. This reaction results in acid production that causes tooth destruction and may eventually lead to necrosis of the pulp with subsequent abscess formation. Generally, the rate of caries was fairly low during most of the pharaonic era, due to the lack of refined sugars in the diet coupled with the fibrous abrasive nature of the food, which tended to inhibit the retention of plaque on tooth surfaces (Rateitshak-Pluss & Guggenheim 1982: 239–44).

However, there were some exceptions, such as the site of Deir el-Medina, where recent evidence indicates that during the New Kingdom the inhabitants of the village demonstrated a higher incidence of caries than many other Egyptian and Nubian populations (Austin 2022). This has been related to the greater socioeconomic access of the villagers, which permitted them a regular supply of state rations as well as the ability to obtain a rich variety of foods. Tomb decorations, food offerings and village texts indicate that foods with a high sugar content, such as dates, honey, cakes and sweetened breads, were consumed. The continual availability of these cariogenic foodstuffs may well explain the higher caries rates. Later, with the invasion of the Greeks in 332 BC, dietary habits gradually began to change, and food items such as fine white bread, honey and dates became more freely available, resulting in increased caries experience throughout the population.

These three major dental disorders would have caused considerable pain and discomfort to the peoples of ancient Egypt and so the question arises – was there a dedicated dental profession or any provision for dental care that could address these problems?

The practice of dentistry in ancient Egypt

Ever since two teeth connected by gold wire were discovered by the Egyptologist Hermann Junker in a mastaba at Giza in 1914, this topic has been debated by both Egyptologists and dentists. To attempt to answer this question it is necessary to review the available evidence on this subject from a variety of resources, such as hieroglyphic inscriptions, human remains, various medical papyri, surgical instruments and ancient writings.

(i) Hieroglyphic inscriptions

In the 1920s Hermann Junker studied the false door of Irenakhty at Giza, where he analysed many of the titles and studied the question of specialisation in medical and dental practice in ancient Egypt (Fig. 2.13). He later expanded his research to other sources and proposed some specific dental titles based on the evidence he had analysed (Junker 1927).

Junker proposed that the hieroglyphic sign of a tusk of an animal, probably derived from an elephant, was *ibḥ* and represented a tooth. The use of an animal equivalent for a human anatomical form is in accordance with Egyptian practice. From this deduction, various titles for a 'dentist' were formulated, with *ibḥy*

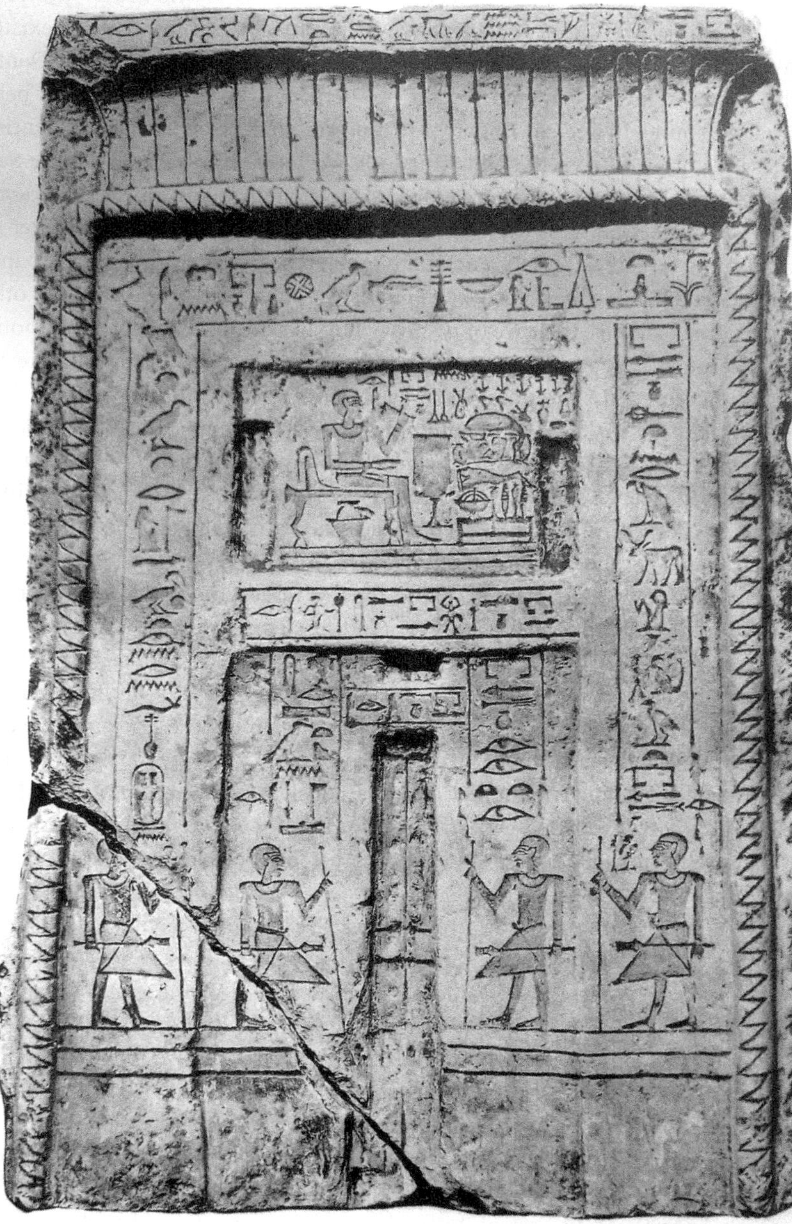

Figure 2.13. Old Kingdom/First Intermediate Period stela of Irenakhty. Hieroglyphic inscriptions relate to a range of medical specialities possessed by Irenakhty in his role of physician at the royal palace. Discovered by Hermann Junker at Giza (Junker 1927: fig. 2).

being 'One who is concerned with teeth' and *iry ibḥy* 'One who deals with teeth'. Other titles linked with *ibḥ* suggest that a hierarchical order in dentistry existed, with *wr ibḥy* being 'Chief of Dentists' and *wr ibḥy pr-ꜥꜣ* being 'Chief Dentist of the Palace'. However, of more than 150 persons who are recorded as being medical personnel in ancient Egypt, only nine are recognised as possible dentists. Of these, eight were from the Old Kingdom, while the ninth was from the Saite Period. Several of the dentists were noted as additionally being physicians, *swnw*.

The various dental titles that Junker originally proposed in 1927 have over the years become largely accepted, and there is reference to them in various papers and books that have subsequently been published on the subject. There is no other corroborating evidence to prove or disprove Junker's original deduction, although many prominent Egyptologists at that time, such as Grapow, Erman, Ranke and Breasted, accepted his proposal. However, more recently other scholars have suggested that the *ibḥ* hieroglyph might not refer to a dentist (Leek 1972; Becker & Turfa 2017: 74). Many of the *ibḥ* were also physicians, so the *swnw ibḥ* may have been a physician treating diseases of the mouth, and not a dentist. There is also a suggestion that the title could denote a different occupation or state office unrelated to dentistry (Kaplony 1963: 583).

The inscriptional evidence relating to the few title-holders of *ibḥ* can perhaps further this discussion. The earliest recorded holder of this title is Hesyre, who lived in the 3rd Dynasty, during the reign of King Djoser (Forshaw 2013). His mastaba tomb (S2405) is located to the north of Djoser's Step Pyramid at Saqqara, and within his tomb were found a number of wooden panels – originally eleven in number, but only six have survived the ravages of time. They are carved from acacia wood, are about 110cm tall and are considered to be among the finest wooden artefacts handed down from antiquity. The hieroglyphic inscriptions on them are beautifully carved and the facial images of Hesyre are particularly lifelike (Fig. 2.14).

Hesyre possessed more than twelve titles: the first of these is *wr ibḥ swnw*, 'Chief of *ibḥ* and Physicians'. Among his other designations were such diverse titles as 'Keeper of the Royal Diadem' and 'Custodian of the King's Property'. Due to this proliferation of titles it would seem unlikely that he actively pursued all these occupations. His role as 'Chief of *ibḥ* and Physicians' may merely have been administrative or ceremonial, although his medical and *ibḥ* titles were the first listed, and so may have carried more weight.

Other 'dentists' similarly held multiple titles. Nyanksekhmet was also a 'Chief of Physicians' and Khuwy was 'Elder of the Physicians of the Palace' and seemingly specialised in gastrointestinal complaints, as attested by his titles of 'Interpreter of the Secret Art' and 'Guardian of the Anus'. Psamtekseneb, who is known from a basalt statue found at Heliopolis, which is now in the Gregorian Egyptian Museum, Rome, was 'Chief of *ibḥ* of the Palace', 'Chief of Physicians' and 'Elder of Physicians'. He lived during the 26th Dynasty, unlike the other

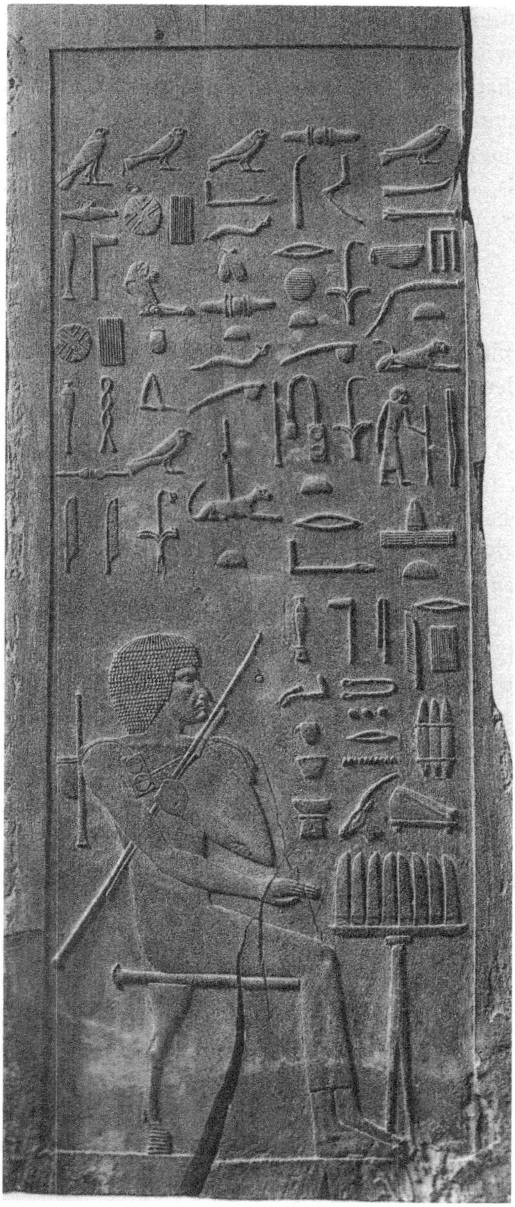

Figure 2.14. Wooden panel of Hesyre (CG 1426) from his 3rd Dynasty mastaba tomb at Saqqara (S2405). Carved from acacia wood, the panel was originally one of twelve. The hieroglyphic inscriptions on the panel list Hesyre's many titles. Discovered at Saqqara by James Quibell. Now in the Egyptian Museum in Cairo (Quibell *et al.* 1913: pl. 31).

known *ibḥ*, who are all dated to the Old Kingdom. However, archaism was a feature of the Late Period, particularly during the 26th Dynasty, and some titles used during this period lacked functional weight and may well have been modelled on older sources. Again, whether the multiple titles held by these individuals indicated that they were engaged in several specialities or that the titles were perhaps administrative or ceremonial is unclear.

So, to consider the evidence that can be deduced from the hieroglyphic titles, the small number of possible dentists for whom we have evidence all date to the Old Kingdom, apart from one. For whatever reason this uncommon title ceased to be used in later periods, and if it did refer to a practising dentist or a physician specialising in oral care then it is uncertain who was responsible for dental treatment in later times.

(ii) Osteological material

It is in the skeletal and mummified remains of the ancient Egyptians that we might expect to find some evidence of interventive dental procedures, if any operative dental surgery was performed. However, from the tens of thousands of remains that have been examined from the entire 3000-year period of Dynastic Egypt the evidence is extremely limited. There is the very occasional instance where a surgical approach for the treatment of a dental abscess is claimed to have been adopted, there are only three cases of possible prosthetic work and a few examples where it has been tentatively suggested that an extraction may have been performed. Much has been made of these cases, with some authors, including Ghalioungui (1971), Iskander *et al.* (1979), Blustein *et al.* (1987) and Chohayeb (1991), claiming, quite categorically in certain instances, that this evidence proves the existence of an operative dental profession. Equally so, other researchers, including Leek (1967a, b), Hoffman-Axthelm (1979), Miller (2008), Forshaw (2009b) and Becker and Turfa (2017), have doubted this.

The first osteological specimen suggested to exhibit evidence of interventive dental therapy was published by Hooton in 1917. He examined an Old Kingdom mandible (PM 59303) excavated from Giza that displayed two small openings in the outer cortical bone below an abscessed tooth. He claimed that, due to the upward angulation of the holes, their artificial symmetrical appearance and the apparent thickness of bone they had traversed, the holes were the result of man-made drillings, effected in order to drain the pus from the abscess below the tooth. Breasted (1930: 9) later supported this view and suggested that they could have been created by a bronze instrument in a bow drill. It is also possible that they may have been created by a hand-held tool (Maccheroni & Fillios 2019). Two other similar cases are documented as exhibiting similar openings, although in the entire 3000 years of dynastic Egypt these are the only examples (Fig. 2.15). Therefore, although it is possible that these perforations were man-made, the infrequency of this procedure does not really support the existence of an operative dental profession.

Another possibility is that the holes could be the result of a normal pathological process caused by the dissolution of bone by pus originating from an abscess. Such canals occur frequently, are found in many different locations

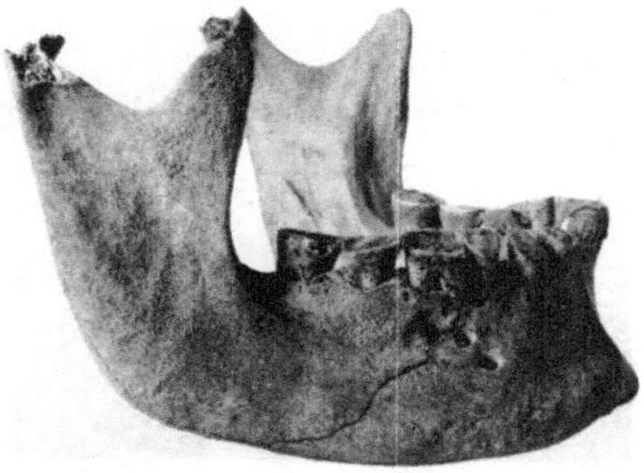

Figure 2.15. Old Kingdom mandible. Excavated by Reisner from a 4th Dynasty tomb at Giza. Displaying two small openings in the bone below an abscessed tooth and originally suggested to be an example of operative dental surgery to drain the abscess. Now in the Peabody Museum of Archaeology and Ethnology, Harvard University, USA, PM 59303 (Hooton 1917: pl. I, 4).

and directions and can be related to any tooth in the dentition. They are often symmetrical and, although giving the appearance of being artificially created, they are not the result of human intervention.

Other finds have been suggested as showing dental bridges, fashioned by ancient Egyptian dentists to replace missing teeth. Unfortunately, the publications relating to these findings often lack a proper description regarding the actual archaeological context and so detailed information and dating is uncertain. One example was found in the Western Cemetery in a tomb shaft of Mastaba G 4840 at Giza and originally dated to about 2500 BC (Junker 1929: 246) (Fig. 2.16). It was not found attached to the teeth or in a skull but among the rubble and skeletal remains of a body. More recently the original Old Kingdom dating has been questioned, as it has been suggested that the piece was not derived from an early tomb but from a later infill deposit that occurred during the Ptolemaic Period (Becker & Turfa 2017: 334).

In this appliance, two mandibular molar teeth were found joined together by a piece of tubular gold wire woven around the teeth at the level of the gum margins. A report at the time suggested that the teeth were from the same individual and that the wiring procedure had been carried out in the mouth of a living person. However, a number of later researchers have concluded that this was unlikely due to such factors as the flimsy nature of the wire and the complexity of the knots, which would virtually make it impossible for them to be manipulated inside the mouth (Leek 1967a; Hoffman-Axthelm 1979; Forshaw 2009b). It is possible that ancient Egyptian embalmers carried out this procedure on a mummified body in order to replace a missing tooth or stabilise a loose one and so make the body whole for the afterlife, a popular belief and practice in ancient Egypt. There are frequent examples of restorations of mummies by embalmers, such as the insertion of false eyes and artificial limbs (Smith & Wood Jones 1910: 214; Gray 1966a; Finch 2011). Alternatively, the device may have been kept or worn as an amulet during life, with the owner perhaps hoping that it

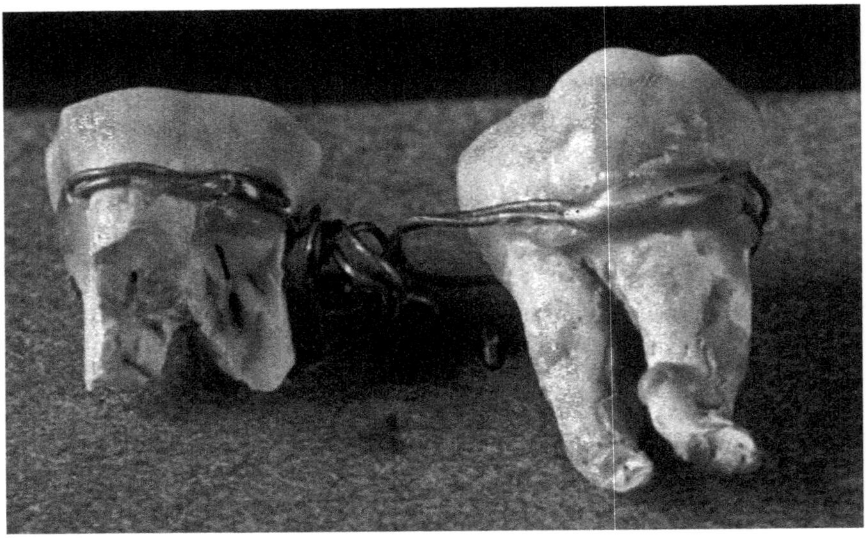

Figure 2.16. 'Giza Bridge' discovered in a tomb shaft of Mastaba G 4840 at Giza. Originally suggested to be a dental prosthetic appliance but this supposition is no longer thought to be the case. Originally dated to about 2500 BC but now considered to be from the Ptolemaic Period. Discovered by Hermann Junker in the Western Cemetery at Giza. Now in the Roemer and Pelizaeus Museum, Hildesheim (courtesy of Roger Forshaw and ©Roemer- und Pelizaeus-Museum, Hildesheim).

would afford some form of power or protection, or the teeth may have been merely kept following their premature loss from the mouth.

No clear examples of teeth being extracted have been reported in the literature. Leek (1967a) examined 3000 skulls without finding a single example of extraction; Miller (2008: 30) investigated some 500 skulls and only found one possible case; Forshaw (2015) investigated 900 skulls from Nubia and found no evidence of extractions; and, more recently, Austin (2022) discovered one possible case among the skeletal remains from Deir el-Medina. The medical papyri are silent on the topic and no ancient Egyptian instrument has ever been discovered that could be utilised for the extraction of teeth, unlike the examples of Greek and Roman forceps that have been unearthed.

In addition, there are many examples of periodontally involved mobile teeth that could easily have been removed by finger manipulation or by means of a simple extraction procedure, but these have been left in situ. The extractions, had they been performed, would undoubtedly have resulted in considerable pain relief. Why these simple extractions were not carried out seems rather strange when you consider the sophistication of the ancient Egyptian civilisation and their knowledge of medicine, although there may have been a reluctance by some individuals to seek dental treatment, just as there is today. So, although it is difficult to comprehend that teeth were not removed on occasions, unless new information is uncovered there is insufficient evidence to support the regular use of such a procedure.

(iii) Dental instruments

One difficulty in the identification of any medical or dental instruments from antiquity is that they were never engraved with their purpose. While a number of finds of supposed medical instruments have been made, their identification as such is debatable.

A celebrated scene that has been suggested as possibly showing dental instruments is depicted on the northern part of the enclosure wall of the Graeco-Roman temple of Kom Ombo (Ghalioungui 1963: 101–04; Nunn 1996: 163–64) (Fig. 2.17). Here there is what appears to be a collection of nearly forty implements or tools and, although different interpretations of their purposes

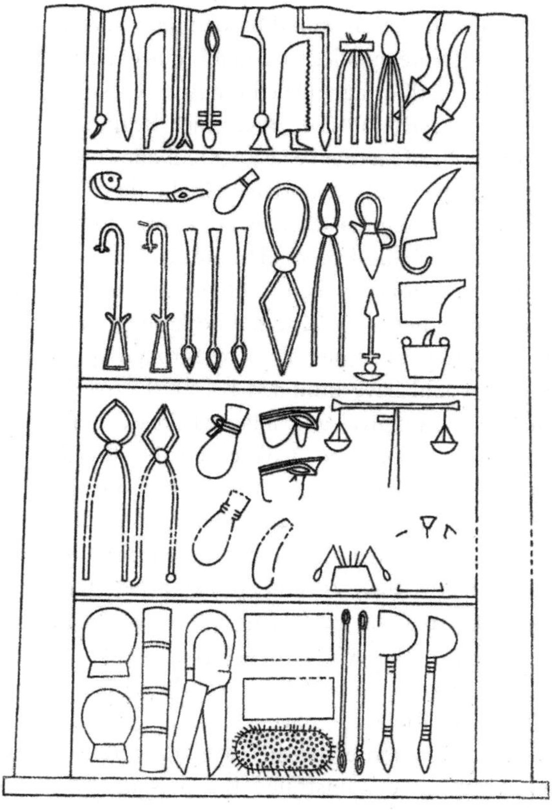

Figure 2.17. Depiction of the instruments/ implements on the enclosure wall of the temple of Kom Ombo. Among the instruments believed to be represented are tooth forceps, cupping vessels, catheters and probes. Redrawn by K. N. White after Nunn (1996: fig. 8.2).

have been suggested, many of the items are contemporary with numerous well-authenticated depictions of Roman and Greek surgical instruments (Cassar 1974; Jackson 1990). Among them appear to be representations of dental forceps.

There are references to surgical instruments and treatment in the Ebers Papyrus (875), but there is no reference to any device used to treat or operate on teeth in any of the medical papyri (see Chapter 5b).

(iv) Medical papyri

An important source of information about dental care in ancient Egypt is to be found in the medical papyri. Although they are silent on all operative aspects of dentistry, four of the papyri (Ebers, Kahun, Berlin and Hearst) include prescriptions for the treatment of dental problems, while a fifth, Edwin Smith, supplies instructions for dealing with a dislocated jaw and fractures to the maxillary and mandibular regions.

In particular, P. Ebers has eleven dental prescriptions, of which five are considered to be for the prevention of tooth loss, either by packing various materials in paste form around the tooth and the surrounding gums, or by using material to fill carious cavities. In the former cases, the theory seems to have been that these materials would harden and serve as a temporary means of stabilising teeth that were mobile, presumably due to periodontal disease, abscesses associated with the teeth or age-related gingival recession (Weeks 1980: 106). An example of such a prescription is P. Ebers 739: 'Beginning of the remedies to consolidate a tooth; flour of emmer seeds; ochre; honey; made into a mass; and the tooth to be fattened therewith' (translated Ghalioungui 1987: 189). Of the components in the prescription, emmer wheat is not known to have any pharmacological action, but ochres, which are iron oxides, are recognised as having astringent and antiseptic properties. Honey, which is a binding agent, is used in more Egyptian medicines than any other ingredient and because of its hypertonicity kills micro-organisms by drawing water out of them through osmosis (Worth-Estes 1993: 69). Thus, honey would have inhibited bacterial growth and helped reduce inflammation in infected gingival and mucosal areas, therefore resulting in some pain relief. However, it would not have cured the disease process, as for this to happen it would have been necessary to treat the source of the infection, such as an abscess, and in addition remove any calculus deposits.

The other possibility is that these materials were utilised to fill carious cavities in the teeth. There is quite an extensive literature, particularly on the internet, claiming that the ancient Egyptians could fill and make gold restorations for teeth, but no specific evidence is provided to support such assertions. Many of these derive from 19th century allegations and even fabrications of evidence (Becker & Turfa 2017: 73).

However, more recently a computerised tomography scan of a Ptolemaic mummy has demonstrated the presence of a 'low-density homogeneous ball of material, possibly linen' inserted into two large carious cavities in adjacent molar teeth. The authors suggest that the material was 'protective, likely medicine-laden', although offer no evidence to support the latter statement (Wade *et al.* 2012). A second mummy, dated from the mid-Ptolemaic to the early Roman Period, has similarly demonstrated a mass of extraneous material between two carious teeth (Pantazis *et al.* 2020). Both papers claim that this is evidence of early dental intervention, although the scans show no evidence of tooth preparation and visual inspection would be necessary to shed further light on this suggestion.

However, one possibility that perhaps needs to be considered is that of self-help or help by another individual, perhaps a family member, who was not necessarily a professional. Extensive carious cavities in teeth are extremely painful to stimuli and they usually cause bouts of throbbing pain that eventually can become continuous. The mere insertion of a linen swab or other such material may provide some short-term relief, as the insertion would prevent the ingress of further foodstuffs. This is recognised in dental surgery today, when individuals break a tooth, lose a filling or generally neglect their dental health and then insert materials such as chewing gum, cotton packing or other sundry materials to relieve the discomfort of the tooth being exposed to the oral environment. This is not really operative dental care or interventive dental therapy, but merely an example of self-help. In most cases such a temporary inclusion would not last for an extended period and would rapidly deteriorate in the oral environment.

More recently Austin (2022) identified a possible filling from the skeletal remains found at Deir el-Medina; unlike the two previous examples, which were dated to the Graeco-Roman era, this case is from the New Kingdom. A molar tooth with a carious cavity measuring some 4 × 4mm was found to contain 'a mass of fibrous material' the form of which suggested that it had been packed intentionally into the cavity rather than consisting of debris accidentally blocking it. As yet the material has not been chemically analysed. Austin suggested that this type of fibrous organic compound may not have been retained long in the mouth, particularly taking into consideration the degrading action of mastication and the soluble effects of saliva. This could explain why such fillings are so rarely discovered and documented, as they would be of a temporary nature and would not survive for thousands of years.

Another group of prescriptions seems to be aimed at treating various ulcers, abscesses and gum infections. An example of such a remedy is P. Ebers 742: 'Another, for the treatment of a tooth that is eating in the opening of the flesh: cumin; terebinth; carob; to be made into a powder and applied to the teeth' (translated Ghalioungui 1987: 189). P. Ebers 745, 746 and 747 are also directed at oral infections, these being in the form of daily mouth washes. It is not certain what is meant by 'eating in the opening of the flesh', although it could refer to a dental abscess. Of components of the prescription, cumin is a carminative, terebinth resin has antiseptic and local anaesthetic properties and carob is a demulcent. Consequently, such a material would be soothing and with antiseptic and anaesthetic properties would provide some temporary relief.

Three prescriptions deal with vaguely defined oral pain and among the various components used to treat the condition is *tjeret*, considered to be willow. Willow contains salicin, a precursor of acetylsalicylic acid (aspirin), but this is present in only low concentrations. However, willow species also contain flavonoids and polyphenols which contribute to an analgesic and anti-inflammatory effect, and so this will have helped to reduce discomfort (Vlachojannis *et al.* 2011).

(vi) Ancient writers

Many ancient authors described the illustrious position that Egyptian medicine achieved in the ancient world, a position it retained, in fable if not in fact, well into the Middle Ages. Homer, in the Odyssey (IV, 231), declares 'Each is a physician with knowledge beyond all men.' The ancient Greeks frequently acknowledged their debt to Egypt's physicians, and it was said that to have studied medicine in Egypt was the highest recommendation a physician could offer (Diodorus Siculus 1, 82; Pliny the Elder, 29, 1). However, it is only Herodotus, writing in his *Histories*, who mentions doctors specialising in diseases of the teeth, a reference which does imply that some form of dental care may have existed.

(vii) Miscellaneous sources

There appears to be little mention of dental matters among the various literary texts from ancient Egypt and no record of non-attendance at work due to dental pain in the many accounts of absenteeism kept by foremen at various building sites and workers' villages (Janssen 1980). There are no depictions of ancient Egyptians experiencing toothache or receiving dental treatment in the various wall scenes – certainly nothing comparable with the Byzantine and late medieval illustrations showing teeth being extracted (Ring 1985: 101–16).

However, one Ramesside text, P. Anastasi IV, refers to a worm as being the cause of toothache. In this text an official in a lonely outpost in the Egyptian Empire describes the deprivations he has to endure and he finishes, rather poignantly, by mentioning the suffering of one of his comrades: 'A *mns*-scribe is here with me, every muscle of whose face twitches, the *wštt*-disease has developed in his eye and the *fnt*-worm into his tooth. I cannot leave him to his fate' (translated Caminos 1954: 189). The worm is also referred to in the medical papyri as a disease agent, although the reference in P. Anastasi IV is the only one suggesting that it was a cause of toothache. The notion that a worm was responsible for dental disorders was widespread among other ancient cultures, with probably the first documented case being a Sumerian text dating to about 5000 BC. This belief continued throughout history and even as late as the 18th century AD an ivory carving of a tooth was produced showing inside it a tooth worm (Suddick & Harris 1990: 142).

Oral hygiene

What about oral hygiene? Did the ancient Egyptians brush their teeth? Hygiene was important in ancient Egypt and, although many cosmetic and toilet articles have been discovered, no evidence of any form of tooth brush has ever been excavated. Possibly some form of wooden tooth pick may have been used, since it is known that other civilisations in antiquity used various implements for oral hygiene purposes, such as chew sticks, tree twigs, birds' feathers, animal bones and porcupine quills (Forshaw 2009b: 423). Perhaps something resembling a miswak was utilised: a twig of the *Salvadora persica* tree whose ends have been frayed. The miswak is reputed to have been used by the ancient Babylonians, is known to have been used for oral care by Muslims since the birth of Islam and, indeed, is still in use today (Bos 1993; Al Sadhan & Alma 1999).

There is evidence that masticatories, materials chewed without an intention to ingest them, were used in ancient Egypt. An example is the betel nut found in Asia, which was used in historic times and is still popular today. A modern, almost universal masticatory is chewing gum. Herodotus wrote that the Egyptians used the root of the papyrus, which was roasted in a red-hot oven. They then chewed it and finally spat out the residue, which is referred to as a quid. Quids have been found to contain inorganic impurities derived from the soil in which the papyrus stems were growing. Such contaminants would have had an abrasive cleansing effect on the teeth. Natron pellets were also chewed, and, with its inherent high pH, natron would neutralise the low pH of saliva that results from eating carbohydrates. This would reduce the risk of caries.

There are two prescriptions in P. Ebers (745, 748) that would appear to be mouthwashes. The remedy uses the Egyptian verb *ẖpꜥ* 'chewing', but the concoction appears to be a liquid preparation, and so its use for rinsing the mouth would appear more likely. It is not obvious whether the prescriptions were directed at the teeth, at the gingivae or at the oral mucosa. Additionally, the specific purpose of the preparations is not clear.

There are no obvious prescriptions for toothpastes in the medical papyri relating to the pharaonic period. A 4th century AD papyrus found near the ancient Egyptian city of Crocodilopolis, written in Greek, describes a 'powder for white and perfect teeth' that, when mixed with saliva in the mouth, forms a 'clean toothpaste'. However, this is a late copy of a Greek medical document and there is no apparent link to earlier Egyptian medicine.

Conclusion – was there a dental profession in ancient Egypt?

In the late 1960s the University of Michigan in co-operation with Alexandria University radiographed the Royal Mummies in the Egyptian Museum at Cairo and, more recently, they have been CT scanned. Mummies of several of the pharaohs, including those of Amenhotep III and Ramesses II, perhaps two of the more celebrated rulers of ancient Egypt, revealed dentitions displaying extremely worn teeth, dental abscesses and advanced periodontal disease. During life they will have experienced dental pain, possibly severe, which must have had some bearing on the quality of their lives. No evidence of any form of dental treatment was found from the radiographic examination, and surely if anyone was to receive dental care it would have been these powerful rulers. If they did not receive treatment, then the peasants, the vast majority of society, would have been unlikely to have had any professional dental care.

Since the 1960s many other mummies from museums around the world have been radiographed and CT scanned. In addition, many thousands of skeletal remains have been examined. Again, no evidence of any operative dental treatment has been found, despite a very obvious need in some cases. Such individuals would very probably have sought and hopefully received dental treatment had it been available.

The evidence would suggest that operative dental treatment, if it did exist at all, was extremely limited, and management of dental problems seems to have been restricted to pharmaceutical preparations that were applied to the soft tissues surrounding the teeth, utilised as filling materials or used as mouthwashes. Such treatments would not have retarded the progress of the dental disease, as they were directed towards the symptoms rather than the cause, and at best may only have provided some short-term relief.

Was there an organised dental profession available to administer the remedies? As reviewed above, there seems to be little evidence to support this proposition. The prescriptions rarely include the name of a specific professional in their wordings. It is quite possible that the *swnw* could have dispensed the various medications, but this is not mentioned in the textual sources. What does seem clear is that many ancient Egyptians suffered from widespread and painful dental disease, which the available treatments can have done relatively little to alleviate.

3

The temple as a location for medical training and practice

The Egyptian temple had several functions, and each was regarded as a recreation of the sacred island where all life forms had originally come into existence; as a home on earth where the Egyptians, through the king's agency, could approach the resident deities for support in their lives; and as a cosmological expression of the land of Egypt. As major landowners and employers of staff, the temples always retained a considerable degree of political and economic power. Here we consider their significance in relation to medical training and the provision of healing treatments.

(a) Professional training

What form of training would the *swnw* and other providers of medical care have received in ancient Egypt? When we consider the case of Hesyre, who lived about 2650 BC and is the first recorded dentist and physician in history, it is difficult to determine or even speculate on the nature of any possible medical or dental instruction that might have been available at that early period. With few predecessors, Hesyre's knowledge of medicine and dentistry may have been acquired through word of mouth or experience obtained by means of observation and trial and error (Forshaw 2013). Indeed, there appears to be little firm evidence regarding the qualifications or requirements for medical training throughout most of pharaonic history.

A survey conducted by Favry (2016) of 1331 different Middle Kingdom titles found examples of direct transmission of function and/or title from father to son. Among these were families where, for example, the titles of 'Lector' (*ẖry-ḥbt*) and 'Chief Lector' (*ẖry-ḥbt ḥry-tp*) were borne by both father and son, but none related to the title of *swnw*.

Diodorus Siculus (I, 81.7) stated that it was commonplace for the sons to follow the profession or trade of their fathers: 'The children of the people receive their education from their father and relatives, who teach them the professions they are to exercise during their lives'. This is perhaps endorsed by an obscure passage in P. Ebers (206): 'You shall prepare for him medicines, secret to who is under the *swnw* except for your own daughter' (translated Ghalioungui 1987: 69). It is not certain why the passage refers to a daughter but it does suggest transmission of knowledge within a family. A late reference in a Coptic papyrus states: 'This is a remedy that I learnt from my father' (Chassinat 1921: 301).

Further evidence for sons following the profession of the father is attested by the Ashmolean stela of Iuny (1885.14), in which are depicted two *swnw*, Huy and Khay, with Huy being the son of Khay. A second stela (Louvre C. 89) also belonging to Iuny features Iuny with another son, Khaemwaset, also a *swnw* (Nunn 1996: 130–31) (see Plate 12).

Similarly, Amenmose, who lived during the reigns of Sety I (1294–1279 BC, 19th Dynasty) and Ramesses II, carried the title of priest of Serket. He is one of the individuals listed on the stela of the foreman Baki (BM EA 265) at the necropolis worker's town at Deir el-Medina. Nearby inscriptions on the tombs of his father and grandfather indicate he belonged to a family of priests of Serket (Pinch 2006: 55; Halioua & Ziskind 2005: 129–30).

The first prescription in the Ebers Papyrus is one recommended to be used when applying a remedy to the body of a patient, and within the text there is a mythical reference to training. The incantation states that the *swnw* is initiated into the sacred texts and imbued with knowledge useful in his practice of healing: 'Thoth; he causes books to speak; he composed compilations of writings; he imparts useful knowledge to the learned, to the physicians his followers … ' (translated Ghalioungui 1987: 9).

Thoth was a significant deity in Egyptian medicine because of his role as god of scribes; his special status of being able to write and recite the written word meant that he was frequently invoked in healing incantations. The House of Life was also under the protection of Thoth and, as referred to below, it is possible that medical texts were stored and copied in the House of Life and may have been used in a teaching capacity.

There is little known about the education and training of medical personnel in other recognised institutions in ancient Egypt, but there are many references to scribal training and scribal schools (Williams 1972). Again, it is possible that some of the writings that were used for teaching purposes in these establishments may have been medical texts.

Did the ancient Egyptian healers study anatomy or other basic medical sciences, an awareness of which would be important in most medical and healing treatments? The medical papyri, especially the Edwin Smith, demonstrate an understanding of anatomy and include a detailed vocabulary of Egyptian anatomical terms, particularly for the external and upper parts of the body. It can be surmised that the same level of knowledge was attained for the lower parts of the body not covered by P. Edwin Smith. This insight would suggest that the ancient Egyptians may have studied anatomy and that at one time a treatise on the subject could have existed. Clement of Alexandria (n.d.; Stromata VI, 6) writing in the 2nd century AD, stated that the ancient Egyptians possessed six books of medical content, one of which related to the structure of the body, although there is no evidence of these texts having survived.

It is known that systematic dissection of the human body was practised at Alexandria during the Graeco-Roman Period by Herophilus and his younger contemporary Erasistratus (see Chapter 7c). From these procedures many anatomical observations were made that enabled a deeper understanding of human anatomy and physiology (Bay & Bay 2010). However, it is usually considered that throughout most of the pharaonic period traditions of respect for the dead would have prohibited dissection, as such procedures would have been deemed a desecration of the body (Baines & Lacovara 2002: 5–36). Nevertheless, descriptions in the medical papyri do indicate that the ancient Egyptian conception of anatomy had some depth.

Battlefield casualties and serious industrial accidents would have offered an opportunity to gain some awareness of anatomy, although it is difficult to observe internal anatomical relationships in vivo. Evidence from mummified specimens indicates that the embalmers possessed a degree of technical expertise, as they were able to remove internal organs through fairly small incisions in the body. They also accessed the cranial cavity via a small perforation they created in the ethmoid bone. This anatomical knowledge may have been passed on to the *swnw* or other individuals involved with medical care by the embalmers (Nunn 1996: 42–43). However, von Staden (1989: 29) cautions that the level of anatomical familiarity required for embalming is closer to that of a skilled butcher rather than a surgeon.

Nevertheless, dressing animal carcasses would have provided a certain level of anatomical know-how, as is evident from the use of animal parts as hieroglyphic signs in references to parts of the human body. On the whole it seems unlikely that the detailed level of anatomical knowledge demonstrated in the Edwin Smith Papyrus could be acquired without some form of dissection experience and anatomical study.

(b) Evidence for the House of Life and the temple

The House of Life is often alluded to in Egyptian texts, but the designation remains vague and difficult to define. It is usually regarded as an institution in which papyrus texts were stored and where scribes and scholars consulted, copied, interpreted and worked with religious compositions and other documents. It was a repository of traditional knowledge, a place of learned discussion and composition and, feasibly, a centre of textual transmission. Jan

Assmann gave it a wider role: 'The House of Life was the centre of cultural endeavour to preserve and ensure the ongoing process of cosmic, political and social life' (Assmann 2003: 73). It seems likely that the institution would have been associated with the temples or palaces, but much of the evidence does not specify a related centre.

The institution is known from as far back as the Old Kingdom and is mentioned throughout the dynastic age, although much of the evidence comes from Late and Ptolemaic Periods. Houses of Life existed in many of the cities of ancient Egypt, with evidence for them at Abydos, Akhmim, Amarna, Edfu, Esna, Koptos, Memphis and possibly Bubastis. It seems likely that, by the Late Period, they existed in the vicinity of many of the ancient Egyptian temples, although the relation between the two institutions is not clear.

There are some suggestions that the House of Life could have functioned as a 'school' or training establishment (e.g., Leblanc 2004), but Gardiner (1938), who assembled an extensive list of sources relating to the House of Life, cautions against such a view. He further comments that only in much later times did education take on a more formal character, citing a papyrus from Tebtunis dating to the 2nd century AD, which states that a candidate for the priesthood had to pass an examination in religious subjects. Considering the academic nature of the House of Life, as well as its function as a repository of knowledge, the documents that were being consulted and composed (including, perhaps, medical texts) may have been indirectly used in a teaching capacity. It is possible that personnel from the House of Life may have trained their own apprentices utilising such texts.

There is some evidence to suggest that the House of Life had an involvement with healing practices. Two royal decrees from the reign of Pepy II (2278–2184 BC, 6th Dynasty), found at Koptos, exempt staff of the Temple of Min from supplying the 'requirements of the House of Life' (Sethe 1903/1933: 286, 10; 289, 8). The requirements or equipment may have included papyrus, reed-pens, ink, medical instruments and medical texts (Gardiner 1938: 160).

An inscription on the statue of Udjahorresnet provides a biographical account of the end of the Saite Period and the subsequent establishment of the Persian 27th Dynasty (see Chapter 4e). From the text it can be seen that Udjahorresnet held a number of titles, among which was that of *wr swnw*, 'Chief Physician', and that he was commanded by Darius I to restore the House of Life at Sais:

> His majesty King Darius commanded me to return to Egypt … in order to restore the department of the House of Life [dealing with medicine] after they had fallen into decay. … His majesty did this because he knew the virtue of this art to revive all that are sick … I equipped them with all their ability and all their requirements which was on record in accordance with their former condition. (translated Gardiner 1938: 157–58)

A similar earlier inscription relates to the House of Life at Abydos, where Peftauawyneith, also a Chief Physician, was entrusted with its restoration during the reign of Haaibra (Apries) (589–570 BC, 26th Dynasty). It is quite likely that the restoration in both these inscriptions referred to re-establishing not only a possible medical department but the House of Life in its entirety.

Further evidence is provided by the Bentresh stela, which dates to the Late or Ptolemaic Period but purports to relate to events occurring during the reign of Ramesses II. Here staff from the House of Life along with the council of the palace were summoned to the king to give advice relating to a foreign princess who had fallen ill (see Plate 13).

The discovery of medical texts among other papyri in the Graeco-Roman Period temples at Dimeh al-Siba in the Faiyum and at Tebtunis suggest a medical function for these institutions. Among the categories of documents that have been published for the latter institution are fourteen medical texts, three of which were discovered within the temple enclosure (P. Tebt. II: 676, 677, 679). The documents date from *c.* 800 BC to after AD 300, and have been translated and published in *The Tebtunis Papyri* (1920–76). Research on the collection continues at the Center for the Tebtunis Papyri at the University of California, Berkeley (www.tebtunis.berkeley.edu). During excavations undertaken by an Italian team in the 1930s, artefacts that were interpreted as possibly relating to the preparation and administration of medicaments were discovered within the temple precinct (Forshaw 2014: 116).

Gardiner (1938: 178) notes an association between healing and the House of Life in a magical papyrus (Cairo 58027) dating to the Roman Period, which is aimed at affording protection to the king during the hours of night. One of the few individuals permitted to view this work was the lector, in his role as a liturgical specialist: '[The book] must not be seen by any eye save [that of] the king himself or the chief lector or the myrrh-keeper of the House of Life' (translated Golénischeff 1927: 126 [3, 14]).

Additional evidence in the same papyrus is a rare reference to a medicament used in the House of Life (Golénischeff 1927: 128 [4, 1]): 'the great mysterious ointment of the House of Life'. It is described as effective 'for a man in danger by night' and among the ingredients listed are fragrant plants (*ꜥnḫ-imyw*), fine oil (*tpt*), honey (*bit*) and goose fat (*gbr*).

In P. Salt 825 (Derchain 1965; Herbin 1988; Ryholt 2019), which is dated to the Ptolemaic Period, there is an indication that the literary compositions of the House of Life were directed at maintaining life, whether that of the gods, the king or mankind generally. This may include a healing function, but is more likely to emphasise the creative power of the texts, the 'sacred books'. Ryholt (2019: 447) develops this theme further by considering the House of Life as a religious institution focused on the maintenance of the cult of Osiris. Details relating to the construction of a House of Life at Abydos are also recorded in P. Salt and this design might have pertained to other such institutions throughout Egypt.

Another possible link between healing practices and temple activities can be construed from a scene carved on the north-western corner of the inner aspect of the outer enclosure wall of the Graeco-Roman temple of Kom Ombo (Nunn 1996: 164). The relief depicts a series of implements often considered to represent surgical instruments (Forshaw 2014: 116–17) (see further Chapter 5a) (see Plate 14).

(c) Temples as centres of healing

There is ample textual evidence, some originating in temple libraries, that some Egyptian temples and personnel were closely involved in healing. In this context, the Tebtunis Papyri provide important information about links between magic and medicine (see above).

The temple sanatoria

By the Late Period, inscriptional and archaeological evidence indicates that some Egyptian temples associated with healing deities provided treatment for patients with physical or mental ailments. This was accommodated either in dedicated chambers inside the temple or in special buildings within the temple precinct (Sales & Das 2018: 17). In these sanatoria, patients would undergo total or partial immersion in sacred water; some also experienced incubation (the Therapeutic Dream or temple sleep). According to the London-Leiden Papyrus (Griffith & Thompson 1904), this involved the patient (or his delegate) sleeping in the temple precinct for one or more nights, with the hope of experiencing a healing dream in which the patient would meet the temple deity and receive direct advice and guidance about a medical problem.

The Greeks are attributed with establishing the earliest centres of temple healing from the 5th century BC, and the Greek god of medicine, Asclepius, had many cult centres throughout the classical world: Epidauros, Kos and Pergamum were particularly important sites (Curnow 2012/13). Indeed, the concept of temple healing may have been introduced from Greece to Egypt. In the later periods, sanatoria probably existed in Egypt at some temple sites (see Chapter 7c). Textual and archaeological sources from the Graeco-Roman Period suggest that several renowned centres existed: Greek graffiti indicate that incubation took place in the Temple of Sety I at Abydos in the Ptolemaic Period; and Strabo (XVII, 1, 17) records that he encountered the practice in the Temple of Serapis at Canopus. There were also sanatoria at Memphis, the Temple of Hatshepsut at Deir el-Bahri, the Temple of Isis-Hathor at Denderah and possibly the Temple of Imhotep at Elephantine.

However, evidence suggests that incubation was practised much earlier (from at least the end of the New Kingdom, *c.* 1000 BC) in the Chapel of Meretseger at Deir el-Medina (Bruyère 1929, 1930). In addition, an inscription on a 19th Dynasty stela from Deir el-Medina relates how the owner, Qenherkhepeshef, apparently refers to the Therapeutic Dream in an address to the goddess Hathor: 'I have spent the night in this forecourt. I have drunk the water … . My body has spent the night in the shadow of your face' (translated Quirke 1992: 136–37).

The Temple of Isis-Hathor at Denderah

A rectangular mudbrick building in the precinct of the Temple of Isis-Hathor at Denderah, discovered and excavated by Baraize, was subsequently identified by Daumas (1957) as a sanatorium. It remains the only almost-complete example still in existence in Egypt today (see Plate 15). Located near the main temple, it stands adjacent to the mammisi (Divine Birth-house), to which it may once have had direct access. The current structure, dating to the Graeco-Roman Period, was possibly erected on top of an earlier sanatorium established in the reign of the 30th Dynasty ruler Nectanebo II.

There is no evidence that this building was ever used for conventional medical treatments (Nunn 1996: 139); however, methods used here to treat sick patients would have included isolation, immersion in baths of sacred water, 'dream therapy' induced through incubation and various magical procedures.

The building contains at least eleven small incubation chambers that were probably windowless; each room had a niche at floor level that may have contained a statuette of a deity. These chambers were arranged around a corridor containing a plinth that probably once supported a healing statue. No complete healing statues were found at Denderah, but they are known from other contexts, such as the black granite example belonging to the priest Djedhor from Athribis (Egyptian Museum JE 46341) (Sherman 1967).

It was customary for healing statues to be inscribed with magical texts. It was believed that water from the temple's Sacred Lake, channelled to flow over these inscriptions, would absorb their miraculous power. Then, when the patients drank or bathed in this water, this potent force would be transmitted directly to them. Once the holy water had been collected from the floor of the corridor it was directed towards a reservoir adjacent to a facility that accommodated a leg-bath, a full-length reclining bath and a seat bath with two seats (pers. comm. K. White). Here, the patients underwent partial or total immersion, perhaps as stand-alone treatments or as ritual ablutions in preparation for the Therapeutic Dream.

The Therapeutic Dream

The Therapeutic Dream – a trance-like state – was induced through silence, sacred songs possibly performed by the *rekhet* (see below, 4d), the use of lamps, and burning perfumed wood. This enabled the patient's soul to enter Nun, where

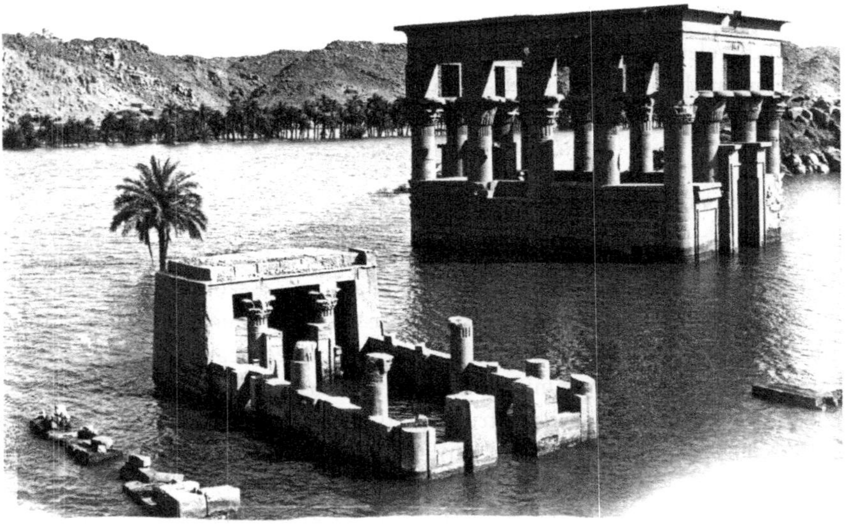

Figure 3.1. An early photograph of the island of Philae showing parts of the temple almost covered by the annual inundation. The temple was dedicated to Isis and was contemporary with her sanctuary at Denderah (Graeco-Roman Period). However, graffiti relate that pilgrims continued to visit the site to worship Isis and her husband Osiris into the 5th century AD, long after it ceased to function as a temple served by its own priesthood (courtesy of The Manchester Museum, The University of Manchester).

the gods dwelt, in the hope of receiving a dream in which the temple deity would provide knowledge of the future and any prospective dangers, as well as cures to heal the patient's physical or mental illness.

The goddess Isis-Hathor was accredited with great healing abilities: according to Diodorus Siculus (1. 25), Isis was regarded as a particularly potent source of healing dreams, while an inscription on the 18th Dynasty stela of Ipuy reports how the beauty of Hathor, glimpsed in a temple dream, had brought him inspiration (Szpakowska 2003: 195). The priests played a major role in the Therapeutic Dream, providing the divine prophetic voices associated with the therapy; they went to considerable lengths to conceal their true identity and deliver a convincing performance. Sometimes they used divine statues that incorporated an acoustic passage through which the priest, hidden behind the image, could deliver the god's words. In some healing sanctuaries architectural devices enabled the priests to conceal their identity and convince the patients that the god himself was addressing them (see below) (Fig. 3.1).

The cult of Imhotep and Amenhotep, son of Hapu, at Deir el-Bahri

There is evidence that by Ptolemaic times the cult of two healing deities, Imhotep and Amenhotep, son of Hapu, was established at the New Kingdom mortuary temple of Hatshepsut at Deir el-Bahri (Milne 1914; Lajtar 2008). These two men were deified and worshipped by generations who lived many centuries later (Wildung 1977). Imhotep (see Chapter 2b), regarded as the founder of medical science in Egypt, was ultimately adopted by the Greeks and identified with their god of medicine, Asclepius. Amenhotep, son of Hapu, was a royal scribe, counsellor and architect of Amenhotep III (*c.* 1450 BC). His reputation was so great that even in his lifetime he was believed to have direct contact with the gods; in later periods, he was greatly renowned for his wisdom and healing powers.

This cult enabled individual petitioners to make offerings to a deified individual in the hope that he would intercede on their behalf and transmit their requests to the gods. Imhotep and Amenhotep, son of Hapu, had other shrines throughout Egypt, but their centre at Deir el-Bahri (which was situated in a small chapel on the upper terrace of the temple and housed the god's statue) was particularly popular. An ostracon from the time of Ptolemy II (285–246 BC) testifies to the healing power of Amenhotep, son of Hapu:

> But I had heard from different sides that the miracles of Amenotes (Amenhotep, son of Hapu) were numerous and that he was merciful and that the hopeless were numerous who had found curing by him. Being a hopeless case, I went along to the sanctuary of Amenotes as a supplicant. Amenotes helped me, and cured by him by a vision and having regained my health, I wish to express to him and the other gods sharing in his altars and cults their miraculous powers in written words for those who visit the temple enclosure of Amenotes that they may see the power of this god when they are taken by any illness. (translated Wildung 1977: 92)

Patients have also left graffiti on the walls of one of the rooms at Deir el-Bahri. Dating to the 2nd century AD, they provide an informal record of personal circumstances and medical expectations. Some are addressed to Asclepius (and sometimes his daughter, Hygia) and Amenhotep, son of Hapu; one provides a personal record concerning the visit of a patient, Andromachos, who was a Macedonian worker for hire; it claims that he was sick but that the god healed him on the same day. This is of particular interest because it suggests that the man was a foreigner who had travelled from another country to seek treatment, and that, despite his relatively lowly status, he had been able to benefit from the medical care provided at the sanatorium.

Oracles in temples

Oracles have been described as a type of consultation that requested 'a deity to answer some practical question through the agency of its public image' (Kruchten 2001). They played an important role in magico-religious practice (Blackman 1925; Baines 1987). A graffito on Stela Louvre C 200 from Deir el-Bahri provides evidence that portable images of gods were included in religious festivals around Thebes from the early 12th Dynasty. However, most information comes from the New Kingdom, when oracular statues became a regular feature of processions accompanying annual festivals on the West Bank. The use of oracles became even more significant as royal authority gradually declined (Ritner 2001a: 325).

Oracular statues were frequently used to deliver public statements, but people also consulted them about a wide range of personal concerns and aspirations. Much of this evidence comes from ostraca and papyri of the Ramesside Period discovered at the royal workers' town at Deir el-Medina. Questions addressed to oracular gods reflect issues relating to legal disputes, religious matters and queries about personal circumstances and provide important insight into people's everyday concerns. Methods of using oracles in a community setting will be discussed in Chapter 4d.

There were different ways in which the laity could engage directly with temple gods. Inscriptions in the courtyards of the Temple of Luxor and the Hypostyle Hall at Karnak demonstrate that they could assemble in certain areas of the complex to praise the gods and experience divine manifestations.

The 'Chapel of the Hearing Ear', built against the northern exterior wall at Karnak in the reign of Ramesses II, provided another opportunity for ordinary people to engage with temple deities (Lesko 2001). Similar arrangements existed in other temples, where ears, engraved on exterior temple walls, enabled the gods to hear peoples' prayers. Petitioners brought offerings of food, flowers and other votive items in the hope of receiving a favourable response.

Oracular statements were sometimes associated with divine statues and iconographic images in wall reliefs situated inside special chambers within the temples. Here, a petitioner could address the god and pose questions relating to their personal medical problems. The ways in which advice was delivered appears to have varied from one temple to another, but from the Late Period onwards mechanical methods were sometimes used to enable the petitioner to 'hear' the deity's voice when the response was given.

In the reign of Ptolemy Euergetes II (170–116 BC) an adjoining room was added to the cult centre of Imhotep and Amenhotep, son of Hapu at Deir el-Bahri (see above). This accommodated patients who came to seek a cure. The two rooms were separated by a door; a window in the vault above this enabled the priest, hidden in the sanctuary, to voice the god's words and deliver the divine healing treatments to the patients, who waited overnight in the exterior chamber.

Discoveries made at the temple at Kom el-Wist in the Delta in 1941 demonstrate another method of managing oracular delivery. Here, a bronze tube hidden in the pedestal of statue of a bull was linked to a small room where the priest would have concealed himself while responding to the petitioner's questions (Brunton 1947).

However, there was always the danger that the priest's true role as divine impersonator might be discovered. They evidently had escape routes to guard against this possibility, as demonstrated in an inscription left behind by one pilgrim, a soldier Athenodorus. This recounts that he heard the divine voice coming from the sanctuary while he was praying in the exterior room; he opened the connecting door in an attempt to catch sight of the speaker, but the inner room was empty. This satisfied Athenodorus that the god himself had spoken, and consequently he received his healing. The priests may have persuaded him to leave this account on the temple walls as a testimony to the authenticity and effectiveness of the therapy (Sauneron 1960: 97–98).

4

Medical treatment and healing in a community context

Although temples made a special contribution to Egypt's complex medical system, most interaction between healers and their patients would have taken place in a variety of other contexts. These included the community care offered by physicians and local healers to families in towns and villages; the medical provision in royal palaces that accommodated not only the royal family but also officials employed in the government and administration; healthcare available to officials and workers at industrial sites and other workplaces; and treatment for the military, with a particular focus on battlefield wounds incurred during campaigns abroad.

(a) Evidence from palaeopathological investigations into disease patterns and treatment in royal workers' towns

Human skeletal remains can be useful in attempting to reconstruct the demographics, lifestyle, diseases and provision of medical care of ancient populations. In ancient Egypt studies have traditionally been directed towards royal and elite mummies, but several more recent investigations have focused on royal workers' communities such as those at Giza, Tell el-Amarna and Deir el-Medina.

The potential for workers of these communities to suffer injuries while engaged in building and industrial activities would have been considerable. Acute injuries such as strains, cuts and fractures, together with more serious crushing injuries, would have been an everyday hazard. In the longer term, chronic conditions may well have been a problem. Repetitive occupational activities promote skeletal responses in areas of stress, such as osteoarthritis caused by persistent load carrying. The physical posture adopted by workers during their occupational activities, such as the squatting position adopted by many trades, would have caused skeletal changes to the knee joints. There is evidence of a high prevalence of squatting facets of the talus and tibia probably directly related to this habitual pose.

As many of these communities and building sites were located in desert conditions, the inhalation of sand particles would have presented an inherent health hazard and predisposed the workers to sand pneumoconiosis (see also Chapter 6a). The presence of sand in the lungs causes the body's natural defences, the inflammatory mechanism, to wrap the particles in collagen, resulting in fibrotic nodules. This process reduces lung capacity and so less air can be breathed in, resulting in breathlessness, especially on exertion and possibly also associated with a severe cough. In addition, pain in the chest, especially when taking a deep breath or cough, may have been a related symptom. Stone working exacerbates this problem by filling the working environment – particularly enclosed quarries – with dust. The quarrying and stone-working activities required for the construction of the pyramids and temples would, therefore, have exposed the workforce to respiratory damage and disease (Tapp 1979; Aufderheide & Rodriguez-Martin 1998: 265–66). Labouring in such hot dusty conditions would have caused the additional problem of dehydration if sufficient fluids were not being imbibed.

(i) Giza

Workers' communities such as those founded at Giza to build the pyramids of the 4th Dynasty were established and maintained as distinct settlements. The inhabitants would not have been representative of other indigenous communities, but were chosen either for their expertise on industrial projects or to provide the support framework necessary for the state-sponsored activity.

Construction work, as noted above, was a hazardous activity, as attested by the high numbers of broken bones recorded among the human remains excavated from Giza. In a study of 272 male and female skeletons of two socioeconomic groups – workers and high officials – a high incidence of fractures was recorded. As many as 44 per cent of the male workers displayed fractures, with the ribs and the ulna being the most affected bones. Many of the fractures of the long bones of the arm – the ulna, radius and fibula – show well-aligned healed fractures, suggesting the possibility of reduction of fractures by manipulation, followed by splinting. The research indicated that the high success rate was equally noticeable both for men and women, and for the officials as well as the workers (Hussien *et al.* 2010). However, it is recognised that some long bone fractures of the arm are relatively easy to treat with simple methods such as slings, and others will heal successfully without access to orthopaedic treatment.

In another study, again from the Old Kingdom necropolis at Giza, two adult male skeletons displaying evidence of amputations perhaps carried out because of previous traumatic incidences were examined. The first of these was a high official, who had his left tibia and fibula removed, while the second, who was a worker, had the right ulna and radius severed. The distal ends of all the amputated bones were well healed, indicating that they lived for some time after the amputations were carried out. In the case of the high official the healing patterns suggest that binding or perhaps therapeutic prostheses were used as an aid in walking. For the worker, who had an amputated upper limb, the distortion and curvature present in the humerus indicates that the arm was used following amputation. Again, evidence for this procedure in two different social classes indicated that medical care was available for all (Zaki *et al.* 2010).

Another potential problem at these sites would have been that the build-up of large populations of people, brought together for corvée duties from different parts of Egypt, may well have precipitated outbreaks of infectious diseases. The close proximity of members of the workforce, demonstrated by the working and living environments at Giza, would have encouraged the spread of disease. Infectious diseases are usually considered the greatest cause of premature fatality among pre-antibiotic societies (Roberts & Manchester 2005: 164).

(ii) Tell el-Amarna

Analysis of skeletal material from the non-elite South Tomb Cemetery at Tell el-Amarna (one of five known cemeteries at this locality) indicates high levels of general, nutritional and workload stress. Trauma, degenerative joint disease of the spine and nutritional deficiencies were found to be commonplace. Among the latter, cribra orbitalia and porotic hyperostosis, conditions commonly attributed to iron and vitamin B12 deficiencies, have been identified. These nutritional deficiencies may have contributed to the extremely short stature noticeable in these Amarna residents. The vertebrae were found to be the commonest area to be affected, with compression fractures and spondylosis identified in some cases. Total trauma rates were exceptionally high, and there was an uncharacteristically high rate of death among older children and young adults.

The overarching picture presented by the bioarchaeological analysis was a population experiencing nutritional stress and workloads physically taxing enough to result in spinal and limb trauma; in addition, there was increased juvenile mortality (Dabbs *et al.* 2015). The data point to occupational injuries and not interpersonal violence. From the pathological evidence available at the site there is little indication of any medical treatment being provided.

(iii) Deir el-Medina

Osteological data obtained from the commingled human remains from Theban tombs 6, 217, and 291 at Deir-el-Medina have provided detailed information about the health of the workers who lived there during the New Kingdom. There is evidence of degenerative joint disease, which can be linked to the workers' role in preparing and decorating the rock-cut tombs in the Valley of the Kings. One atypical finding among all adults was a high incidence of osteoarthritis in both knee and ankle, suggesting an increased pressure on these joints in daily life. This may be due to Deir el-Medina's relatively remote location in a topographically diverse area. Constant climbing in the Theban hills in conjunction with a rocky landscape would place undue stress on the joints. The workers as part of their daily life had to routinely undertake a steep climb from their village to their workplace in the Valley of the Kings (Austin 2017).

Unlike the communities at Giza and Tell el-Amarna, relatively few traumatic injuries have been found among the human remains at Deir el-Medina. A dataset of 127 of these remains yielded three compression fractures of the vertebrae; one fracture of the ulna, which was found to be well aligned and fully healed; and a possible peri-mortem fracture in a male adult femur that displays little evidence of healing and was probably related to the ultimate cause of death.

Evidence for infection in the workers is attested by the number of cases demonstrating periostitis of the tibia, a condition present in 19 per cent of adult bones, 60 per cent of which were male. When this is correlated with the numbers of and reasons for the sick days that the workers took it could suggest that infectious diseases were the dominant cause of patterns of short-term illness.

A survey of the palaeopathological evidence indicates that, on the whole, the health of the workers at Deir el-Medina was relatively better than those at Giza and Tell el-Amarna. This would seem to have been due to a reduced level of occupational stress in their daily lives and fewer episodes of malnutrition and disease. In addition, there appears to have been better access to health care provided by the state (Austin 2017).

(b) Kahun: the site and its archaeological significance

To the south-west of Cairo lies the Fayoum, a region of remarkable fertility fed by local springs and the Bahr Yusef, a tributary channel that joins this area to the Nile. Today, the lake at the centre of the Fayoum – known in antiquity as Lake Moeris – is called Birket el-Qarun. In pharaonic times kings and courtiers visited the Fayoum to enjoy its excellent hunting and fishing opportunities and in the 12th Dynasty some of these rulers chose to build their pyramids nearby, on the fringes of the desert.

This brought unprecedented activity and employment to the region, as exemplified by the pyramid and temple complex that Senusret II (1877–1870 BC, 12th Dynasty) built for himself at Lahun (Illahun). The pyramid, which incorporated several innovative design features, was plundered in antiquity, but, beneath mounds of sand, the adjacent town built to accommodate the families of royal workers engaged in constructing this complex survived almost intact.

In antiquity, the town and temple were called 'Hetep-Senusret' ('Senusret is satisfied'). Today, the site is known either as Kahun or Lahun (after the pyramid);

it is particularly significant because of the wealth of everyday items that have been discovered there (Quirke 1998). These provide a unique insight into the domestic conditions and practices of a particular community; some items, too humble to be placed in tombs, are known only from this particular domestic context.

Kahun was designed as a rectangular unit surrounded by a massive brick wall; another internal wall separated the two sections of the town. Blocks of houses for the workers' families occupied the western area, while the eastern part contained large houses to accommodate the officials who supervised the royal works.

This town site was one of the most significant discoveries made by the British archaeologist William Flinders Petrie. His overall plan for the years 1888 and 1889 was to excavate several sites in this area simultaneously (Fig. 4.1). Petrie's excavations in the Fayoum included the Pyramid of Senusret II at Lahun; two small adjoining temples; Gurob, a royal residence town dating to the New Kingdom; and Kahun, situated to the north of the larger Lahun temple (Petrie 1891). As a previously unexcavated site, Kahun was of particular interest to Petrie, especially as it offered the first opportunity to investigate a complete plan of an Egyptian town. However, results of the excavation exceeded all expectations as, in addition to the substantial remains of buildings and a wide range of everyday items, Petrie also discovered a significant number of papyri that cast light on the

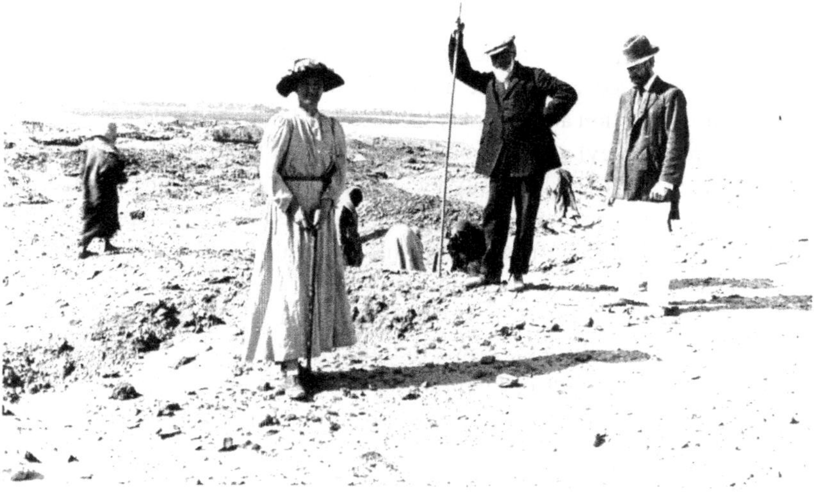

Figure 4.1. Photograph taken at Kahun showing W. M. F. Petrie (centre), his wife Hilda, and a visitor to the site, C. T. Campion. Petrie had just finished excavating the enclosure immediately around the Lahun pyramid and his group had walked across to Kahun (courtesy of The Manchester Museum, The University of Manchester).

social, religious, medical and educational activities of the community (Collier & Quirke 2004). According to his journal, Petrie started to excavate at Kahun in April 1889. Altogether, he cleared some 2000 chambers in the town, although this accounted for only about two-thirds of the site, as the remainder lay under cultivation.

Although palaeopathological evidence is not available from the site, archaeological and inscriptional material offers a unique opportunity to study aspects of community medicine practised there. As well as the Kahun Gynaecological Papyrus (a document of considerable medical and social significance), equipment belonging to a local healer was found in one of the private houses (Petrie 1890: 30, pl. VIII). This unique group of items was associated with healing practices and protective magic performed for ordinary women in the local community (see Chapter 5e).

Much of the funding to excavate Kahun came from Jesse Haworth, a Manchester textile manufacturer and one of the longest-established members of the Manchester Royal Exchange. Haworth's enthusiasm for Egyptology probably began around 1877, when he and his wife read Amelia Edwards' book *A Thousand Miles up the Nile*, which inspired them to make the same journey in the winter of 1880–1881. They became acquainted with Amelia Edwards when she lectured in Manchester in 1887, and she subsequently introduced Haworth to Petrie. As a devout nonconformist Protestant, this wealthy industrialist was interested in the role Egyptian archaeology could play in illuminating the Bible and was readily persuaded to become a major sponsor of Petrie's excavation, thus emerging as one of the first patrons of scientific excavation in Egypt.

Almost all the discoveries made at Kahun were eventually divided equally between Petrie's collection at University College London (now the Petrie Museum of Egyptian Archaeology) and Haworth, who donated them to The Manchester Museum, located at The University of Manchester. Here, they formed the nucleus of the Egyptology collection, which expanded and developed over the following years, benefiting from Haworth's continued funding for many of Petrie's excavations at sites throughout Egypt.

Haworth also made a substantial contribution to a subscription fund opened to enable an extension – the Jesse Haworth Building – to be added to the museum to house his many donations of Egyptian antiquities. When this was opened in 1912 the artefacts from Kahun were displayed to the public for the first time as the central feature of a new gallery.

(c) The Kahun Gynaecological Papyrus

The Kahun Papyrus, also known as the Kahun Gynaecological Papyrus, was discovered at Kahun and now forms part of the collection of the Petrie Museum (Griffith 1898; Stevens 1975; Bardinet 1995: 221–29, 437–43; Quirke 2002; Strouhal *et al.* 2014). On the reverse of the document is a reference to the 29th year of Amenemhat III, dating the papyrus to about 1825 BC. It is thus one of the earliest known medical papyri (see Plate 16).

The document, which covers three sheets, is badly fragmented and although extensive restoration work has been carried out some of the descriptions are still difficult to understand. The earliest known manuscript on gynaecology in the world, it includes thirty-four cases concerning gynaecological matters, but nothing relating to the closely allied topic of obstetrics.

Because of the breaks in paragraphs of the document some of the text is missing, but the manuscript provides a fascinating insight into ancient Egyptian gynaecology, contraception methods and ideas relating to conception. The various prescriptions comprise fumigations, pessaries and a variety of oral medications. However, there are no surgical procedures for gynaecological conditions in the Kahun Papyrus or indeed in any of the other medical papyri.

Although there are no exact parallels with the Kahun Papyrus, the Berlin, Carlsberg, Ebers, London and Ramesseum papyri contain substantial gynaecological elements and similarities between the various documents may indicate a common source. The papyrus provides a major contribution to our understanding of medical care and social organisation at Kahun.

Opening section

The first two pages of the papyrus encompass several cases involving assorted symptoms and signs, seemingly having their origin in primary disorders of the uterus. Although attempts have been made to identify the conditions being described, the exact nature of the disorders is not always clear.

Fertility

The next section, which relates to the important topic of fertility, is better preserved. Bearing children was very important in ancient Egypt and the Kahun and other medical papyri contain a large number of tests for fertility, pregnancy and determining the sex of the unborn child. In some cases, it is difficult to ascertain whether the test was for fertility or pregnancy. Both P. Kahun (Case 26) and P. Berlin (Case 196) give closely related instructions for the examination of a woman's breasts in order to ascertain whether she would conceive. The two papyri are damaged, but a study of both texts allows for the missing sections to be filled in:

> For distinguishing who will conceive from who will not conceive: when she lies down, spread fresh oil on her breasts, both of her arms and her shoulders. Get up early in the morning to examine her. If you find her veins (*metu*) fresh and good, not sunken, she is one who will give birth readily.

> If you find them collapsed like the skin over her limbs it is unhealthy (?).
> If you find them dark and green when you see her, she will give birth later.

Dilated vessels over the breasts are a commonly accepted indicator of pregnancy (Bastian & Piscitelli 1997).

In P. Kahun 27 it is recommended that a woman should sit over a mixture of beer and dates. If she begins to vomit, it is an indication that she will conceive; if she does not, she will not. Moreover, the number of times she vomits is supposed to correspond to the number of children she will have. P. Berlin 193 includes a similar test relating to sickness (Strouhal *et al.* 2014: 126, 163).

P. Kahun 28 describes another test that recommends that a woman should insert an onion into her vagina. If her breath smells of onions the next day, she will conceive. If not, she will never give birth. This seems to be based on the idea that there was a communication between the womb and the mouth. If the womb was open, then the odour of the onion would come out through the mouth, but if she was pregnant then the womb would be closed, preventing the odour penetrating upwards through the body to the mouth. A very similar test is recorded in P. Carlsberg VIII, 4 (Strouhal *et al.* 2014: 125, 162).

P. Kahun 30, another prescription for determining fertility, is introduced by a magical invocation, the only incantation in the Kahun Papyrus. The text refers to the god Horus and the calf of Horus, but the wording is not clear because of the many tears in this section of the papyrus.

Some of the tests described in the papyri are similar to those recorded in the *Greek Hippocratic Aphorisms* and *On Sterile Women* texts, which are dated to about 400 BC and so may suggest a link between Greek and Egyptian medicine (Stevens 1975; Nunn 1996: 192).

Conception

Should a woman prove to be fertile then P. Kahun provides advice on how to conceive. P. Kahun 18, an incomplete text, states: 'Another for unveiling a woman from [...] half a scoop of milk [...] scoop, solidify (?), sprinkle in her womb'. Some sources have suggested that this could be an aphrodisiac, although it may well be a prescription for a treatment of some disorder of the womb (translated Stevens 1975; Watterson 1991: 86).

Some tests documented in the papyri could be used to confirm a woman's pregnancy. Physical observations mentioned include the condition of the eyes, skin and breasts. More specific tests are described in P. Kahun, but the section referring to this is again defective. Quotations from other medical papyri are helpful in understanding pregnancy testing and perhaps the most celebrated of these is P. Berlin 199, with a less well-preserved parallel text given in P. Carlsberg III:

> Another [determination] whether a woman will give birth or will not give birth: barley and emmer, the woman should moisten with her urine every day, like dates and like sand in two bags. If they all grow, she will bear a child. If the barley grows, it means a male. If the emmer grows, it means a female. If they do not grow, she will not give birth. (combined translation of both papyri by Nunn 1996: 191)

A laboratory experiment that reproduced this test found that in 70 per cent of cases the urine of pregnant women caused the seeds to sprout, while the urine of non-pregnant women and men did not cause germination in any of the cases (Ghalioungui *et al.* 1963). The unique blend of hormones, particularly chorionic gonadotropin, in a pregnant woman's urine, promoted seed germination (Ravagan & Grossi 2009). The test was accurate in determining sex in only 48 per cent of cases, so only equivalent to chance. The barley and wheat pregnancy test has survived over the millennia, being taught in the Salerno medical school in the Middle Ages and still reputedly being in use in the Near East in the 1960s.

The medical papyri also describe a method that attempts to influence the sex of an unborn child: for this, milk from a woman who had been delivered of infant boys was given to a woman who wished to become pregnant. The liquid used for this was stored in jars shaped like a mother nursing her baby, although human milk had other uses in general medicine.

Contraception

Pregnancy and childbirth in an ancient society were undoubtedly accompanied by many physical dangers, and many infants would have died at an early age. The problems caused by frequent pregnancies would have encouraged the Egyptians to consider and develop contraceptive measures. There may also have been a need to limit family size because the land available for domestic settlements and supporting families was scarce. Housing accommodation in purpose-built towns such as Kahun was particularly restricted.

The medical papyri describe a range of preparations to prevent conception, which utilised various ingredients of herbal, animal and mineral origin, some of which may have had some efficacy. These were applied either by smearing externally on the vulva or internally as a tampon of plant fibres. P. Kahun 21 recommends crocodile dung dispersed in sour milk and, while appearing repellent, the mixture is not unlike a sponge soaked in weak acid, and would have had a similar spermicidal effect (Watterson 1991: 88–89). Similarly, P. Ramesseum IV.C II also recommends the use of crocodile dung, this time placed on moistened fibres inserted at the orifice of the uterus. Another contraceptive prescription, P. Kahun 22, includes honey and natron as its active agents, which again would have some spermicidal effects.

Pregnancy

Once pregnant, it was important for the ancient Egyptian woman not to bleed, since it was often an indication of a miscarriage or premature birth. Attempts at preventing this were based on magical acts as well as more practical solutions. The causes of the bleeding were usually attributed to harmful powers and the solution was to magically close the birth canal with a knot constructed out of plant fibres, the *tyet*, usually known as the magical knot of Isis (Robins 1993: 79–80; see Chapter 6c).

Procreation was a crucial element of ancient Egyptian culture and so it is not surprising that considerable emphasis was placed on the health and care of women. The many prescriptions devoted to women's health in the Kahun and other medical papyri testify to a high level of care and attention.

(d) 'Wise women' and local healers

Women's role in community-based medicine

Community-based medicine played an important role in Egyptian society, whether undertaken for the elite in the royal palaces (see Chapter 4e) or for the non-elite residents of towns and cities. This healthcare would have included physical and pharmaceutical remedies for a wide range of ailments, but there are also interesting examples of magico-medical treatments (Borghouts 1994).

Much of the focus was on problems encountered by almost all women, regardless of status. These related to fertility and to pregnancy and childbirth, which were often accompanied by physical dangers, including a high death rate among neonates and infants. In the palaces, assistance was provided by physicians, magicians and female assistants, while within domestic communities lower-status healers offered similar protection and treatment for the non-elite. The royal workmen's towns of Kahun, Deir el-Medina and Tell el-Amarna provide particularly interesting inscriptional and archaeological evidence of healing methods available within these communities.

The role of the *rekhet* ('wise woman')

Both men and women practised as local healers (see Chapter 2c), although relatively little evidence has survived of women's role in magic and community treatment. However, they do appear to have played a particular role in divination, being attributed with the ability to detect spirit possession. The various non-elite groups from which seers were drawn probably included dwarfs, children and women; among the latter, the primary role of the *rekhet* ('wise woman' or 'knowing one') was to contact the dead and identify spirit possession.

It was believed that a 'wise woman' had a special awareness of the divine presence, and this enabled her to mediate between the gods, the dead and the living. The role may have been inherited within the family, and a woman perhaps became involved in these matters once her childbearing years were over (Pinch 2006: 56).

Divination and healing

By the New Kingdom, oracles came to play an increasingly significant role in religious practices. They demonstrated that the gods took a personal interest in the lives of the laity, and could provide them with advice and guidance about a range of matters, including property and personal disputes; the guilt or innocence of individuals accused of crime; and the health concerns of petitioners and their families.

The term that described the procedure of approaching or petitioning an oracular deity is *pḥ-nṯr* (Ritner 2001a: 324–25). Sometimes this was specifically associated with temples (see Chapter 3c), but it also occurred as an important element in many religious processions that were part of the social fabric of communities in many parts of Egypt. At these events, statues of deities believed to possess special oracular powers were paraded by *wꜥb*-priests, either hidden in portable shrines, carried in a portable bark or open palanquin or mounted on vertical poles (Kruchten 2001: 610).

Oracles provided an opportunity for personal interaction with the gods, when petitioners could present their queries and requests to the statue through the agency of a senior priest accompanying the procession. Approaching the god's statue, the petitioner would either make his request orally or write it down on a scrap of papyrus or flake of pottery or limestone, which the priest then read out to the statue (Wente 1990: 184). In some instances, the god would select a reply from two opposing statements written on a pair of petitions. The god's response would be ascertained through specific movements made by the statue. Assent might be conveyed by the statue 'nodding' or, for a negative answer, 'walking backwards'.

The spoken delivery of a message through a divine statue was another oracular method: here, the priest, impersonating the deity, would deliver the god's response to the petitioner (see Chapter 3c). A god could also issue an amuletic decree, which its owner could use to provide personal protection against a series of dangers and diseases listed in the document.

Centuries later, Herodotus (II, 83) stated that there were various methods of consulting oracles in different regions of Egypt. Their use became widespread throughout the country from the New Kingdom onwards, but the most famous examples are known from the Theban region, where the image of Amun of Karnak was transported in a barque as the centrepiece of processions taking place in Thebes and on the West Bank during the Opet and Valley Festivals.

Amun of Karnak's overlordship of all the Theban oracular deities is well documented, but ostraca and papyri from Deir el-Medina provide evidence of more localised events. One cult celebrated at Deir el-Medina over a period of four days commemorated the death of the deified king Amenhotep I (Černy 1927: 183; Kitchen 1983: 104, 370). An important feature of this event was an oracle through which Amenhotep I, the patron god of the royal workforce, could be approached for answers and advice about local disputes, administrative issues and general problems affecting the community (McDowell 1999: 107–15).

The cobra goddess Meretseger also had an important oracular presence at Deir el-Medina. Prayers and images carved on stelae and wall surfaces in the goddess's rock-cut shrine indicate that petitioners offered prayers to express gratitude for her help and to ask for protection, wealth and good health.

It is possible that 'wise women' played a part in oracular proceedings in community settings, as well as perhaps serving in temples (see Chapter 3c), where they may have enacted the role of a goddess who delivered speeches and sacred songs to patients visiting for medical treatment or foretold the future of those who came to the temple to know their fate.

Because of their presumed ability as seers, 'wise women' may also have been accredited with the power to detect which god or evil power was responsible for personal affliction or illness (Teeter 2011: 100). Magico-medical texts mention these spirit-induced illnesses, but do not usually provide information about methods of diagnosing them. Nevertheless, people perhaps assumed that the *rekhet*'s contact with the dead enabled her to make these diagnoses, especially in sick children. Exorcism, undertaken to remove evil spirits from patients, may also have been part of the *rekhet*'s role. An unusual scene in the tomb of Ankhmahor at Saqqara, depicting dancing women and men and women fainting in a state of collapse, may illustrate some of these rites (Pinch 2006: 140).

'Wise women' formed a distinctive group at Deir el-Medina, where they may have exercised multiple and overlapping roles. Some researchers have used ostraca discovered at the site to support the claim that the *rekhet* had a dual role in the community, as both diviner/exorcist and healer (Borghouts 1982: 25; Lesko 2002: 236; Pinch 2006: 56). References to 'wise women' are also found in letters dating to the late 2nd millennium BC (Vercoutter 1980, 127–33; Pinch 2006: 56), and a tale inscribed on the 4th century BC Metternich stela relates how a local 'wise woman' was able to advise the goddess Isis that the illness suffered by her son Horus had probably been caused by a scorpion sting or snake bite (Klasens 1952: 54–58; Allen 2005: 49–63).

However, not all researchers agree that the *rekhet* fulfilled this dual role. Janssen & Janssen (2007: 6) suggest that divination, rather than healing, was her prime role, although a letter in the Deir el-Medina archive is ambiguous on this point. The letter, Ostracon Letellier, may have been written by a father to his sons' nurse (Janssen & Janssen 2007: 148). The author was a necropolis workman named Qenherkhepeshef, a 19th Dynasty scribe in charge of administration at Deir el-Medina. He addresses a village woman, Inerwau, asking her why she has not consulted the local 'wise woman' who would provide insight into the deaths of two children who had been in her care: 'Why did you not go to the "wise woman", on account of the two boys who died in your charge? Ask the "wise woman" about the death the two boys have incurred'. The letter does not confirm whether the 'wise woman' was expected to offer any medical advice or treatment or simply provide some information about the events around the children's deaths.

The precise role of 'wise women' within the community setting thus remains unclear. However, it may have included midwifery (see Chapter 2d). The *rekhet* had a relatively low social status, but this may not have prevented her from taking up this occupation because, although some midwives certainly achieved privileged positions in wealthy households (see Chapter 2d), this may have been generally regarded as low-status employment because it involved procedures considered to be 'ritually impure' (see Chapter 2d).

The healer's equipment

There is no textual information about any potions and remedies that the 'wise women' may have used to treat their patients, or any magical equipment they may have possessed. However, items found in a house at Kahun were probably owned by a local healer and used in her magical rituals (see Chapter 4b). Unusual grave goods found in the Tomb of Madja (TT1370 at Deir el-Medina) may also have belonged to a 'wise woman'. The collection, which dates to the 18th Dynasty, includes animal dung, coloured stones, shells in a basket and small ceramic coffins containing winged insects (Meskell 1999: 180).

Sin, disease and salvation

Not all magico-religious community treatment focused on women and children. A remarkable set of inscriptions occur on papyri and memorial stelae set up by workmen, mostly in local chapels at Deir el-Medina but also in a few other places (Gunn 1916; McDowell 1999: 91–126). The workmen directly address various gods in these prayers, sometimes expressing a special kind of personal piety and awareness of the concepts of confession and salvation. These ideas appear to have been very rare in Egypt, and were perhaps brought in at this time by Asiatic immigrants; alternatively, they may have been a long-standing feature of popular faith within Egypt but perhaps not usually expressed in writing. Evidence of these beliefs possibly survived at Deir el-Medina only because the workmen had better-than-usual literacy and chose to record their prayers in writing.

These prayers were addressed to deities by petitioners who acknowledged their undefined sins (perhaps blasphemy or impiety). It was believed that these sins had incurred divine wrath and punishment in the form of health afflictions. Showing suitable contrition, the petitioner offered thanks to the deity for forgiveness and for a consequent recovery either for himself or for a sick relative.

Some prayers, including that offered by the necropolis scribe, Nekhtamun, mention that the deity has caused the petitioner to see 'darkness by day'. However, it is not clear if this term describes a physical condition – perhaps the result of long hours spent working in badly lit tombs – or if it relates to an emotional state of depression (Gunn 1916).

(e) How palaces fitted into the healthcare system

Palace complexes: the background

Many royal palaces were located in cities and included space to accommodate state functions, a residence for the king and his family, and some sections for state administration. Every town associated with a pyramid complex also had its own palace where the king stayed when he visited the site to inspect progress on his funerary monuments. Relatively little evidence of these palaces has survived, largely because they were constructed from mudbrick and wood; however, excavation has revealed that they were originally impressive, spacious buildings with a very high standard of decoration. This is demonstrated by painted fragments from the walls, ceilings and floors at Malkata (Thebes) and Tell el-Amarna, and by faience tiles and inlays from Ramesside palaces in the Delta. There would have been a wide variation in the age, status and individual healthcare requirements of people living in the palace complexes, and a range of medical personnel and treatments was employed to address these needs.

Medical staff

Physicians

Medical knowledge and expertise were sometimes attributed to those who held the highest political offices in the country. Notable examples are Imhotep (see Chapters 2b, 3c) and the 1st Dynasty ruler Djer, who, according to Manetho's *Aegyptica*, was a physician and anatomist. This royal association with medicine and healing doubtless reflected a much earlier tradition when local rulers provided community leadership in socio-political, religious and magic-medical matters (see Chapter 2a).

Inscriptional evidence indicates that, generally, the royal court was served by a variety of physicians whose titles give some indication of their hierarchical status and medical specialisations (Nunn 1996: 117–19, Tables 6.1–6.3). In the Old Kingdom almost half of the physicians and dentists identified in inscriptions were members of the royal court, but in later periods there is more inscriptional evidence relating to physicians who served the wider community. This is because their existence and career paths were increasingly recorded in the more elaborate tombs and funerary assemblages they acquired as result of the democratisation of religious beliefs and funerary practices in the First Intermediate Period and Middle Kingdom (Nunn 1996: 118).

The titles held by royal physicians provide some indication of the medical hierarchy that existed in the palaces. This was headed by a 'Controller or Administrator of Physicians of the Palace' (*ẖrp swnw pr-ꜥꜣ*) – a position held in the Old Kingdom by an ophthalmologist, Medunefer. The next level included the 'Inspector of Palace Physicians' (*sḥḏ swnw pr-ꜥꜣ*), 'Inspector of Physicians to the King' (*sḥḏ swnw n nsw*) and 'Overseer of the Two Sides of the Boat of Physicians of the Palace' (*imy-r gswy dpt pr-ꜥꜣ swnw*). Other titles included the 'Chief of Palace Physicians' (*wr swnw pr-ꜥꜣ*), 'Chief of Physicians to the Lord of the Two Lands' (*wr swnw n nb tꜣwy*), 'One with authority over the Physicians to the Lord of the Two Lands' (*ḥry swnw n nb tꜣwy*) and 'Chief of Physicians to the King' (*wr swnw n nsw*).

In the next tier came the 'Physician of the Palace' (*swnw pr-ꜥꜣ*), 'Physician to the Lord of the Two Lands' (*swnw n nb tꜣwy*) and the 'Physician to the King' (*swnw n nsw*). Elite women in the palaces were attended by the 'Chief of Physicians to the House of the Royal Wife (Queen)' (*wr swnw n pr-ḥmt nsw*) and 'Physician to the House of the Royal Wife (Queen)' (*swnw n pr-ḥmt nsw*).

Titles of some Old Kingdom royal physicians indicate that they specialised in a particular condition or area of the body, such as ophthalmology, gastroenteritis and proctology. However, as exemplified by Irenakhty (Nunn 1996: 127; see Chapter 2f, ii), it was possible to simultaneously hold roles associated with a variety of specialisms.

Some of those with the highest titles in medicine and healing (who sometimes had close familial ties to the king) may not have been practising physicians, but perhaps functioned entirely as administrators within the court medical system. One example, Mereruka, was identified in wall inscriptions in his well-known Tomb at Saqqara as a vizier and relative of King Teti (2345–2323 BC, 6th Dynasty), but he also held the title of 'Overseer of the two sides of the Boat of Physicians of the Palace' (*imy-r gswy dpt pr-ꜥꜣ swnw*). However, Egyptologists remain undecided over whether this was an honorary medical title or whether he actively practised as a royal physician (Jonckheere 1958; Ghalioungui 1983).

The inscription on the green basalt naos-statue of Udjahorresnet, which was originally set up in the Temple of Neith at Sais during the reign of Darius I

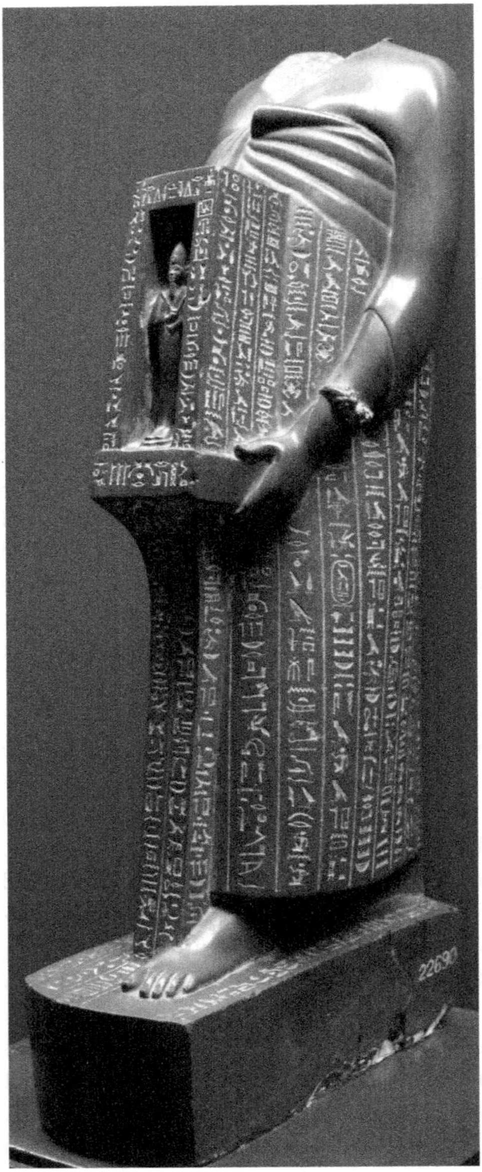

Figure 4.2. Statue of Udjahorresnet holding a naos (shrine) bearing the image of Osiris. Udjahorresnet lived between the end of the 26th Dynasty and the beginning of the 27th Dynasty. Provenance unknown, thought to have come from Sais. Black basalt. Now located in the Museo Gregoriano Egizio, Rome, 22690 (photograph: Aidan Dodson).

(522–486 BC) and is now located in the Gregorian Egyptian Museum, Rome, records that in the 26th Dynasty he pursued an early career as a naval officer (Lichtheim 1980: 36–40; Lloyd 1982; Lopez 2015; Wasmuth and Creasman 2020) (Fig. 4.2). He was subsequently promoted by the Persian kings who ruled Egypt during the 27th Dynasty. Cambyses (525–522 BC), the Persian ruler, appointed him as a senior administrator in the royal household, chief physician and priest of Neith, and later Darius I asked him to undertake the restoration of the House of Life at Sais (see Chapter 3b). His statue inscription emphasises that this was a major achievement of his career, and he clearly carried considerable responsibility and authority at the highest level in medical matters. However, it is unclear whether this involvement was limited to a supervisory and administrative role or whether he also practised as a court physician in Egypt. He may also have worked as a healer when he visited Persia, in the tradition of Egyptian and Greek physicians who held prominent positions at the Persian court.

This continued a tradition pursued over many centuries. Egyptian physicians had early attained an international reputation and court physicians contributed to a well-documented exchange of medical concepts that enhanced the high-level diplomacy pursued by Egypt with neighbouring lands. The Amarna archive records instances of requests for medical help from foreign rulers and there is also an appeal by the Hittites later in the 19th Dynasty (see Chapters 2c, 7b).

Magicians

Midwives and nurses who supervised royal pregnancies and births (see Chapter 2d) would have been in regular attendance at the palaces. In addition to this practical support, women and children of the royal household also received magico-religious and ritual treatments and protection. This was provided by magicians (*s3w*) (see Chapter 2c) who were engaged to undertake a variety of duties for the royal family. Magicians who performed these rites for royal women may include a group of three women who were buried close to the royal women in the funeral temple of Mentuhotep II (2055–2004 BC, 11th Dynasty) at Deir el-Bahri (Pinch 2006: 131).

One particularly important group of palace magicians, attached to the 'House of Nurses', were known as 'Magicians of the Nursery' (*ḥk3yw n k3p*) (see p. 51). They (and perhaps lectors) were responsible for reciting the 'Spells for Mother and Child' that occur in Papyrus Berlin (3027, recto 2.2–7, 3.8–4.2) (Borghouts 1978: 42–43, nos 67, 68). These incantations offered help to neonates and protection in childbirth and against childhood diseases caused by spirit possession. The spells have some parallels with those found in papyri from a burial assemblage discovered near the Ramesseum (see Chapter 5e, i).

Other healthcare therapies

The royal household would also have had access to a range of therapies intended to improve general health and well-being, and doubtless employed physiotherapists, manicurists, pedicurists and hairdressers. However, evidence of these procedures is rarely found in the archaeological, iconographic or inscriptional record.

A unique scene in the tomb of Ankhmahor and Khentika at Saqqara depicts two seated men whose toes and fingers are being manipulated by two therapists

(Capart 1907: 51, pl. 66). One recipient says: 'Do not let it be painful' and the therapist replies: 'I do as you please'. Various interpretations of this scene include surgery, physiotherapy, massage, reflexology or manicure and pedicure (see further Nunn 1996: 133; Ghalioungui 1963: 97, pl. 10).

Inscriptions also attest the existence of royal manicurists: Niankhkhnum and Khnumhotep, the owners of a 5th Dynasty tomb discovered at Saqqara in 1964 (Moussa & Altenmüller 1977), carried the titles of 'Manicurist of the King' and 'Overseer of Manicurists of the Palace'. Similar titles of 'Manicurist' and 'Manicurist of the Palace' are listed in Jones (2000: 308).

(f) Healthcare provision at industrial sites and for the military

Industrial sites

The large workforces at the construction sites throughout pharaonic Egypt would have fallen victim to many diseases and occupational accidents. Their healthcare would have been an important consideration in the efficient workings of these industrial operations. Texts from communities such as Deir el-Medina indicate that individuals within the village had access to medical knowledge and that the workers also practised medicine. Many of the healers, such as the *swnw*, the 'Controllers of Serket' and the 'wise women', are represented at these sites. Professionals such as the *swnw* were state employees, some of whom may have been appointed from among the existing workforce, and these employees would then have been able to supplement their rations by taking on this additional healing role.

A wall painting in the 20th Dynasty tomb of the chief sculptor Ipuy at Deir el-Medina displays some examples of what appear to be accidents in the workplace (Davies 1927: 31–76; Nunn 1996: 56–57, 127, 178–79) (Fig. 4.3). One of the craftsmen depicted in the scene has been described as undergoing treatment for a foreign body in his eye. Eye injuries may well have been a frequent occurrence among tradesmen such as carpenters and stone masons, particularly working without eye protection. Another eye condition, nystagmus, a disorder of uncontrolled eye movement, would have constituted a complication for those labouring under the poor lighting conditions associated with quarries, mines and tombs (Miller 1991).

A pair of figures placed in the top right-hand corner of the Ipuy scene has been interpreted as representing an attempt to reduce a dislocated shoulder by the classic Kocher method, which involves pulling the affected arm in the direction of the arm's longitudinal axis, followed by external rotation of the limb. The arm is then adducted until a pop is heard or felt, signifying that the shoulder has relocated back to its normal position (Chitgopkar and Khan 2005). It is quite

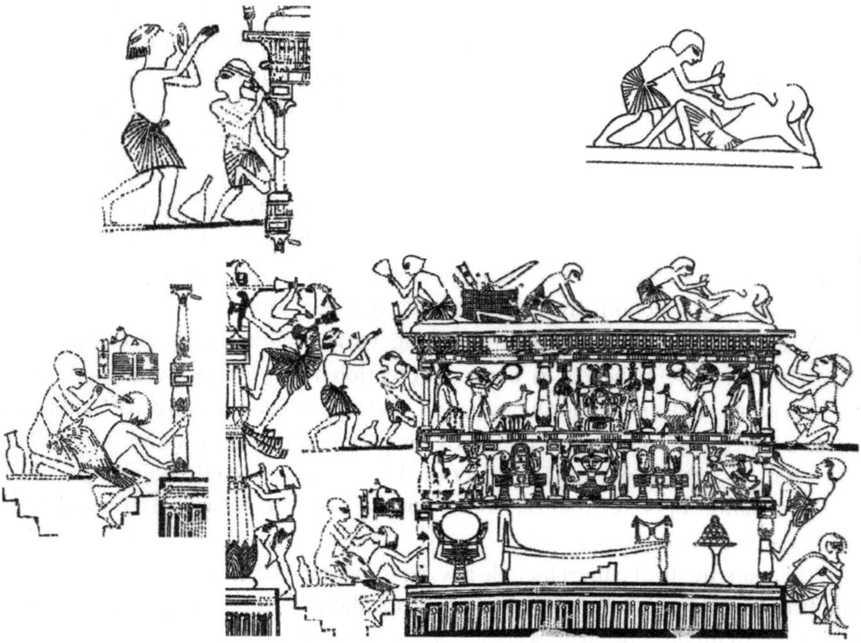

Figure 4.3. Composite of the catafalque scene from the 20th Dynasty tomb of the chief sculptor Ipuy (TT 217) at Deir el-Medina. The scene shows a number of occupational injuries. Redrawn by K. N. White after Davies (1927: pls 37–39) and Blomstedt (2014b: fig. 3).

likely that dislocations of this nature were common occurrences among manual workers. However, a simpler explanation for this scene is that the depiction may simply represent a craftsman pulling to his feet a reluctant resting colleague.

Finally, there is a depiction of a workman with a mallet positioned or falling on one of his feet. The craftsman appears to be raising his arms in the air in a gesture of pain and surprise. Alternatively, he may merely be gesticulating and calling to one of the workmen, seated on top of the furniture.

Snake and scorpion bites would have been a constant problem at these industrial sites. Ostraca found at Deir el-Medina relating to workers' attendances have entries for workers who had time off as a result of scorpion stings. Ostracon BM EA 5634 records that during the reign of Ramesses II Seba had one day off due to a scorpion sting, and Ostracon Cairo 25519 records that during the reign of Siptah (*c.* 1194–1188 BC, 19th Dynasty) Roma had a day off, as did the workman Nebnefer. In general, scorpion stings seem to warrant only one day off from work, although it is known that on occasions the severity of the sting can result in death, particularly in more vulnerable groups (Collier 2016). Evidence suggests that the sick and injured were entitled to time off from work at Deir el-Medina, and possibly this situation may have applied at other industrial sites.

Some textual sources contain incantations aimed at protection against snakes and scorpions. The recto of P. Chester Beatty VII, discovered at Deir el-Medina, invokes the protection of the goddess Serket against scorpions and includes remedies to treat bites. From incantation 13, 6.6: 'To be recited over barley-bread crumb, onions and ochre, heated and placed at the side of the sting. It can't spread'. This would appear to be a magically infused poultice aimed at preventing the spread of the venom through the body (Collier 2016).

Many shrines, particularly in the Late Period, contained stelae known as *cippi*, which were believed to confer protection from attack by animals such as scorpions and snakes (see pp. 3, 111). *Cippi* provided a range of texts and incantations that could be recited both for prevention of attack and for relief in the event of a sting or bite. The effect of the incantation could be reinforced by the application of water that had been poured over the stela, thereby absorbing its magical texts and scenes (Price 2016).

The main medical papyri include few details about snakes and scorpion bites but the Brooklyn Museum Papyrus (in two parts), dated to the Late Period, resembles a manual to guide those who were called upon to treat individuals suffering from such bites (see Chapters 2C, 4F). The logical rationale that is adopted to manage these injuries resembles that of the methodology apparent in the Edwin Smith Papyrus. The second part of the papyrus (47.218.85) is mainly concerned with treatment, which is threefold: local treatment for the bite, administration of drugs (mainly herbal) and magical incantations, some of which were specific for certain types of snake. The remedies are listed according to the species of snake and the signs and symptoms that developed as a result of the wound.

Within the Brooklyn Papyrus the *swnw* are not referred to but in the second section there is documented a remedy intended for the use by the 'Controllers of Serket'. It would have been these healers who would have specialised in medical treatments related to poisonous bites and stings, and would have acted as intermediaries to the deities when reciting the various incantations (Austin 2014: 93–97). The 'Controllers of Serket' examined snakes by description, toxicity and the reptile's divine associations (Sauneron 1989: 180–88; Ritner 2001a: 326). Amulets protecting against such bites and stings, a dominant concern in these sites, would have been a further safeguarding measure utilised by the workmen.

Labouring in external environments would undoubtedly result in skin abrasions and wounds and thus expose workers to the risk of tetanus. Tetanus is a bacterial infection caused by the bacterium *Clostridium tetani*, which is commonly found in soil, dust and manure. Although there is no direct evidence of tetanus from skeletal material or mummified tissue, Case 7 of P. Edwin Smith describes the classic symptoms of tetanus: a rising fever, sweating, lockjaw and spasms. Case 5 of P. Kahun may also describe this condition (Sanchez & Meltzer 2012: 83). Although tetanus, if untreated, is often fatal, the treatment recommended in Case 7 was the insertion of a wooden wedge wrapped in linen between the teeth, which was intended to keep the mouth open in order that fluids could be administered. With the prognosis of 'a medical condition I will fight with', the hope was that the condition might improve (Sanchez & Meltzer 2012: 71–85).

Mining expeditions

There is a considerable body of surviving archaeological and inscriptional evidence that provides an insight into how mining and processing operations were undertaken in pharaonic Egypt. Unlike modern mining techniques, where long-term mining communities are the norm, pharaonic mining was predominately short-term, with the concept of the 'expedition' being the overriding impression of mining activities (Seyfried 1981: 4).

Conditions on mining expeditions must have been challenging. The work was hard, the climate extreme and all supplies required transportation from the Nile Valley by members of the expedition. It would be expected that casualties and fatalities on desert-based quarrying and mining expeditions would have been considerable. Dehydration, disease and injuries would have taken their toll. The procurement of adequate supplies of water for the expeditions would have been a major concern. An inscription from the reign of Ramesses II relating to gold mining at Wadi Allaqi in Nubia (Quban Stela) stated that previous expeditions lost half of their personnel and donkeys due to dehydration (Zibelius-Chen 1994; Klemm and Klemm 2013: 294).

Inscriptions were frequently left on rock faces and stelae by members of these state-organised expeditions, and some included the title of *swnw* as well as other healers within their subject matter. These inscriptions are found not only within the boundaries of Egypt but also at Sinai, Hatnub, Wadi Hammamat, Wadi el-Hudi and other sites. The texts range from simple inscriptions that merely list a name and title(s), often with an offering (*ḥtp-di-nsw*) formula, to more elaborate texts that may include self-laudatory epithets, biographies and appeals to the living.

In the Sinai, turquoise, copper and malachite were mined, although much of the surviving epigraphic evidence relates to the extraction of turquoise. Stelae dating to the Middle Kingdom list the names of various *swnw*; for example, Renefseneb was a 'Chief Physician' and Akmu, who was a *swnw*, also carried the title of *s3w*, 'magician'. Imunefer was a 'Controller of Serket', who would have treated bites and stings from snakes and scorpions, which were particularly widespread in the Sinai desert.

At the travertine quarries of Hatnub, which are located in the Eastern Desert, a graffito dated to the 12th Dynasty shows two healers: Heryshefnakht, who was unique in bearing the triple qualification 'Great of Physicians of the King, *wʿb*-Priest of Sekhmet and Overseer of Magicians', and Ahanakht who was a *wʿb*-Priest of Sekhmet and also a *rḫ k3w* (one who knows oxen) and therefore perhaps could be referred to as a vet (Nunn 1996: 128–29).

In 2010 four sets of human remains were excavated from the necropolis of Deir el-Bersha, adjacent to an ancient quarry. The necropolis was in use from the late Old Kingdom to the New Kingdom. Three of these individuals display amputations with evidence of successful healing, while the fourth died shortly after a traumatic incident and then associated attempted amputations. Differential diagnoses indicate that these pathologies were probably due to trauma and not disease, and so probably related to mining activities (Dupras *et al.* 2010).

Military

Anthropological evidence for warfare can potentially provide evidence for medical treatment that may have been given to those suffering injuries in battle in ancient Egypt. Analysis of the various battle scenes portrayed on New Kingdom temple walls, textual information (particularly the medical papyri) and palaeopathological studies are all useful additional sources.

The earliest evidence for armed conflict in Egypt, and possibly the world, comes from Jebel Sahaba, now in northern Sudan. Here Cemetery 117 was found to contain the human remains of about sixty-one persons dating back approximately 13,000 years. At least 45 per cent of these individuals died of inflicted wounds, making this the earliest evidence for inter-communal violence in the archaeological record. Chips and flakes of chert, the remnants of arrows or other weapons, were found mixed with, and in some cases still embedded in, the bones of twenty-six of these individuals, while cut marks were found on the bones of others (Hoffman 1993: 91–99; Crevecoeur *et al.* 2021).

Two Old Kingdom private tombs, those of Inti at Deshasha and Kaemheset at Saqqara, portray siege scenes featuring walled Asiatic towns. Some of the scenes from the tomb of Inti depict armed conflict between the Egyptians and the Asiatics. Arrows are being released at the combatants and there are representations of battle-axes and swords (McDermott 2004: 20–22).

There are numerous depictions of battle injuries and killings in the large-scale scenes of warfare specifically adopted as decoration for temple walls in the New Kingdom. These scenes had their forerunner in the early 18th Dynasty, but only fragments of these now survive. This common theme, adopted particularly during the 19th and 20th Dynasty, had major symbolism, and by the reign of Sety I Egyptian craftsmen were competent in the depiction of the human body. The scenes representing specific campaigns were designed to demonstrate the power of the king and his success in defeating chaos and perpetuating Ma'at (the natural order of the universe). Noticeably, these tableaux do not depict injuries sustained by the Egyptians, as that would contradict this ideology.

Sety I fought a series of wars in western Asia, Libya and Nubia in the first decade of his reign. Scenes of four of his major battles are inscribed on the exterior face of the Hypostyle Hall at the Temple of Amun at Karnak. Together with the accompanying hieroglyphic records, they provide extensive information about the events leading up to the wars, the battle scenes and the victory that followed. Among the scenes are wounded and dead enemy soldiers. Injuries to the head, chest and abdomen are common, with portrayals of penetrating wounds caused mainly by arrows but in a few instances by spears.

The depiction of the injuries in the wounded enemy soldiers, particularly those involving trauma to the head, neck and limbs, are shown with great realism, so much so that details such as loss of consciousness and limb paralysis can be identified. It seems probable that such scenes may have been witnessed by the artist who worked on these images (Sanchez 2000).

Ramesses II's battle against the Hittite king Muwatalli II and his coalition forces at Kadesh in *c.* 1275 BC is the best-documented military event in ancient history and an important source of information relating to warfare in the New Kingdom. Scenes of the conflict can be seen at the temples of Karnak, Luxor, Abydos, Abu Simbel and at the Ramesseum. As with Sety I's reliefs, injuries are depicted only among the Hittite soldiers. Again, the Egyptian artists' power of observation and faithfulness to reality are manifest in their detailed portrayal of injuries. The artists seem to accurately depict the body's reaction to being struck by arrows and other weapons.

There are very few examples of physicians being depicted in the various battle scenes, but one scene in the Abu Simbel version of the Battle of Kadesh has been interpreted as a representation of an injured soldier undergoing treatment for his leg. The soldier is depicted sitting on a sack while his colleague holds his foot on his own knee and appears to be scrutinising the injured limb. There is no indication of whether the examination is being conducted by a *swnw* or merely by another soldier (Sanchez 2003). Equally, there is little direct textual or iconographic evidence of physicians being attached to the army, although it is almost certain they would have been part of the forces that Egypt would send on campaigns.

By the New Kingdom Egypt had extensive battlefield experience and would have had significant medical knowledge of the effects of injuries. This is evident in P. Edwin Smith, which provides considerable information on the treatment of traumatic injuries, particularly to the head and cervical spine, injuries that were seen much more frequently in warfare than elsewhere.

The Egyptian *swnw* would have had to treat arrow wounds as well as many slash and stab injuries. They were aware of the poor prognosis related to deep cranial and cervical wounds, and so attempted to alleviate symptoms and provide palliative care. Gaping wounds associated with the head and face were treated with the application of fresh meat, oil and honey. Other injuries to the nose, ears, lips, throat and shoulders are described in the papyrus, and bone fractures were treated with manipulation and splints. Many passages in P. Edwin Smith are devoted to such wounds and for this reason it has often been suggested that the text may well have been written by a *swnw* with military experience.

Medical complaints could also arise in encampments, particularly those occupied for long periods of time, such as during siege warfare. Lice infestations, dysentery, diarrhoea and infections are but some of these problems. P. Ebers (44–49) has various remedies to treat diarrhoea, one of which states (44): 'Remedy to stop evacuation: Fresh *djaret*-plant, fresh porridge, fat/oil/honey, wax, water. Cook and eat for four days in a row' (translated Ghalioungui 1987: 21).

5

Methods of treatment

A wide range of treatment methods were available to the Egyptian healers. These included some surgical procedures for a limited range of conditions, and a significant tradition of pharmaceutical remedies that come down to us in the medical papyri.

(a) Surgical treatment

Herodotus (II, 84) commented that in ancient Egypt there were specialists within the field of medicine, but he did not specifically mention surgeons as being among them, and there is no other indication that surgery was considered a separate branch of general medicine. While there is considerable evidence for the management of injuries and trauma (see Chapter 5c), there is less support for surgical procedures relating to conditions that did not result from trauma. Overstated claims of surgery in ancient Egypt have been published in international peer-reviewed publications. Such information is secondarily spread through the literature and on the internet, although these publications do not usually claim to possess a detailed knowledge of ancient Egypt. This incorrect dissemination tends to distort the picture of the actual surgical attainments of the ancient Egyptians.

The medical papyri refer to minor surgical procedures such as incisions to drain or excise swellings, cauterisation, sutures to close wounds, bandaging and the reduction of dislocations. There is also palaeopathological evidence of amputations and the setting of fractures with splints. However, cases of advanced surgical techniques have not been found from examinations of skeletal and mummified remains. Surgery, for example, is not prescribed for the treatment of gynaecological conditions; the remedies recommended are either oral or local medication. This is despite the fact that gynaecological problems are well represented in the medical papyri, particularly in the Kahun Papyrus. The medical papyri and other literary sources lack detailed descriptions of extensive surgery comparable to operations performed in ancient Rome and portrayed by Aulus Cornelius Celsus (VII, VIII), for example.

Rowling (1989: 316) stated that of the estimated 30,000 mummies and skeletal remains from all periods of ancient Egyptian history that were investigated in the closing years of the 19th century and the first two decades of the 20th century, no certain instance of a surgical scar was ever observed. However, Sullivan (1998: 113) noted that it is extremely difficult if not impossible to identify a therapeutic incision in mummified specimens, particularly in view of the use of embalming materials and the state of preservation of many of the mummified bodies.

'Knife treatment'

The medical papyri provide few details of any operating techniques undertaken, but do make reference to the 'knife treatment' (*ḏwꜥ*), presumably some form of surgical procedure. This is illustrated by most of cases 857–77 in the Ebers Papyrus, which describe the surgical removal and treatment of various swellings (*ꜥꜣwt*), some of which may have been tumours (see Chapter 6d). There is no reference to the 'knife treatment' in P. Edwin Smith, a text where this term might be expected to be found.

For this procedure, different knives are referred to and the various cases follow the same methodology of examination, diagnosis, prognosis and treatment. This differentiation into logical component parts is also evident in cases 188–207, 831–33 and 857–62 in P. Ebers, and is a characteristic again obvious in the trauma cases listed in P. Edwin Smith. In the remainder of the sections of the Ebers Papyrus, the indication is that the diagnosis has already been made and the text merely provides a remedy to treat a named disease. This obvious split between the two styles of case presentation reinforces the notion that the Ebers Papyrus is a collection of medical texts from different sources that have been combined into a single document and arranged in a seemingly random manner (Nunn 1996: 32; David 2008b: 190).

An example of treating such a swelling is P. Ebers 865, which refers to an enlargement of the lower part of the abdomen in which 'the water rose and dropped'. It has been suggested that this is a case of ascites (a condition in which fluid builds up in spaces within the abdomen). The treatment is to puncture the swelling with a knife while taking care not to damage the anatomical structures below the puncture site.

P. Ebers 872 describes a swelling of the vessels (*metu*) that is rounded and solid on palpation. The treatment recommended is cauterisation followed by the knife treatment. This suggests that the ancient Egyptians realised that cauterisation would reduce excessive bleeding, and perhaps supports the diagnosis of a haemangioma. This degree of caution in anticipating the danger of severe haemorrhage is also conveyed in P. Ebers 873, which similarly describes a swelling of the *metu*: 'you must not lay a hand on anything like this' (Nunn 1996: 165–67; Strouhal *et al.* 2014: 75–79).

P. Ebers 864 describes a bulge under the skin on top of the abdomen and above the navel. The examination consists of palpating the enlargement while asking the patient to cough and then determining if it had increased in size. This appears to be a description of a typical umbilical hernia, a number of apparent depictions of which can be seen in paintings and reliefs of servants and workmen in various tombs. The advised treatment for the condition is the application of heat, but it is unclear whether this was cauterisation to occlude the neck of the hernia or the application of gentle heat to relax the abdomen (Nunn 1996: 165–67).

A closer examination of some of these and other cases in the Ebers Papyrus suggests that the procedures were carefully planned and executed, and, while they are not examples of major surgery, they would, nevertheless, have required some anatomical knowledge as well as a degree of skill and experience. P. Ebers 871 provides guidance for operating on a 'swelling of pain-matter' (*ʿꜣt nt wḥdw*), which is considered by Nunn (1996: 167) to be an abscess. The instructions involve taking care to avoid an adjacent major vessel and ensuring that no remnants of the swelling are retained. Similarly, in P. Ebers 875 the advice is to take care to avoid damaging the tissue boundaries and surrounding anatomical structures. Although this could be described as basic treatment, nevertheless the instructions provided in the papyrus follow a logical sequence and advise care in completing the various procedures. This suggests some knowledge of anatomy and an awareness of possible complications and also tends to indicate previous experience.

Some of the cases in the papyri recommend that the operator re-examines the patients periodically after completion of treatment. This would allow him to determine what further therapy, if any, was necessary and would have provided opportunities to evaluate the results of his treatment. Such an approach would permit the physician to gain experience and ultimately to improve outcomes.

Wound care and dressing

For the treatment of wounds the medical papyri make no mention of preliminary wound washing or debridement, but P. Edwin Smith frequently recommends the initial application of fresh meat. Covering a wound with fresh meat would maintain tissue moisture, form a protective barrier, provide some coagulating factors and may afford beneficial enzymatic effects (Sanchez & Meltzer 2012: 37). However, bacteria (*Salmonella* and *Escherichia coli*, which are present in raw meat) could potentially cause a serious infection, though the ancient Egyptians may well have used meat as they considered that 'flesh heals flesh'.

An essential part of any wound management is wound dressing, and bandages and dressings composed of linen were frequently recommended in the medical papyri, being used to apply medicaments as well as to bind wounds. One possible example of an ancient Egyptian dressing has recently been demonstrated in a Ptolemaic/Roman Period female child mummy. A CT scan revealed a bandage-like structure on the mummy's left leg, the dense radiographic appearance of which was suggested to have been due to its being impregnated with natron (Panzer *et al.* 2022).

The ancient Egyptians were experienced in the use of bandaging, as attested by the elaborate bandaging present in many of their mummies. This tradition had resulted in the development of a class of specialists in bandaging (*wt*). Whether the *wt* were involved in the treatment of patients is uncertain and they may merely have supplied bandages for use by an operator.

Linen, with its tight weave structure and subsequent strength, was ideally suited for bandaging gaping wounds and supporting fractures. It was capable of holding dressings in place and providing mechanical stability. If the sides of a wound needed to be approximated, then paired strips were used to close the injury, as in P. Edwin Smith, Case 10, which describes a laceration above the eye. It would seem quite likely that the linen strips had adhesive properties, perhaps being impregnated with compounds such as gum resin or a 'glue type material', and functioned much as 'steri-strips' do today. It is known that the ancient Egyptians produced a 'glue' from animal by-products that were ground up into a gelatinous mass that was boiled and then dried by evaporation (Halioua & Ziskind 2005: 38).

Lint made from linen or vegetable fibres was used to absorb secretions, as in P. Edwin Smith, Case 28, which describes an infected throat wound. The lint could also be impregnated with medicaments such as oil and honey for local application, as in P. Ebers 767, which describes a wound to the ear.

Infection

Bacterial infection is a normal consequence of an open wound and a probable sequel to surgical procedures in a pre-antibiotic society. Although many infections leave no mark on the surviving skeletal and mummified soft tissue, a recent CT study of twenty-one child mummies indicated that in three of the mummies there were structures that were considered to resemble dried pus, indicative of a purulent infection during life (Panzer *et al.* 2022).

There is further evidence of what appears to be infection in the medical texts. Although the ancient Egyptians would not have understood the bacterial origin of infection, they were familiar with the concept of something evil entering the body. In P. Edwin Smith, Case 8B reads: 'As for "that which enters from outside" it means the breath of god from outside, or a dead man, that is to say, that which his flesh produces has caused to enter' (translated Sanchez & Meltzer 2012: 88). In this context there is also reference to the term wekhedu (*wẖdw*) (see Chapter

1b) and ryt (*ryt*), which is translated as pus; the latter word is associated with an abscess, and wekhedu also appears in the same context.

The classic signs of infection are pain, swelling, redness and heat around the site of the wound, and there are references to such indicators as a secondary occurrence in P. Edwin Smith. Case 7 describes a head injury associated with a compound skull fracture and mentions symptoms: 'his forehead being clammy with perspiration', 'his face being flushed', 'his flesh having developed heat' and 'the odour of the chest/vault of his head being like the excrement of goats' (Sanchez & Meltzer 2012: 77–85). This latter symptom refers to the smell of an infected intracranial wound. The smell of wounds is caused by a mixture of organic acids and amines produced by bacteria (Thomas *et al.* 1998).

Case 41 describes a chest wound, not affecting the bony structure of the chest, which has become infected:

> If you examine a man for a wound-infection in his chest when that wound is inflamed, with a concentration of warmth flowing from the mouth of the wound to your hand, and the lips of the wound are red, and when that man is feverish from it, his flesh does not accept a bandage, and that wound cannot acquire a margin of (new) skin, while the crust that is in the mouth of that wound is watery and feverish and the drops that fall from it are clear. (translated Allen 2005: 97)

Similarly, inflammation and infection are also described in other cases in P. Edwin Smith, such as Case 24, a mandibular fracture; Case 28, an anterior neck wound; Case 39, an infected chest wound; and Case 47, a gaping wound in the armpit. Case 39 describes the important principle of treating an abscess – that of drainage – and also recommends the use of cauterisation, which would facilitate haemostasis. Such examples demonstrate that the ancient Egyptians understood and established sound clinical reasons for their treatment plans as well as recognising the existence and nature of possible complications.

Suturing

Suturing is not referred to in P. Ebers, but in seven cases in P. Edwin Smith (3, 10, 14, 23, 26, 28, 47) suturing of the wounds is recommended for the treatment of lacerations and 'gaping wounds'. The threads used for this purpose may have been made from plant fibres or animal material, such as tendons or the intestine of an animal cut up into thin strips. Traces of surgical suturing have not been found in any mummy, although there is a celebrated example of a 21st Dynasty mummy, that of a priest of Amun, in which an embalmer's incision has later been sutured (Smith & Dawson 1924: 119, fig. 36) (Fig. 5.1).

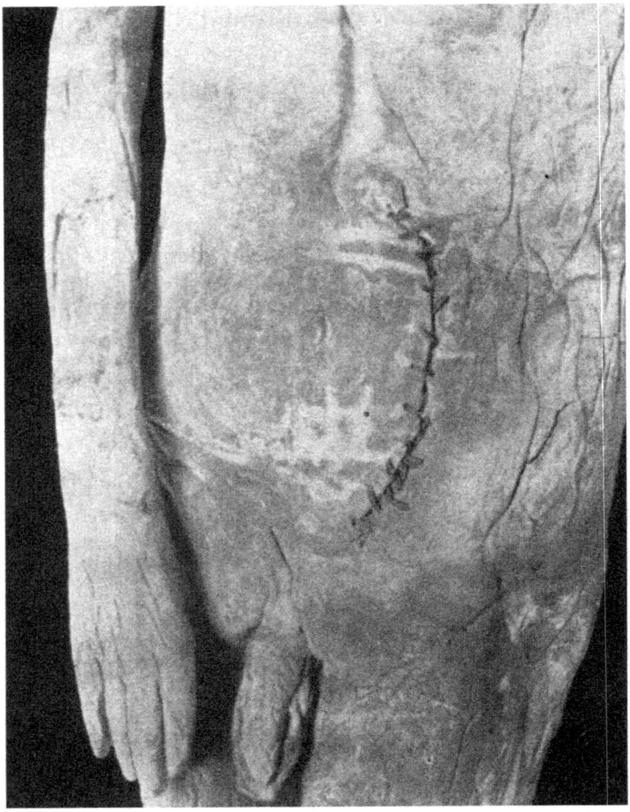

Figure 5.1. Sutured embalming incision in a 21st Dynasty mummy of a priest of Amun (Smith & Dawson 1924: fig. 36).

Anaesthesia

Whether the ancient Egyptians made use of any drugs or chemicals for anaesthesia, sedation and analgesia is a topic often debated. Many of the plants from which drugs such as opium and cannabis were obtained were known of, although there is no real evidence that the ancient Egyptians were aware of their psychotropic properties. Nor is there mention of any kind of anaesthesia or analgesia being advised for the surgical procedures detailed in the medical papyri. However, it is possible that various chemicals were utilised.

Opium

Opium is derived from the capsule of the poppy *Papaver somniferum*, a plant not native to Egypt. The poppy is frequently shown in tomb and temple scenes in the New Kingdom, but this depiction is usually considered to be the red poppy, *Papaver rhoeas*. Cultivation of *Papaver somniferum* within Egypt is not thought to have occurred until sometime later (Counsell 2008).

Opium is known to have been in use in Crete and Cyprus during the 2nd millennium BC, but is thought to have been used for religious purposes rather than for recreational or medicinal applications. Merrillees (1962; 1979) suggested that opium was imported into Egypt from Cyprus during the New Kingdom. He based this on the distinctive shape of Cypriot ring ware juglets, which he suggested resembled the head of a poppy, and also upon the supposed identification of morphine in a similar Egyptian juglet from the 19th Dynasty tomb of Kha (Fig. 5.2).

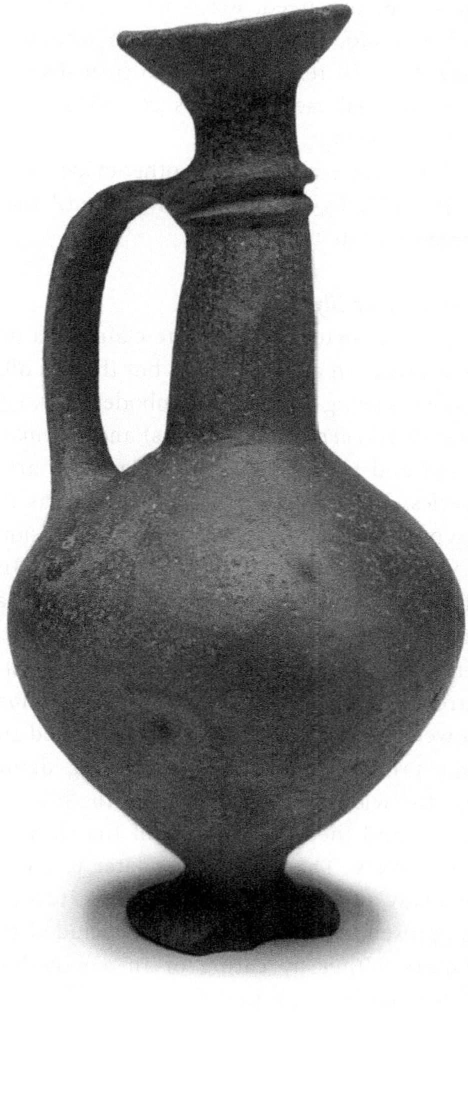

Figure 5.2. Distinctive ring ware juglets were imported into Egypt from Cyprus during the New Kingdom, but scientific studies have not supported the theory that they were used for opium. A foreign origin, based on stylistic criteria, has also been attributed to other pottery. This vessel, imported from the Levant, was discovered at Gurob, a town in the Fayoum where textiles were produced for the Royal Court. 18th Dynasty. Now in The Manchester Museum, 2146 (courtesy of The Manchester Museum, The University of Manchester).

Early analytical work attempting to verify the opium trade hypothesis was carried out on residue samples from the Cypriot juglets but was inconclusive. Koschel (1996) produced a positive result in his assays, but this was for only one unprovenanced pot. Counsell (2006, 2008) carried out a detailed analytical study into the general use of narcotics in ancient Egypt. To test for opium, he obtained residue from thirteen Cypriot juglets in the Manchester Museum collection and investigated them with modern analytical tests, chiefly liquid chromatography/mass spectrometry. He failed to detect opium in any of his samples.

It is considered that *shpn* and *shpnn* are the ancient Egyptian words for poppy and poppy seeds (Lefebvre 1956: 110; Charpentier 1981). Ghalioungui (1987) accepted this translation, although Grapow *et al.* (1954–1973: IV, 490) and Germer (1979: 236) disagreed. References to *shpn* and *shpnn* appear in, for example, P. Ebers 440, 443 and 445, which recommend its application externally as a constituent in remedies used to treat disorders of the scalp. The sole reference to its internal use is P. Ebers 782, where it is suggested as a medication to stop children crying.

There appears to be little other evidence to support the narcotic use of opium in Dynastic Egypt and it was not until the Roman Period that there is more evidence of its use.

Lotus, water lily

There is an extensive literature claiming a narcotic and aphrodisiac role for the lotus flower in ancient Egypt, but there is often confusion as to which botanical species is being referred to (Emboden 1978, 1979, 1989; Bertol *et al.* 2004) (Fig. 5.3). *Nymphaea caerulea* (blue lotus) and *Nymphaea lotus* (white lotus) are native to Egypt and widely depicted in Egyptian art and decoration (Fig. 5.4). A third species, *Nelumbo nucifera*, also known as the pink lotus, was introduced into Egypt about the time of the Persian invasion (525 BC).

Some researchers (Emboden 1979, 1981; Harer 1985) state that both the blue and white lotus contain alkaloids that are present in both the flower and the rhizome of the plant, which are capable of producing a narcotic effect. In contrast, the pink lotus is known to contain more alkaloids and its narcotic effect is well described (Wróbel 1977). Harer (1985) proposed that the flowers of the blue lotus were immersed in wine to extract active alkaloids, thus producing a more intoxicating drink. Among the evidence he cited was the widespread depiction of the blue lotus in New Kingdom banqueting scenes and the common use of the flower as decoration on drinking bowls and goblets. This theory was later tested by Counsell (2008: 204–09) using an array of analytical investigative techniques. He was unable to identify the presence of alkaloids and concluded that the consumption of blue lotus flowers, either by eating or in a wine-based infusion, would not give an additional intoxicating effect.

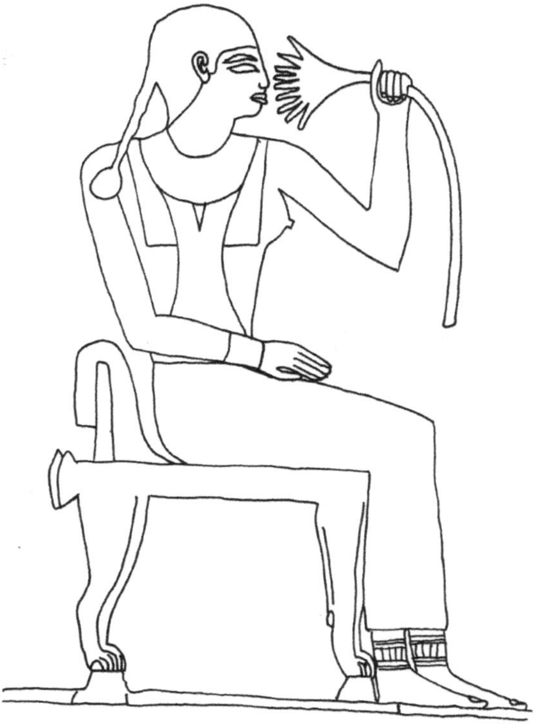

Figure 5.3. Representation of an elite woman sniffing a lotus blossom. Currently there is no evidence that this produced a psychotropic effect. Drawing based on New Kingdom examples of tomb wall-scenes depicting guests attending banquets (courtesy of R. David).

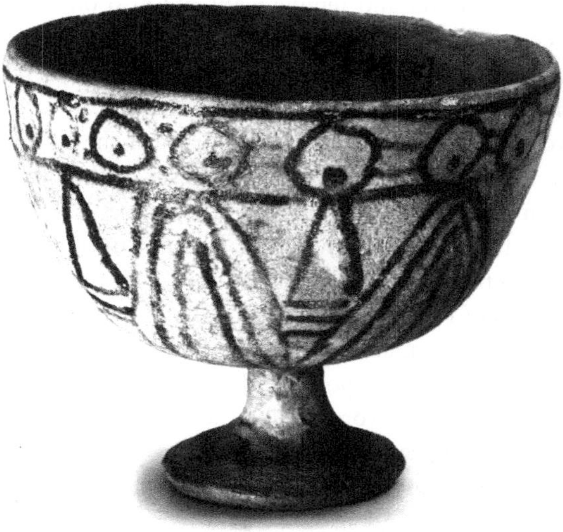

Figure 5.4. Blue faience drinking cup with lotus flower decoration. Scientific tests have not supported the theory that blue lotus flowers were immersed in wine to produce a more intoxicating drink. 18th Dynasty. From Riqqeh, now in The Manchester Museum, 5784 (courtesy of The Manchester Museum, The University of Manchester).

Although the blue lotus has a pleasant aroma, there appears to be little evidence to support the suggestion of a psychotropic effect by merely sniffing the lotus blossom, as is often depicted in scenes from ancient Egypt. At present there appears to be little other scientific evidence relating to a narcotic role for the 'lotus' in ancient Egypt.

Cocaine and nicotine

Initial reports of the discovery of cocaine and nicotine in mummies (Balabanova *et al.* 1992; Parsche *et al.* 1993) were later criticised, as the very low levels of the drugs that were detected made the results somewhat unreliable. Modern contamination of the mummies seems a more likely explanation and it seems improbable that the ancient Egyptians were exposed to cocaine during their lifetimes.

Cannabis

Shemshemet is considered to be the Egyptian word for cannabis and it appears a number of times in the medical papyri. In P. Ramesseum III it is recommended as an eyewash and in P. Ebers 617 and 618 as a poultice for a sore toenail, and there is a description of a rectal application in P. Chester Beatty Bt 24. However, the remedies do not provide clear evidence that the ancient Egyptians were aware of the effects of cannabis on the central nervous system.

Mandrake

Mandrake is not a typically Egyptian plant and has its origin in the Mediterranean basin. Mandrake plants were cultivated in Egyptian gardens, however, as depicted in several wall scenes from the mid-18th Dynasty onwards. The Egyptian word for mandrake is believed to be *rrmt* and there are frequent depictions of the fruit and plant not only on palace, tomb and temple walls but also on objects such as coffins, pottery and cosmetic spoons. Additionally, there are references to the plant in Egyptian literature (Casini 2018).

Mandrake (*Mandragora officinarum*) belongs to the botanical family Solanaceae and contains several alkaloids. An alcoholic extract of the root has powerful sedative properties and is able to produce anaesthesia. Although the narcotic effect is mentioned in Classical Greek sources (Theophrastus 9, ix-1), reference to *rrmt* is lacking in the medical papyri, and it is not until the 3rd century AD that its narcotic effect is mentioned in an ancient Egyptian source (see the Demotic Magical Papyrus of London (BM EA 10070) and Leiden (NMA I, 383) (Griffith & Thompson 1904: 150–51, col. XXIV, 18)).

As the mandrake is widely depicted, it is possible there is another term in the medical texts that refers to mandrake, a word that has not yet been identified (Germer 2008: 294). At present there appears to be no convincing indication that the ancient Egyptians were aware of the psychotropic properties of the mandrake plant during the Dynastic Period.

'Memphite Stone'

Dioscorides (5, 158) and Pliny (36, 11) state that the Egyptians practised a form of local anaesthesia utilising stone from the vicinity of Memphis. The technique involved grinding the stone into powder, mixing it with vinegar and then applying to the part of the skin where a surgical procedure was to be performed. Both Ghalioungui (1963: 104) and Nunn (1996: 169) assumed the stone was either limestone or marble, which, mixed with vinegar, would produce carbonic acid, but commented that this acid would not produce a local anaesthetic effect when applied to the skin.

Conclusion

There seems to be no real evidence that the ancient Egyptians possessed any drugs or chemicals, other than alcohol, that would have been able to produce the depth of anaesthesia required for a painless surgical procedure. Similarly, there is no real indication that the ancient Egyptians had any effective analgesics, although in P. Ebers 293 one of the constituents of the prescription is willow, which may also be mentioned in a badly damaged section of P. Kahun (Case 33). The bark of the white willow contains, as noted above, low quantities of salicin, a precursor of acetylsalicylic acid (aspirin) (see Chapter 2c).

Ophthalmology

Eye injuries occupy a prominent place in the medical papyri, perhaps suggesting that they were not an infrequent occurrence. Diseases of the eye would have been commonplace, as the hot, bright sun, dust, insects and poor hygiene are all apt to favour ocular disorders. In particular, trachoma, caused by the bacterium *Chlamydia trachomatis*, may well have been a cause of conjunctivitis and ultimately blindness in ancient Egypt.

The sensitive ocular structures, especially the retina, decompose fairly quickly after death and so archaeological evidence of eye disease is often lacking. In addition, mummies sometimes have artificial eyes placed in their empty sockets, covering the shrunken remnants of the eyeballs, further obscuring any disorders. Intact eyes found in situ in mummies provide rare opportunities to use histological techniques to detect eye disease. Ruffer's study (1911) of an optic nerve was compromised by the poor state of preservation of the sample. However, an autopsy carried out in 1990 on the Leeds Mummy, Nesyamun, was able to examine the ocular structures: the eyeball, optic nerve and muscles contained in the orbit (which control the eye movements), along with their accompanying nerves, were all well preserved. In this case, the examination of histological sections of one of the larger nerves supplying these muscles indicated partial degeneration of the oculomotor nerve, which supplies some movements of the eye. One possible cause is peripheral neuritis, a condition that may occur as a result of vitamin deficiency, diabetes mellitus or even poisoning by heavy metals – substances known to have been used therapeutically in ancient Egypt – although these would not selectively affect the oculomotor nerve (Tapp & Wildsmith 1992: 146–48).

Of the four medical specialists listed by Herodotus (II, 84), 'Doctor of the Eyes' appears to be the commonest. Some seven individuals are known to have possessed this and other related titles such as *swnw irty* (Physician of the Eyes, Oculist); *swnw irty pr-ꜥꜣ* (Oculist of the Palace) and *wr swnw irty pr-ꜥꜣ* (Chief of the Palace Oculists) (Ghalioungui 1983: 43–44). One such example is found on the stela of Irenakhty, an Old Kingdom/First Intermediate Period *swnw*, where appended to his name are a remarkable number of medical specialities, including 'Ophthalmologist of the Royal Palace' (see Chapter 2f, ii). A further mention of oculists by Herodotus (III, 1) refers to the Late Period, when Cyrus, the Persian ruler, asked Ahmose II (Amasis) for the services of the best oculist in Egypt, an event that, according to Herodotus, contributed in part to the Persian invasion of Egypt in 525 BC.

Considerable space is allocated to remedies for diseases of the eyes in the Ebers Papyrus (prescriptions 336–431), an important source of information on this subject. Of the many conditions described, some are difficult to identify, but some of the prescriptions detail medicaments for conditions including blindness, cloudiness and watering of the eye, troublesome eyelashes and spots and blood on the eye. The preparations mainly involve topical treatments consisting of ointments and eyedrops formulated from a wide variety of mineral, vegetable and animal products. P. Ebers 424 and 425 describe remedies 'to eliminate an inward bending of hair in the eye' (perhaps trachoma), making a reference to the eyelash having been pulled out. Possibly this may be a minor surgical procedure, but, as with many such practices, the technique is not described in any detail.

Further evidence comes from religious and literary texts, where there are references to eye complaints, mainly blindness, which is frequently attributed to divine punishment for an individual's sins. In artistic sources there are many representations of blindness often relating to harpists, which may imply that a special employment opportunity existed for the blind (see Chapter 6d).

Although there is no mention in the medical papyri of surgical intervention for the treatment of eye conditions, there have been some suggestions that cataracts were treated surgically (Hickson 1971; Millar & Lane 1988). The main foundation for this proposal is the scene in the tomb of Ipuy where an 'operator', possibly a fellow worker, is holding an injured person's chin while directing what appears to be a long-pointed implement to the eye area. It has been suggested that this depicts a surgical procedure (see Chapter 4f). However, this seems unlikely when the setting of the scene is considered, as the site is a busy workplace where a number of workmen are manufacturing a catafalque. It would seem very strange that one of the workers would decide to have cataract surgery while continuing with his work, although it might have been the only opportunity if the surgeon was itinerant. There seems little other evidence to support the assertion that cataract surgery was performed in pharaonic Egypt (Blomstedt 2014a). This scene has also been interpreted as a depiction of a kohl-painter attending to the craftsman as a preventative measure to reduce irritation from dust and the sun's glare, or of the application of an eye medication with a quill. Many of the eye remedies were in the form of ointments, consisting of both black and green eye paint mixed with fatty matter, honey and various minerals. A basket behind the operator in this scene has sometimes been interpreted as containing instruments and drugs belonging to an oculist (Anderson 1997).

Circumcision

Herodotus (II, 37) noted that the ancient Egyptians practised circumcision, although the medical papyri make no mention of this procedure. There is very little direct evidence of the practice itself, although several tomb scenes appear to depict it. An early example is to be seen in a relief fragment discovered in the

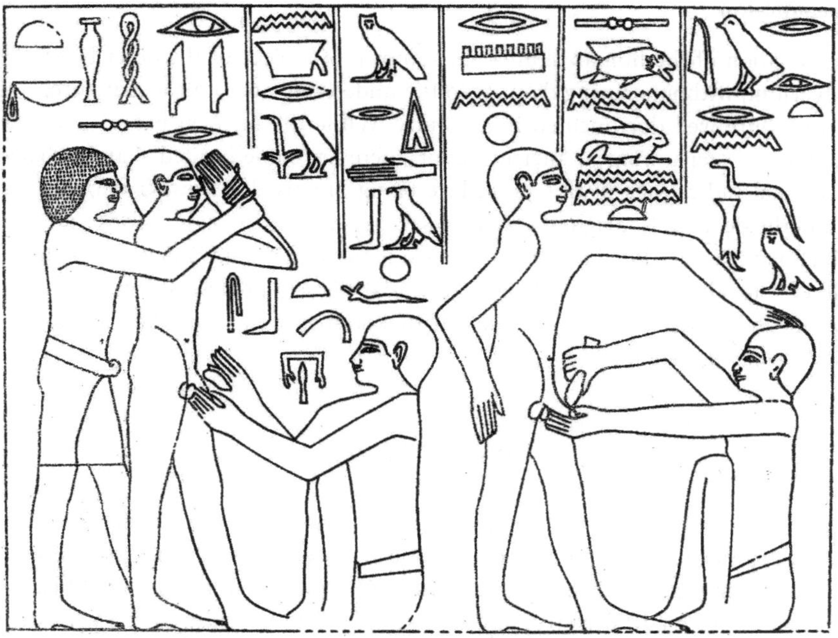

Figure 5.5. Circumcision scene in the tomb of the 6th Dynasty vizier Ankhmahor at Saqqara. Redrawn by K. N. White after Badawy (1978: pl. 27) and Worth Estes (1993: 57).

pyramid complex of the 5th Dynasty king Djedkara (2414–2375 BC) (Megahed & Vymazalová 2011). There is a celebrated relief in the tomb of the 6th Dynasty vizier Ankhmahor at Saqqara (Fig. 5.5), with a possible parallel scene found in the nearby tomb of Khentika. In a First Intermediate Period stela from Naga ed-Deir a certain Wha claims to have been circumcised along with 120 other men, which could suggest a ritual nature to the proceedings (Roth 1991: 62–72). The procedure is also depicted in a wall relief in the Temple of Mut-en-Asheru at Karnak.

Herodotus (II, 37) refers to the hygienic advantage of male circumcision, but it is possible that circumcision was commonly undertaken for ritual initiation into manhood or for acquisition of temple phyle membership, rather than for medical reasons. The procedure was probably performed in the temple by priests, as attested by a *hem-ka* priest in attendance in the scene portraying the circumcision of Ankhmahor. Evidence from mummified remains and wall scenes indicates that this practice was by no means universal, although Elliot Smith, when examining the remains from a prehistoric cemetery at Naga ed-Deir, excavated by the Hearst Expedition, observed that all the men had been circumcised (Smith 1908).

Trepanation

Trepanation of the human skull – the removal of a piece of the outer bone, the calvarium, without causing damage to the underlying anatomical structures – is a procedure well documented in antiquity. While the medical papyri make no mention of trepanning in ancient Egypt, there are some limited – and debated – skeletal indications of this procedure being practised (Lisowski 1967: 651–72; Aufderheide and Rodríguez-Martín 1998: 31–34; Nerlich *et al.* 2003: 191–201; Martin 2013: 545–56). The purpose of trepanation in any ancient culture is difficult to identify, but relief of intracranial disease processes, injuries, ritual significance and release of negative spiritual entities are among the motives that have been suggested.

(b) Instruments

There are references in the medical papyri, particularly the Edwin Smith, to surgical procedures, but the texts include few details regarding the methods employed or types of instrument utilised. One difficulty in the identification of any ancient medical instrument is that they were never engraved with their purpose, nor have any been found in a context in which they might be positively identified as surgical equipment.

A number of finds of supposed medical instruments have been made, however. One example is the copper implements found in the mastaba tomb of the royal physician Qar, located north of the pyramid of Sekhemkhet at Saqqara. The mastaba has been dated to the 6th Dynasty, although the tomb was reused during the Late Period. The implements have been variously suggested as model tools, engraving equipment or surgical instruments. It has been suggested that medical devices may be shown in the celebrated scene depicted on the northern part of the enclosure wall of the Graeco-Roman temple of Kom Ombo (see Chapter 2f, ii). In addition, many museums have collections of implements often labelled as possible embalming tools, as instruments or as of unknown purpose, some of which may have had a medical function (see Plate 17).

The medical papyri refer to instruments when mentioning the 'knife or cutting treatment' (*ḏwꜥ*), in which different types of blade are listed: the *ds, šꜣs, khpt, ḥmm* and *swt*. Particular functions and differences between the knives are not obvious, although the use of one rather than another is often recommended. The *ds, šꜣs* and *khpt* knives have a knife determinative at the end of the word, whereas the *swt* instrument has a reed determinative. *ds* is also the word for flint, sometimes with and, on occasion, without a stone determinative, suggesting that the *ds* knife was made from this sedimentary rock. Blades fabricated from obsidian and flint were in use by predynastic times. The *ḥmm* knife has a copper determinative and in P. Ebers 865 a puncturing action for this knife is implied, perhaps suggesting a pointed metal instrument. Small pointed copper knives excavated by Petrie at Kahun and designated as foundation deposits could be examples of such an instrument (see Plate 18). In addition, the archaeological record has many other examples of knives of different shapes and materials, but it is difficult to attribute a specific function for many of these.

The *swt* instrument described in P. Ebers 876 appears to relate to the management of something resembling a haematoma: 'you should then incise it with a reed that is used to make a knife treatment'. There are other references to knives fabricated from organic materials in antiquity. The *Tale of the Two Brothers* is a complex and vivid tale in which the wife of the elder brother attempted to unsuccessfully seduce the younger brother, which resulted in a feud between the siblings. The tale ends happily but not before Bata cuts of his own phallus with a reed knife to emphasise his innocence. In ancient India bamboo blades were utilised in surgical procedures (Majno 1975: 90; Lichtheim 1976: 206).

P. Ebers 875 refers to the removal of a 'swelling on any body part', considered by some sources to be a guinea worm. The case describes the use of several different instruments during the procedure. A *ds* knife is used to make the initial incision, after which a *hnw*-instrument, which may be a type of forceps, is used to grasp the worm. A *šꜣs* knife is then utilised to extirpate the remnants, while taking care to avoid damaging the tissue boundaries and surrounding anatomical structures. The change to the *šꜥs* knife implies a different stage in the procedure and this knife may be something resembling a curette (Ghalioungui 1987: 251–52; Miller 1989: 249–54).

Other than the *hnw*-instrument mentioned above and the Kom Ombo scene, there are few other references to forceps in the textual and inscriptional records. However, there are many surviving examples in museums worldwide, but it is difficult to conclude whether their function was medical, cosmetic or for use in mummification procedures (see Plate 19).

In P. Ebers 504 a thorn is used 'to eliminate white spots in a burn ... it is cut up with a thorn' (translated Ghalioungui 1987). It is difficult to determine the procedure that is being described but perhaps it could relate to aftercare in debriding scar tissue or piercing blisters.

Cauterising the wound was advised in some cases following surgical procedures. In P. Edwin Smith, when treating a chest abscess, a hot 'fire drill' or 'firestick' is recommended, whereas in P. Ebers 872 a heated *ḥmm* knife is the instrument of choice for cauterising a swelling of what appears to be blood vessels.

Many of the prescriptions in the medical papyri indicate precise measurements for each constituent of the preparation, particularly for those remedies prescribed for internal administration. Weights were seldom used and it was volume that was the main measure. Two units, the *ro* (approximately 14ml) and the *henu* (around 450ml), were commonly used. However, many prescriptions merely recommend proportional amounts of the various ingredients. A number of vessels have been discovered that would be suitable for the measuring of pharmaceutical ingredients, such as conical measuring cups, some of which have measurements engraved on the sides (Pommerening 2010: fig 6).

A set of seven 18th Dynasty cylindrical bronze volume measures with handles were discovered at Kom Ombo, each double the capacity of the previous. Various functions have been attributed to these vessels, such as measuring gold dust, but a pharmaceutical purpose is just as likely (see Plate 20). In addition, many examples of glass jars and containers are evident in the archaeological record, which again may have been containers for pharmaceutical ingredients (see Plate 21). Similarly, there are examples of spatulas constructed out of various materials, including metal and bone, some of which have a rounded end with a trough-like cut that could potentially be used for measuring and mixing medicaments (see Plate 22).

A convex glass lens made from perfectly clear man-made glass dating to the 1st century AD was found at Hawara and is now located in The Manchester Museum (2090). A lens such as this could be used for activities such as writing, but might also be used for medical procedures where a degree of magnification was required, such as surgery (see Plate 23).

(c) Trauma and miscellaneous other treatment

Sophisticated though it was by the standards of its time, life in ancient Egypt would have presented many hazards. The population lived in close proximity to dangerous animals: crocodiles and hippopotami inhabited the Nile and its banks, and snakes and scorpions encroached into the arable land upon which the population lived and worked. Manual workers in the many quarries and construction projects would have risked life and limb on a daily basis. As a consequence, traumatic injuries would have been a frequent occurrence in the life of the ancient Egyptians, necessitating a rapid response.

P. Edwin Smith is often referred to as a surgical papyrus and is a valuable resource for understanding ancient Egyptian trauma care. The papyrus's forty-eight cases commence at the top of the head and progress downwards in a systematic manner, terminating at the upper part of the thorax and arms. They end mid-sentence in Case 48 and it would seem likely that at one time there were further parts to this treatise that would have related to examples of trauma to the lower parts of the body, but to date such texts have not been unearthed (see Plate 5).

Each of the forty-eight cases has a coherent structure, beginning with the title, which is followed by the diagnostic procedure, in which relevant clinical signs are detailed. This is followed by a prognosis, which consists of one of three verdicts related to the treatment potential in the circumstance: 'favourable', 'uncertain' or 'unfavourable'. The unfavourable verdict is translated by Breasted (1930: 46) as 'an ailment not to be treated' (*mr nn irw.ny*), with the implication that the case was hopeless and no treatment was to be provided – perhaps an early form of triage. This translation has been followed in later publications (Majno 1975: 91; Ghalioungui 1980: 57; Nunn 1996: 28). However, each of the three verdicts can be interpreted as an expression of the practitioner's expectation of the individual's progress using the treatments that are available.

A more recent translation of the unfavourable verdict is 'a medical condition that cannot be handled/dealt with', which perhaps means that a successful outcome was not anticipated from the prescribed treatment (Sanchez & Meltzer 2012: 3). This was not, therefore, a decision to withhold treatment, merely a recognition that the treatments available would be unlikely to help this condition. This suggestion is supported by the fact that in the majority of these unfavourable cases some form of care was provided. In Case 5, a head injury with an associated depressed skull fracture, the treatment consisted of not bandaging the wound, which would have been contraindicated, but placing the patient on bed rest and observing progress. Similarly, in Case 6 the advice was not to bandage, but to gently apply oil to the wound and monitor the progress of the condition. Further support for the provision of such palliative care is provided by a remedy in P. Ebers (200), where the recommendation for a stomach ailment is to provide treatment and not abandon the individual: 'Go against it, do not abandon'.

Such verdicts and treatment advice in some of the cases imply a hope of recovery, while in others, those perhaps regarded as hopeless, the instructions provided are observation, care and attention. This humanitarian concept is supported by a passage from a New Kingdom text, *The Instruction of Amenemope*, in which it is recommended not to ridicule people with impairments (see Chapter 5d).

At the end of each case are the explanatory sections, the glosses or footnotes, in which definitions and alternative interpretations are discussed. These include a dictionary of terms, which might imply that some of the terms used were no longer in the language and so required an explanation, giving some credibility to the suggestion of a date of origin for the papyrus before the 1500s BC, although it is possible that certain archaic features were deliberately introduced into the text to give the appearance of antiquity, a concept held in esteem by the ancient Egyptians. The papyrus has been dated on stylistic grounds to about 1650–1550 BC but may be a copy of an older text, although opinions vary on this point (Breasted 1930: xiiv–xv, 9–10; Nunn 1996: 27; Allen 2005: 70; Sanchez & Meltzer 2012: 12).

What sets this papyrus apart from other medical texts is that it states whether an ailment can be treated or not, something not seen in other medical papyri. It is also objective and scientific, devoid of theories, and in only one case is there reference to an incantation and mention of a deity. The recommended instructions are attentive to the patient, there are repeated assessments of the condition being treated and the clinical observations are listed in a methodical manner.

That the ancient Egyptians understood the principles of trauma care are illustrated by many of the case descriptions recorded in the document, which incorporate detailed anatomical, clinical and therapeutic information. For example, Case 6 describes a severe head wound with a depressed skull fracture that has exposed the surface of the brain. The explicit and detailed anatomical descriptions of the brain and the dura mater membrane enveloping it, and the recognition of the existence of cerebrospinal fluid, are quite exceptional for this early date in history (Sanchez & Meltzer 2012: 65–70).

As well as these detailed explanations and treatment regimens for trauma, there are also examples of traumatic injuries and their treatment evident in the surviving skeletal and mummified remains. The most notable are fractures, the usage of splints and amputations.

Fractures

There is evidence that the ancient Egyptians understood the principles involved in diagnosing and managing bone fractures. They used the method of 'closed treatment', a procedure that does not require surgical intervention. The technique consists of manipulation or 'reduction' followed by the application of a device, a splint, to maintain this reduction until healing occurs. The Edwin Smith Papyrus describes fractures and their treatment in some detail, and there is also widespread palaeopathological evidence of well-healed fractures. Case 35 of

P. Edwin Smith describes a reduction of a fracture in a clavicle that is similar to the procedure described in a modern textbook on surgery, although the details regarding the use of splints in P. Edwin Smith are slightly confusing.

In 1908 Wood Jones published an account of the occurrence of fractures that he and his team discovered during the First Archaeological Survey of Nubia. He noted a high incidence of fractures of the forearm and clavicle, which he attributed to blows from sticks. Although the results were variable, some of the healed fractures were well aligned, suggesting human intervention. Similarly, as described in Chapter 4a,1 broken bones were detected among the community of workers who built the pyramids of the 4th Dynasty, and these often-displayed well-aligned healed fractures again indicated the reduction of the fractures by manipulation followed by splinting. However, Schultz (1967: 50–51) questioned the role of medical intervention in the management of fractures when he observed healed fractures with correct alignment in wild primates, suggesting that certain fractures could heal well without assistance.

Splints

The archaeological record contains a few examples of splints that were used to immobilise these long bone fractures. Grafton Elliot Smith describes two cases from Naga ed-Deir, both dating to the 5th Dynasty and the oldest known in the world (Fig. 5.6). One of these splints was applied to a compound fracture of the forearm involving both the radius and ulna. It consisted of pieces of bark, a linen bandage and coarse grass packing, a device which Elliot Smith noted had been carefully prepared and which would have supplied effective support. He based this conclusion on his study of many similar examples of fractures that displayed excellent healing patterns. The second example was a fracture of the right femur to which four wooden splints wrapped in linen had been fixed. The wood had been shaped in two of the splints and they were all held in place on the leg by bandaging. Although the splints appear to have been placed carefully, they would have been of little value as the powerful leg muscles would have produced a tendency for the fragments to override, thus resulting in rotation and shortening of the healed limb (Smith 1908).

Other cases in the Edwin Smith Papyrus mention the use of various materials to provide support and splinting. Case 7 advises the use of 'a wedge of wood, padded with cloth' inserted in the patient's mouth to hold open the jaws as the patient was unable to open his mouth on his own. Case 35 describes a clavicular fracture in which splints or supports, fabricated from double strips of linen, were bound on the inside and outside of the upper arm. Finally, Cases 11 and 12 describe 'stiff rolls of cloth' being used to restrict and support the nose following a fracture of the nasal septum (Sanchez & Meltzer 2012: 107–19).

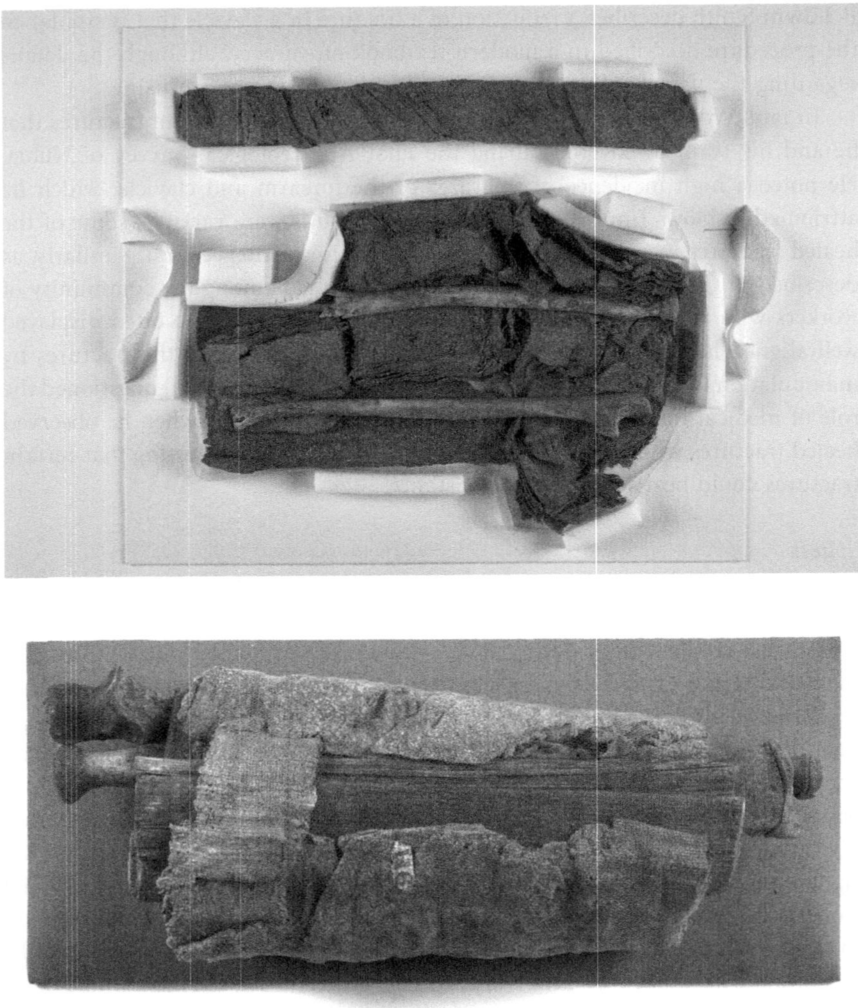

Figure 5.6i, ii. Ancient Egyptian splints (5th Dynasty) discovered at Nag-ed Deir by the Hearst expedition to Egypt (1907–1908). After suffering a fracture, this person's arm was splinted with a piece of palm-wood and wrapped in bandages. Recently restored and housed at the Royal College of Surgeons, London (photograph and permission by the Royal College of Surgeons, UK).

Amputations

Descriptions of amputations are lacking in the medical texts but they may have been described in the 'missing' sections of the Edwin Smith Papyrus, which would probably have included the extremities of the body. There is now an

increasing amount of palaeopathological evidence that amputations were carried out in ancient Egypt, many of which appear to be associated with traumatic incidents.

Amputations displaying successful healing patterns are recognised among the skeletal remains of the Old Kingdom pyramid builders excavated from the Giza necropolis (Hussien *et al.* 2010; Zaki *et al.* 2010). Brothwell & Møller-Christensen (1963) published details of an 11th Dynasty skeleton displaying an amputation of the forearm and subsequent distal fusion of the radius and ulna. Dupras and her co-workers (2010) describe four cases of skeletal remains excavated from the necropolis of Deir el-Bersha that display amputations with successful evidence of healing and are thought likely to have been the result of traumatic incidents (see Chapter 4a, i and iii). Finally, Nerlich *et al.* (2010b) describe two cases of amputation dating from the New Kingdom to the Late Period. These particular amputation sites are covered by layers of soft tissue and skin, indicating that the procedures were performed some time before death. In a general review of the original textual evidence as well as modern literature relating to surgery in ancient Egypt, Blomstedt (2014b) considers that limb amputations were not routinely performed, although they might have been carried out under extraordinary circumstances.

There is evidence of amputations being carried out on the battlefield in ancient Egypt, where it is known that the victors removed the right hand of their enemies to present to the king as evidence of their success. A relief inscribed on the inner southern wall of the second courtyard of the Temple of Ramesses III at Medinet Habu depicts amputated hands and penises being counted, and the biography of Ahmose son of Ebana (Lichtheim 1976: 12–14) describes how on a number of occasions Ahmose presented to the king an enemy hand as a trophy, for which he was then rewarded with the Gold of Valour. Recently archaeological evidence of this practice was discovered at Tell el-Daba (ancient Avaris), where sixteen skeletonised hands were unearthed (Bietak 2012).

Other examples of traumatic injuries as attested in the medical papyri

Dislocations

The ancient Egyptians were able to recognise joint dislocations and understood the need to correct such an injury, as attested in cases in P. Edwin Smith. Many of these demonstrate a considerable understanding of the anatomical and functional aspects of particular joints. In Case 31, a dislocated neck vertebra that had resulted in a spinal cord injury, the text indicates that the physician had some knowledge of the physiology and function of the spinal cord. He was able to relate the injury to the neurological symptoms he observed, which included paralysis and urinary incontinence.

Again, this depth of knowledge is displayed in Case 34, a dislocation of the articulation between the ribs and the sternum probably caused by thoracic wall

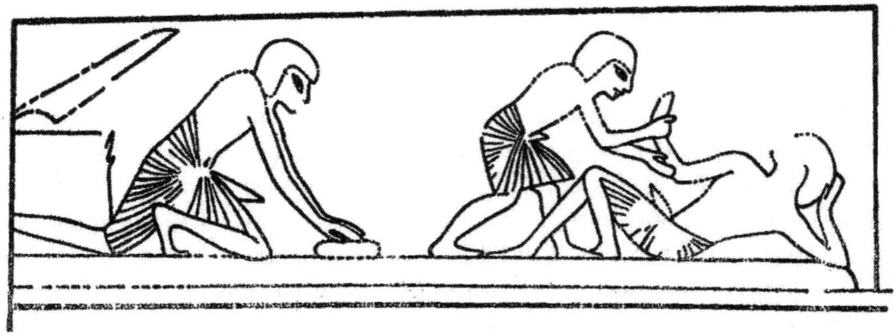

Figure 5.7. Possible attempt to reduce a dislocated shoulder. Part of the catafalque scene in the 20th Dynasty tomb of the chief sculptor Ipuy (TT 217) at Deir el-Medina. Redrawn by K. N. White after Davies (1927: pls 37–39) and Blomstedt (2014b: fig. 3).

blunt trauma. These types of injury would have been frequent in falls from construction scaffolding and chariots, and also as a result of direct blows in warfare (Sanchez & Meltzer 2012: 261–65).

Case 25 provides simple advice for correcting a dislocated mandible showing a clear logical approach differing little from that practised today. The technique used is still very popular and is routinely employed in surgeries, dental practices and hospital emergency departments. As such, it is the earliest description of a surgical procedure still in use in the modern world, a technique that has stood the test of time (Forshaw 2020).

It now seems to be commonly accepted that the earliest evidence relating to the reduction of a dislocated shoulder dates back to ancient Egypt and is portrayed in the tomb of Ipuy, although, as previously mentioned, there may be a simpler explanation for this depiction (see Chapter 4f). Nevertheless, the scene has been adopted as the emblem of the Egyptian Orthopaedic Association (Blomstedt 2014b) (Fig. 5.7).

Burns

P. Ebers incorporates a section (482–509) describing medicaments for the treatment of burns, some with recognisable beneficial properties, although for others, including plant and herbal products, no health benefit has been demonstrated.

P. Ebers 482 and 493 recommend black mud, probably Nile mud, which might cool the burn for a short period and so relieve pain, although today water would be used. The mud brought down by the inundation from the Ethiopian Highlands includes quantities of sedimentary clay containing a high concentration of minerals, which may have some beneficial properties. Today treatments involving the application of mud are popular in spas and at therapy centres in places such as the Dead Sea region and Italy. Other agents recommended include honey; oil, which would be soothing; copper flakes, which have a bactericidal effect; and red ochre, an iron oxide, which has mild astringent, antiseptic and healing properties (Nunn 196: 182–83).

P. Ebers 504, which reads 'Another to eliminate white spots in a burn', addresses the scarring left by burns and is an early attempt at cosmetic treatment: similarly, 501 reads: 'Another to blacken a burn'. The medicaments listed in P. Ebers 509 have the personal recommendation of the author, who states that he used it personally: 'Truly effective. I have seen [the success], it has often happened to me' (translated Ghalioungui 1987).

Bites

The bites and stings of scorpions, snakes, crocodiles and other animals would have been a common hazard in ancient Egypt, causing acute traumatic injuries that would have required prompt attention.

The priests of Serket were known to be responsible for treating snake and scorpion bites (see Chapter 2a). One particular magico-medical treatment, popular in the Late Period, involved reciting an incantation that was available from a range of texts inscribed on a healing statue or stela (*cippus*) (Price 2016: 169–82; Chapter 3c). The 30th Dynasty Metternich stela is particularly informative in this respect, as inscribed on the back of the stela is an incantation directed against a scorpion sting (Nunn 1996: 107–10; Allen 2005: 49–63): '"Isis, Isis come to your Horus. You who know her spell, come to your son", so say the gods in her area, "since a scorpion has stung him, a spiny scorpion has hunted him, an insect has rubbed him"' (Fig. 5.8). There are similar incantations in P. Chester Beatty and P. Berlin (Case 78).

Other than these incantations and invocations to the gods, there is little else in the way of treatment for snake bites in the main medical papyri, apart from in the second section of the Brooklyn Papyri (see Chapter 2c), which is a guide for the management of snake bites. The logical approach adopted in the papyrus resembles that seen in P. Edwin Smith. The recommended treatment involves local measures such as the 'knife treatment', which in this case is probably aimed at incising and enlarging the wound in order to allow the venom and tissue fluid to ooze out, so limiting the absorption of the venom. Bandaging, advised in several cases, was used to retain specific medications rather than as a tourniquet to prevent the spread of venom. Natron was one of the agents recommended, and would have been a logical compound to utilise as it has the capacity to reduce swelling by means of osmosis. In addition, almost 100 prescriptions are listed in the papyrus, many of them of herbal origin. Onion is the most common ingredient of these remedies, probably because the sulfonic acid present in onions, the same chemical that causes

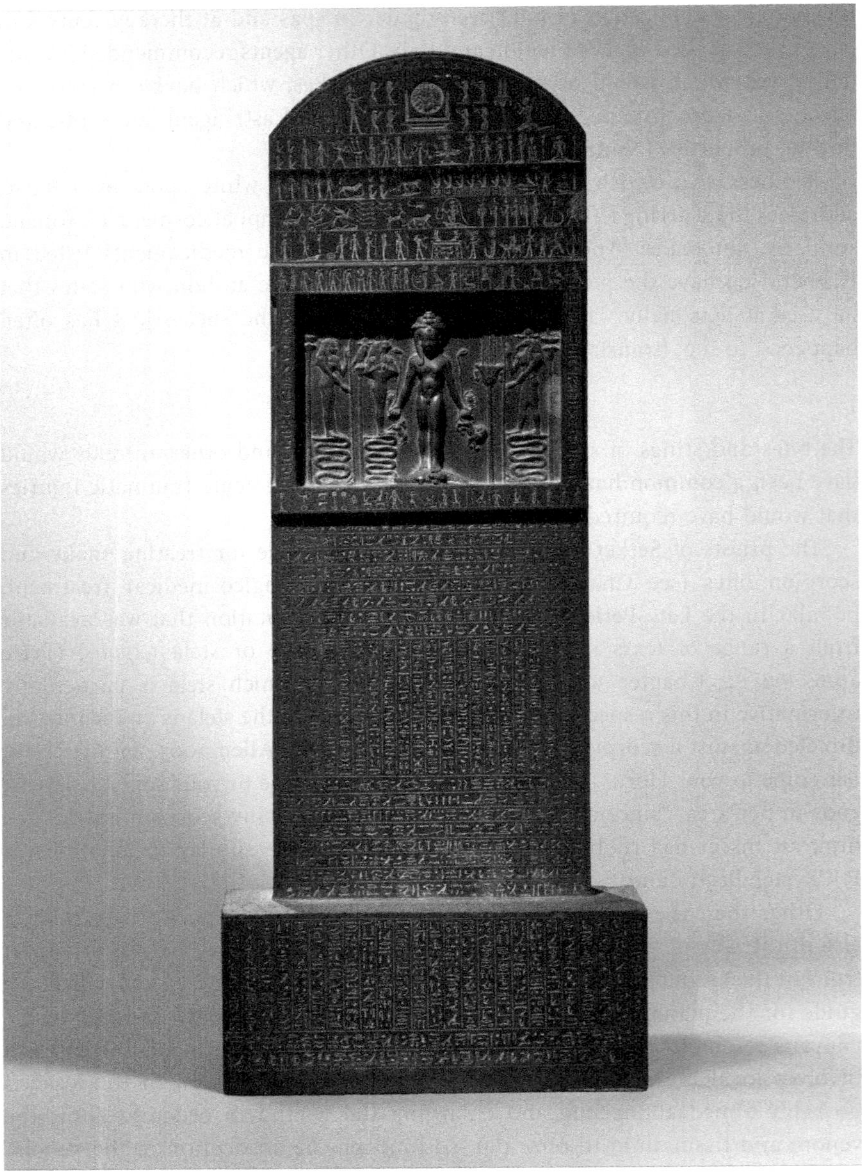

Figure 5.8. The Metternich Stela. A healing stela (*cippus*) on which are engraved many magical texts for protection from bites of venomous animals. The front includes a representation of the child Horus. Discovered in Alexandria. 30th Dynasty, reign of Nectanebo II. Greywacke. Metropolitan Museum of Art, New York, 50.85 (courtesy of the Metropolitan Museum of Art, New York, Fletcher Fund, 1950).

tears when onions are chopped, has a deterrent effect on snakes. In addition, the papyrus includes other incantations, most of which are intended for use with a particular remedy.

P. Ebers has four prescriptions (432–35) seemingly directed at a 'human bite' (*rmṯ*). Grapow *et al.* (1954–1973: IV 2, 161) consider that *rmṯ* may be a scribal error for *rr*, meaning pig, while Ghalioungui (1987: 124) is uncertain. Although human bites could occur in altercations and warfare, the bites of animals would have been more frequent. P. Ebers 436 is aimed at treating a crocodile bite. Ghalioungui (1987: 5) considers that P. Ebers 432–36, with parallel prescriptions enumerated in the Hearst Papyrus (H. 21–23, 239–44), are the remains of a lost 'Book of Bites'.

(d) Deformity and disabilities: prosthetic and other treatments

The ancient Egyptian attitude to deformity and disability

Inscriptional evidence suggests that the ancient Egyptians had a complex and somewhat ambivalent attitude towards disability and deformity. According to official teaching, all people, including those with disabilities or deformities, had been created by the gods and should therefore be treated with respect. However, the *Instruction of Amenemope* (BM 10474, Chapter 25, II. 8–12), one of the *Wisdom Texts* used to educate young people, indicates that, at least in some instances, behaviour fell far short of this ideal: 'Do not laugh at a blind man, nor tease a dwarf, nor cause hardship for the lame, don't tease a man who is in the hand of the god, nor be angry with him for his failings' (Lichtheim 1976: 160).

Methods adopted to address the impact of deformity and disability

The personal impact of deformity and disability was addressed in various ways. The medical papyri do not discuss diseases or malfunctions specifically associated with these conditions, although they contain references to symptoms sometimes linked to afflictions such as arthritis, blindness, deafness, paralysis, joint pain and old age (David 2017b).

Magic was generally employed to maintain good health and protect against debilitating illness (see Chapter 1a), and spells acquired to cure disabling conditions were carried around in special small containers (Pinch 2006: 142–43). Magical powers believed to be intrinsic in some manufactured items could be transferred to the owner's body to replace and restore the functions of the original limb or organ (Pinch 2006: 108). To this end, petitioners sometimes placed models of perfect limbs or organs outside temples or tombs associated with healing, or wore or carried amuletic jewellery representing idealised body parts.

More practical aids, such as sticks and staves, were available to assist walking (Finch 2011). More than 130 examples were discovered in Tutankhamun's tomb, and some iconographic images depict him leaning on a stick. This unusual representation has prompted speculation that he used these walking aids because of ill-health. However, the finds are not unique: whole or fragmentary sticks and staves exist in other royal burial assemblages and are depicted in other sources. They may have been part of a king's insignia rather than being associated with medical care (Brown 2017). The sticks and staves in Tutankhamun's assemblage may represent a mixture of uses, ritual and functional, and an ongoing project documenting and assessing this material will perhaps clarify this matter (Veldmeijer & Ikram 2020).

A reassessment of the radiographic reports and a study of his footwear suggests that Tutankhamun was not perhaps the frail, disabled monarch presented in some publications. In fact, a survey of his tomb contents, including the worn leather armour, the bows and the hunting fan, as well as iconographic evidence from the wooden chest and the blocks depicting battle scenes, reputed to having been part of Tutankhamun's mortuary temple, could even suggest that Tutankhamun may have been active on military campaigns (Johnson 1992; Brier 2023).

The Egyptian attitude compared with those of neighbouring societies

The Egyptians' perception and treatment of disability and deformity differed greatly from attitudes in contemporary neighbouring societies. Actions taken by the Babylonians, Greeks and Romans included barring people with physical differences from holding religious offices, and even exposing and killing infants born with deformities (see Chapter 7a). This divergence was probably at least in part due to different religious beliefs and concepts. Egyptians and Greeks both believed that the human body reflected their gods' own physical appearance. However, whereas the Greeks attributed an idealised physical perfection to all their deities, regarding any human physical variation as ungodlike and therefore unacceptable, the Egyptians took a different view. Their pantheon included a dwarf-god, Bes, and in none of their religious writings is there any suggestion that those with physical anomalies should be stigmatised. Without any expectation that universal perfection should exist in this world, they may have been more ready to accept people with disabilities and deformities and to integrate them into everyday life.

The Egyptians did, however, anticipate an idealised afterlife, for which the preservation and integrity of the body was considered essential. They attempted to achieve this through mummification and by replacing any missing body parts that had been lost during life either through embalmers' carelessness or because of congenital deficiency, surgical intervention, accident or trauma.

Prosthetic devices: the funerary context

Modern prosthetic medicine addresses patients' total or partial absence of body parts by providing a range of artificial options. For example, an orthosis such as a walking stick or shoe support can assist or support the function of a body part, while a cosmesis (e.g., a false eye) has aesthetic importance for the wearer, although it will not have the functionality of the missing part. A prosthesis, however, may provide a properly functioning replacement for the missing body part, and should also integrate visually with the patient's overall bodily appearance.

The Egyptians developed a range of funerary 'prostheses' to replace body parts missing at the time of mummification, and it was believed that these could be 'magically activated' for the owner's use in the afterlife. However, these were not properly functioning replacements. Examples include the false feet incorporated into a Ptolemaic Period mummy in the Archaeological Museum, Naples (Guiffra *et al.* 2006). Another Ptolemaic mummy in the Oriental Museum, Durham (DUROM 1999.32) contains a prosthesis that replaced the left forearm (Gray 1966a; Finch 2012/13). In a mummy in the Manchester Museum collection (1770), missing limbs were replaced at death with two false legs and feet formed from mud, wood, reeds and linen (David 1979).

Prosthetic devices: for use in life

There is convincing evidence that prosthetic medicine was practised in the ancient world (Wilson 1992). Evidence of prosthetic medicine in Greece and Rome comes from references in Classical writings as well as the example known as the Capua leg. For many years, this was identified as the oldest surviving prosthesis (Sudhoff 1917; Bliquez 1996: 2667). Discovered in 1884 at Santa Maria di Capua and dated to *c.* 300 BC, it was found attached to a skeleton from which one leg was missing. The prosthesis, which consisted of a hollowed-out wooden core overlaid with bronze sheeting, was probably attached to a bronze waistband. No research was ever carried out on the functionality of the item. Acquired by the Royal College of Surgeons, London, the leg was destroyed during World War II bombing in 1941, and the only existing information about the piece is now preserved in early studies, photographs and a replica in the Science Museum, London.

More recent studies have now convincingly confirmed that the earliest extant extremity prosthetic devices – two great-toe restorations – come from Egypt. Although the earliest examples of prostheses were probably developed for funerary use, at some point the concept was adapted for living amputees, perhaps sometimes associated with surgical procedures (Nerlich 2010b). This enabled physicians to provide practical solutions for patients whose limbs were missing (Reeves 1999; Finch 2012/13). Loss of a great-toe seriously impairs balance.

Examples of prostheses for the living

Only two prostheses with evidence of everyday wear have been found in Egypt; both are restorations for great-toe amputations, and have been the subject of the detailed studies briefly outlined here.

An unprovenanced example (BM EA 29996) (Reeves 1999: pl. XVII) representing a great-toe with a portion of the right foot, was purchased by the British Museum in 1881. Made of cartonnage, it incorporates a series of holes for attachment to the foot; a red coating applied to the inside of the piece is possibly the gum of the Dragon's Blood tree, imported in antiquity from Socotra off the coast of Yemen. Dragon's Blood is still considered by some to have antiseptic and magical powers: for example, it is used in Socota as a treatment for many ailments and in African-American folk magic. There is evidence of wear in several areas, and the materials and construction indicate that the restoration dates from a period before 600 BC.

The second example, now in the National Museum of Egyptian Civilization, Cairo (JE100016a), was discovered by a German–Egyptian mission to study Tomb TT95 at Thebes (Nerlich *et al.* 2000b). This is also a restoration of the great-toe and a portion of the right foot, with some evidence of wear on the underside of the toe (see Plate 24). It was attached to the foot of a mummy of a woman, Tabaketenmut, and has been dated to the 21st–22nd Dynasty. The mummy and prosthesis have been extensively studied (Nerlich *et al.* 2000a; Finch *et al.* 2012; Burzacott 2017; Loprieno-Gnirs 2020) and it has been concluded that the toe was removed – probably surgically – during the owner's lifetime, perhaps as a response to ischaemic gangrene. The prosthesis consists of three sections: two are carved from a dense hardwood (probably elm) and have twenty-nine drilled holes; the third part – a woven leather strap with eleven holes – was used to attach the restoration to the foot. A twining technique was used in the manufacture of the strap, which has been identified as rawhide, and horn was used for the inlaid toe. The item was repaired and readjusted several times in antiquity.

The experimental archaeology approach at Manchester

Within the overall context of the wide-ranging Manchester Mummy Project, one researcher, Dr Jaqueline Finch, produced a study to determine whether the artefacts described above had actually been worn and used as true prostheses when their owners were alive. This built on her previous research on a mummy in the Oriental Museum, Durham (see above, p. 147).

Finch's type of investigation, often complex and involving a multidisciplinary approach (Finch 2018), exemplifies 'experimental archaeology'. This concept was first formulated by Professor Robert Ascher (1931–2014) and designed to increase knowledge and the meaning and use of an artefact by demonstrating how it works.

Finch's project on the two great-toes involved the application of biomechanical testing to assess the functionality of the artefacts: did they have the correct design, construction and fit to make them usable in life?

Volunteer unilateral amputees with a similar foot presentation were approached through the appropriate channels and co-opted for the study. However, they could not wear the rare, irreplaceable original restorations, and so were fitted with replica prostheses which simulated as closely as possible the materials, construction and details of the originals. The volunteers then tested the functionality of the replica restorations in a gait laboratory. This trial generated vast amounts of complex data that had to be collected and analysed in order to assess the level of performance, stability and comfort experienced by the wearer. Some tests showed that the addition of a sandal improved the action of the right toe and had a stabilising effect on the volunteer's right side. When the volunteers were finally given the opportunity to assess the comfort and stability of each design, they awarded a much higher rating to the wood and leather device in the Egyptian Museum, Cairo.

There were some strong underlying similarities between the two restorations, although they were quite different in design and materials. They were both unique items and designed for individual personal use; they fitted closely to the foot and each had the structural addition of a great-toe. Although they are rare examples, they indicate the existence of a well-established tradition of prosthesis production and demonstrate that the makers had a clear understanding of foot anatomy and the nature of the materials used in these products. There is no inscriptional or archaeological indication of the makers of prostheses for the living, but some may have been produced by embalmers who already had significant experience of preparing funerary restorations for burial assemblages (Györy *et al.* 2020: 103).

The study of the two great-toe restorations has shown that both functioned well as prostheses for living patients, perhaps being worn with a sandal to provide stability. The research also confirms that, even if only for a limited clientele, prosthetic medicine was being practised in Egypt centuries before it developed at Capua.

These rare, sophisticated examples were evidently produced to meet the needs of wealthy clients, but simpler, perhaps homemade, versions made from materials available locally probably existed. They may have been widely used throughout society but, because they could be readily discarded or destroyed, they would be unlikely to survive in the archaeological record. However, anthropological evidence, such as the patterns of healing seen in skeletal remains from Giza, confirms the opinion that prosthetics were not restricted to elite use (Zaki *et al.* 2010).

By addressing the functional, cosmetic and even religious requirements of the living, prosthetic replacements may have contributed significantly to individual well-being. Research has shown that these aids assisted standing and walking and, as in the funerary context, were believed to reinstate a person's physical 'wholeness'. For example, the priest's daughter who owned the Cairo toe may have performed some religious rites herself in the presence of a god and worn the prosthesis so that her body was whole and complete when she encountered the divine image (Finch 2018).

(e) Performative aspects of healing

Evidence discussed in the previous sections has enabled researchers to reconstruct the main techniques that comprised the ancient Egyptian medical system and to gain some idea of the equipment and materials that were used. However, two groups of items, almost all of which are now housed in The Manchester Museum, probably provide unique insight into some of the performative aspects of healing. Both groups were possibly owned and used by individual healers, and date to the same period, but they were discovered in very different contexts. One comprised a burial assemblage from a tomb while the other was excavated from a house in a royal necropolis workers' town.

i) Ramesseum collection

The Ramesseum collection of artefacts was discovered on the West Bank of Thebes in a Middle Kingdom shaft tomb located underneath the storerooms of the Ramesseum, the mortuary temple of Ramesses II (see Plate 25). A recent suggestion is that the chamber where the assemblage was discovered may have been the underground section of the Chapel of Sehetepibre (Miniaci 2020: 7–13). The objects were uncovered at the bottom of the tomb shaft and comprise a white plastered wooden box one-third full of poorly preserved papyri, beside which were items including figurines, clappers, worked tusks, beads and writing tools. Over the years the assemblage has attracted much scholarly debate as to the function of the collection and the identity and occupation of the tomb-owner (Quibell *et al.* 1898: 3; Kemp & Merrillees 1980: 166; Bourriau 1988: 110–11; Ritner 1993: 220–33; Forman & Quirke 1996: 106–07; Quack 2006; Lorand 2009: 13–22; Parkinson 2009: 142–44, 2019; Forshaw 2014: 30–46; Miniaci 2020).

Perhaps the most distinctive piece within the grouping is a nude wooden female figurine measuring some 200mm in height with a divine face or mask. The figurine, which holds a bronze serpent in each hand, is similar to a figure holding serpents portrayed on one of the magic wands in the collection (see Plate 26). One suggestion is that it represents either a female Aha or Bes, a goddess often depicted as protecting women and children, or someone acting as this goddess (Parkinson 2009: 144). It has also been proposed that the statuette may denote a *s3w*, a 'female magician', who is acting as a divine helper (Pinch 2006: 56). This particular piece is unique owing to its size, material and type of representation. The only other vaguely similar wooden figurine, smaller in size but less detailed, was found at Kahun, but has been missing since it was excavated (see Chapter 5e, ii).

Also among the collection are several fragments of worn ivory wands, often referred to as apotropaic wands or birthing tusks. These wands occur from the Middle Kingdom through to the Second Intermediate Period, and are usually made of hippopotamus ivory, although examples in faience, ebony or calcite are also known. Those in this collection are fashioned from hippopotamus ivory and engraved upon them is a range of creatures, symbols and hieroglyphs and an array of 'composite animals', which can be defined as creatures not found in nature but products of human imagination. The purpose of the apotropaic wands seems to have been to confer protection by warding off evil forces, and they often seem to have been directed at the most vulnerable in society, such as children, as well as pregnant and nursing women. Many of them show evidence of wear, which is considered to have been caused by the action of drawing out a defensive perimeter or magical circle around the bed of a mother or a child. They are attested in the hands of wet-nurses and women entrusted with the rearing of children. (For a full discussion of apotropaic wands see Quirke 2016.)

The collection also contains three bluish green faience animal statuettes shown in a squatting or standing position; they have disproportionately large heads, and are similar in appearance to those inscribed on apotropaic wands. It has been suggested that the statuettes could be three-dimensional versions of the protective demons that appear on the wands, and their additional presence may have been necessary to ensure success during the enactment of a ritual (Bourriau 1988: 116). Among other items in the collection is a group of naked miniature female figurines, objects common in Middle Kingdom burials. Their place among the grave goods is considered to be one of fertility and protection.

The papyri found within the assemblage were confined within the wooden container, suggesting that they probably constituted an intentional collection and were deliberately deposited in the burial. Many of the texts relate to healing and protection (see Chapter 1c), but in addition there are literary, theological, liturgical and administrative papyri.

All the items within the corpus are considered to be chronologically homogeneous and have been dated to the mid-13th Dynasty. None of the finds bears a title with a personal name, leaving the identity of the owner(s) and user(s) uncertain. Although the assemblage shares features common in other burials of the period, the presence of a large number of papyri on a variety of subjects, together with the presence of uncommon artefacts such as the lion-faced female, make the assemblage unique within late Middle Kingdom funerary material culture (Miniaci 2020: 87).

To fully comprehend the Ramesseum burial assemblage in its entirety is difficult, as there are a number of problems and unanswered questions associated with the objects. The original excavation report by Quibell *et al.* (1898: 3–4) is fairly brief, very few photographs were taken and as a result the contextual evidence is incomplete. There are no inscribed items, the burial was disturbed at least twice in antiquity and it is not completely certain that all the objects came from the same burial. These factors make it difficult to assess the occupation or social status of the artefacts' owner or indeed if the assemblage had a unifying theme.

Nevertheless, it is possible to make certain inferences. The majority of both the texts and the objects appears to be of a healing and protective nature and, importantly, they had been used in life, as is evidenced by the wear, alterations and repairs that are visible on the artefacts. The presence of the papyri and reed pens indicates an individual with scribal knowledge, and its wide-ranging subject matter suggests someone who perhaps had links with the administration and the temple, while also having knowledge of healing and protection.

Suggestions as to the occupation of the Ramesseum tomb-owner include magician, local storyteller and entertainer (Gardiner 1955: 1); sage, priest and healer (Bourriau 1988: 87, 110); or perhaps a practitioner of magic with specialist knowledge of rituals associated with feminine fertility and protection (Ritner 1993: 231). Overall, the range of material correlates to a learned individual with ritual and scribal experience, and more recently a lector has been suggested as someone who might have utilised such equipment (Pinch 2006: 131; Parkinson 2009: 157; Forshaw 2014: 46). While it is possible that such a collection could be placed in a tomb to provide protection for a deceased person, who may not even have been the owner of the items, it is equally possible that these items record the labours of that person during life.

(ii) The Kahun collection

A unique group of objects discovered in one of the houses at Kahun (see Chapter 4b) provides some insight into the healing practices and protective magic performed for ordinary women in the local community. The items date to *c.* 1900 BC and appear to have a particular association with birth, and perhaps with rites to promote the fertility of local women and protect them and their children from illness and danger (David 1996: 137; Quirke 2005: 83). They may have belonged to a professional female healer – a local magician or 'wise woman' – who resided in this house (see Chapter 4d). However, an alternative explanation is that the items may have been owned by a wealthy household in order to provide magical protection for its own members (Quirke 2005: 840).

The group originally included a wooden figurine of a female dancer wearing a tail and a head-dress or mask. This may have represented the healer herself, or

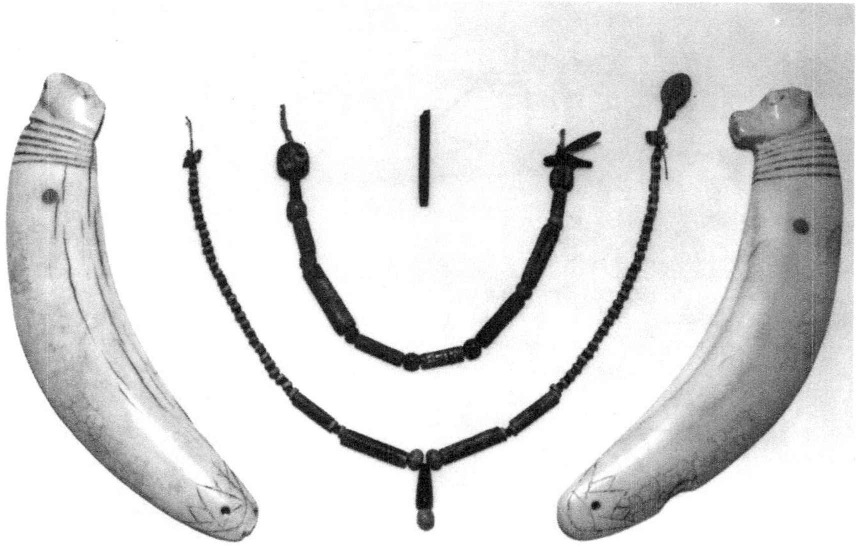

Figure 5.9. Selection of faience and carnelian beads and a pair of ivory clappers or apotropaic wands, probably used in rites to protect mother and baby, and discovered in a house with other ritual equipment that probably belonged to a community healer. From Kahun, now in The Manchester Museum, bead strings 155, wands 124 (courtesy of The Manchester Museum, The University of Manchester).

the god Bes or his consort, Beset (Pinch 2006: 131–32) (see Chapter 5e, i). A pair of ivory clappers or apotropaic wands, probably associated with pregnancy and the protection of mother and baby (see Chapter 5e, i), was found with the statuette (Fig. 5.9). Many examples of these wands have a variety of demonic creatures incised on the flat (convex) surface (see below), but this pair is undecorated.

In another room of the house Petrie discovered a full-size canvas mask that was part of the same set of equipment. It is made of three layers of canvas stuck together and moulded to form the face of a deity, either the household god Bes or his consort Beset. The mask is painted black, and details such as the arches above and under the eyes, spots on the cheeks and red lips are also depicted. Holes have been made at the eyes and nostrils to allow the wearer to see and breathe. The mask shows signs of wear: some of the surface is missing, probably as a result of frequent use, and there is evidence of some repainting (Fig. 5.10).

Overall, the Ramesseum and Kahun groups seem to have some common features: for example, both contained apotropaic wands and, originally, a wooden figurine of a masked female deity (the Kahun example reportedly disappeared soon after excavation). However, the two owners of these collections

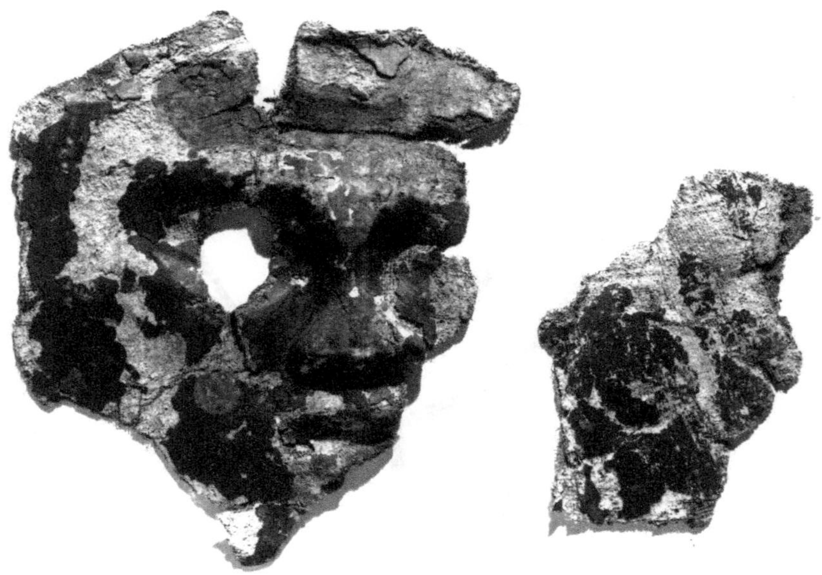

Figure 5.10. Stucco and linen mask perhaps representing the goddess Beset; possibly worn by a female healer when performing rites. Found with a pair of ivory wands and a wooden figurine. Holes are made at the eyes and nostrils to allow the wearer to see and breathe. Some of the surface stucco is missing through use, and the mask has been painted black to cover up this damage. 12th Dynasty. From Kahun, now in The Manchester Museum, 123 (courtesy of The Manchester Museum, The University of Manchester).

perhaps fulfilled different roles: the Kahun practitioner probably acted as a local community healer, specialising in magical rites, while the papyri collection included in the Ramesseum burial may indicate that the owner was literate and provided medical care at a different level.

(f) The Ancient Egyptian pharmaceutical tradition

Pharmacy in ancient Egypt

Ancient Egyptian medicine combined magical incantations and performative rituals with the utilisation of a wide range of surgical and pharmaceutical treatments. In the medical papyri, the pharmaceutical prescriptions outnumber the surgical procedures.

The Greeks are customarily acknowledged as the founders of the pharmaceutical tradition, and pharmaceutical treatments were an important element of Greek and Roman medicine. However, one of the aims of the 'Pharmacy in Ancient Egypt Project', a multidisciplinary study set up at The University of Manchester in 2005, was to produce evidence that the ancient Egyptians practised a rational, reproducible system long before the Greeks.

Although there is no extant evidence that the ancient Egyptians had a pharmacopoeia as such, the medical papyrus prescriptions can be regarded as a formulary. They show that pharmaceutical ingredients were obtained from animal, mineral and plant sources (Győry & Blázovics 2020; Argilés *et al.* 2021). Some of these substances are extensively discussed in Aufrère 2021.

The Pharmacy in Ancient Egypt Project

This project, which concentrated on the use of plants and herbs in ancient Egyptian medicine (Pain 2007; David 2010), involved an international, interdisciplinary group of Egyptologists and scientists and had unprecedented access to relevant scientific facilities and to collections of modern and ancient plants held in institutions in Britain and Egypt. Previous studies in this field had focused exclusively either on translation of the therapeutic regimes prescribed in the medical papyri or on botanical studies of ancient and modern Egyptian plants. However, this interdisciplinary research adopted the 'Manchester Methodology', an interdisciplinary system that combines historical and scientific analytical techniques previously employed to investigate diseases in mummies.

Aims of the project

A key aim was to provide the first scientific assessment of the contribution that ancient Egyptian pharmacy has made to modern science. The intention was to demonstrate that the Egyptians had developed an effective pharmacy tradition alongside a medical system that was at least partially science-based. Another focus was to determine the efficacy of the treatments prescribed in the medical papyri (Campbell *et al.* 2010). To achieve this, the textual evidence from the papyri was evaluated and the component drugs and method of preparation of the remedy were considered and compared with modern pharmaceutical protocols relevant at a time when drugs were regularly made in a dispensary. The *British Pharmaceutical Codex* (BPC 1973) and the *British Pharmacopoeia* (BP 1973) were used as the basis for this comparison.

The study also sought to trace the geographical sources and trade routes for some of these ancient pharmaceutical ingredients and to produce an accurate identification of the plants used in ancient Egyptian pharmacy. For this, it was necessary to determine the accuracy of existing translations of the pharmaceutical ingredients listed in the medical papyri, many of which have been disputed (Germer 1998; Montserrat 2021).

Translators of Egyptian texts often have to rely heavily on the context of a word in order to infer its meaning. However, in the medical papyri, many of the words used for plant or mineral ingredients do not appear elsewhere in the literature, so early translators had to rely on some educated guesses. They consulted contemporary pharmacopoeia to find an ingredient with the same presumed medicinal use that best fitted the description given in the papyri. However, some of these ingredients would not have been available for use in the ancient medicines because they are derived from plants that either did not exist in Egypt or were not imported at that time (but see below re: climate change in Egypt). Pharmaceutical analysis has provided an opportunity to assess the translations and validate them in terms of contemporary pharmacological application.

Initial studies

A pilot scheme was set up to make a scientific comparison between the substances and usage recorded in four medical papyri (Ebers, Edwin Smith, Kahun and Chester Beatty) and examples known from 20th century pharmacy. A thousand ancient prescriptions were analysed and compared with modern standards and protocols. This involved checking Egypt's flora (well documented in geological and archaeological sources) to see whether the plant named in the ancient text grew or was traded in Egypt at the time when the document was compiled. Then the named ingredient (as given in the translation) was checked to see if it could have worked in the way the prescription indicated. To do this, a sample was prepared from each recipe in the papyri that made available all the information required to reproduce a remedy, namely the ingredients, method of preparation and dosage.

The initial study produced a plausible identification of 284 ingredients derived from plant species (134), animals (24) and minerals (28), providing a first step towards compiling a pharmacopoeia that would have been available to the ancient Egyptians. The research demonstrated that 64 per cent of the ingredients prescribed in these ancient papyri were still included in Martindale's *Extra Pharmacopoeia* (Martindale 1977) and on a par with modern usage over the period of the past fifty years, while 67 per cent of the Egyptian remedies complied with the *British Pharmaceutical Codex* (BPC 1973), the modern source of standards and protocols for major medicines. These findings contradict earlier opinion (for example, Nunn 1996: 162) that Egyptian remedies were largely 'magical' and sympathetic, and unlikely to have produced major therapeutic effects.

Further investigations

The research was extended to assess the efficacy of remedies in other medical papyri. This concluded that symptoms and appropriate treatments (drug, dosage and method of administration) are the main foci of the papyri and that, although the Egyptians were generally unaware of the causes of disease where they were not obvious, many of the prescribed drugs were therapeutically viable.

Examples of effective treatments include castor oil, Balanites oil and figs as laxatives; kaolin and powdered carob for diarrhoea; liniments for musculo-skeletal disorders; resins and metals (with antimicrobial properties) and honey for wounds; extract of pomegranate and Balanites oil as powerful anthelminthics for parasitic infestations; celery (recognised as a modern anti-rheumatic) for pain relief; and saffron for back pain (Campbell 2008).

However, 'magical' remedies are also featured. For example, advice to anoint the head with concoctions including hedgehog quills and black lizard are included in a series of prescriptions to cure baldness (Ebers Papyrus 464–74). A different prescription (250) in the same papyrus had originally been interpreted as a 'magical' cure for migraine: 'Another [remedy] for suffering in half the head, the skull of a cat-fish, fried in oil. Anoint the head therewith' (translated Ghalioungui 1987). However, this may represent a rational treatment. Migraine is a common neurological disease that causes a variety of symptoms, most notably a throbbing, pulsing headache which can be severe. It often characteristically occurs on one side of the head only and so the mention of 'half a head' in P. Ebers 250 provides a possible clue to the condition being treated in this case. A natural remedy for migraine involves massaging with oil and the word 'anoint' in the remedy could refer to massaging. Additionally, the skull of the catfish, when fried, would produce a viscous oil that would be suitable for use in massage.

The transmission of pharmaceutical traditions

A rare opportunity arose as part of the project to combine Egyptological and ethnographical research. In order to explore the possibility of any direct continuous pharmaceutical tradition from ancient to modern times, the Pharmacy in Ancient Egypt Project developed a partnership with the Medicinal Plant Conservation Project at St Katherine's in Sinai. The latter project had been set up by the Egyptian government in 2002 to protect biodiversity in the area and to identify medicinally important plants used by the local Beduin. The Pharmacy in Ancient Egypt Project was able to compare the traditional Beduin remedies with ancient Egyptian treatments and establish any similarities and possible methods of transmission.

The geographical sources of medicinal ingredients

The project also explored various possibilities regarding the sources from which the Egyptians may have obtained their medicinal ingredients (Campbell & David 2010). This established that, locally, plants were derived from agriculture, animal products from animal husbandry and hunting and minerals from mining, smelting and building. However, other ingredients, including some resins, waxes, frankincense, cedar and coriander, came through trade with the Near East, Libya, Nubia and the southern Mediterranean.

The project used minimally invasive analytical techniques (for example, visible light microscopy, environmental scanning electron microscopy (ESEM) and Fourier-transform infrared spectroscopy) to investigate Egyptian and Nubian non-indigenous materials found in predynastic graves. This work confirmed that a wide range of organic materials was present in these burials and indicated that some were imported into Egypt as early as the 4th millennium BC via trade and contact with the Near East. Since some of these substances occur much later as ingredients in recipes found in the medical papyri, they may have had a similar use in early Egyptian communities (see Chapter 2a).

Molecular studies on plant-based medicines

The project took initial steps to lay the foundation for a future study that could attempt to identify whether the remains of a particular plant, described in the medical papyri as a treatment for a specific condition, are present in a mummy where that disease had already been identified through palaeopathological investigation. This might indicate that the plant had been administered for medicinal purposes. As a basis for future research, likely plants of medicinal importance were identified and protocols developed to detect their aDNA in mummified remains (Metcalfe 2010).

Some outcomes of the project

Based on the climatic and environmental conditions required by the botanical materials identified in the medical papyri, they are likely to have been derived from two main sources: imports from the Levant, Mesopotamia and North Africa; and locally within Egypt, where a phytogeographical study of the herbs and plants mentioned in the medical papyri has identified thirty sites of origin. However, current studies are exploring the possibility that periods of climate change within Egypt may have had a direct and dramatic impact on the local flora and fauna, greatly affecting the range and types of source material available locally for medicinal ingredients (pers. comm. Judith Bunbury).

Overall, the project reached several important conclusions. Analysis showed that in the ancient Egyptian prescriptions the arrangement of the formulae was consistent throughout and was remarkably similar to that seen in 20th century medicines. Additionally, the combination of ingredients in the ancient prescriptions was similar to modern examples: most included 'the active ingredient, ancillary drugs which may alleviate some of the severe side effects of the therapeutic drug (such as flavourings to disguise a bitter or unpleasant taste) and a vehicle to carry the ingredients in even distribution and permit measurement of a suitable volume' (Campbell *et al.* 2010). As noted above, the analysis demonstrated that 67 per cent of the Egyptian remedies examined are compliant with the protocols for formulation described in the *British Pharmaceutical Codex* (BPC 1973), indicating that ancient Egyptian formulations met the standards of modern pharmaceutical scrutiny.

However, evidence has not yet been found that narcotics were used in Egypt before the Roman Period (Counsell 2008) (see Chapter 5a). The Egyptians lacked knowledge of toxicity or contraindications, although their prescribing, formulation, preparation and dosage methods suggest that they were aware of the potential dangers and benefits of individual treatments. In addition, there is no indication that they understood the concept of sterilisation, although antiseptics and disinfectants (myrrh, frankincense, pine resin, onions, garlic and honey) were used.

Although it is unlikely that pharmacy was a distinct profession in Egypt (see Chapter 2f), the project has been able to demonstrate that a therapeutic and reproducible pharmacy existed there some 1800 years before it did in Greece. 'Magical' remedies certainly continued in use over the millennia, but they were outnumbered by rational, therapeutically viable treatments, and the Egyptian tradition clearly provided the basis from which modern 'Western' medicine was later developed (Héthelyi & Győry 2020).

6

Recipients of healthcare: the patient's perspective

In any society, health and well-being are influenced and defined by individual perception and circumstances. A key aim here is to reach some understanding of how the ancient Egyptians regarded personal health problems and acquired treatment for them. Some causative factors, including climate, geography and environment, may have had significant health impacts across the whole society. However, some conditions were more specific to individual circumstances, being caused or influenced by factors such as genetics, age, living and employment conditions, and dietary choices.

(a) Geographical and environmental conditions: their impact on health and disease

Diseases linked to environmental conditions

Geographical and environmental conditions were causative factors in some diseases that occurred widely throughout the population (see Plate 1). General health hazards included the toxic bites and stings of local fauna, particularly snakes and scorpions. Locally grown cereals and pulses formed the basis of the diet, with the addition of varying quantities of meat and fish. For most people, the diet was quite well balanced, but some foodstuffs were unhealthy for particular sections of the population (see Chapter 6b). In addition, intermittent famines and more general malnutrition, particularly among certain sectors of the population, were likely to increase the impact of epidemic disease, including typhoid and dysentery.

The impact of a sand-laden atmosphere

The proximity of the desert played a major role in some diseases. For example, particles of sand and grit were traditionally added to the grain to facilitate the bread-making process, but eating the contaminated bread caused the wear observed in the teeth of many mummies and skeletal remains (see Chapter 2f). Sand was also a major causative factor of the lung disease sand pneumoconiosis, which results from inhaling particles of sand, stone or wood (see Chapter 4a). This is one type of a group of diseases known generally as pneumoconiosis; the other types are silicosis pneumoconiosis and anthracosis pneumoconiosis; all are classified according to the causative factor, which is either geographical/environmental or occupational, and all have been identified in Egyptian mummies.

Silicosis pneumoconiosis is usually associated with specific occupations such as mining and stone-working, where large amounts of crystalline silica dust are inhaled over many years (see Chapter 4a). The disease has been identified in the mummy of Nakht (ROM I), where analyses have indicated that birefringent particles in the lung tissue are granite, suggesting that Nakht perhaps worked as a stone-mason (Reyman *et al.* 1977). Anthracosis pneumoconiosis (characterised by a carbon pigment) usually results from exposure to dust or wood smoke. This condition, described in mummies (Ruffer 1910a; Shaw 1938; Isidro *et al.* 2014), can probably be attributed to the domestic use of fires for cooking.

Sand pneumoconiosis would have had a greater impact on the population as a whole. This form of the disease was caused by the intermittent but recurrent sandstorms that were an integral feature of the Egyptian landscape. During these events, people exposed to them inhaled particles of silica (sand) that became embedded in the lungs, causing inflammation and scarring. This condition is still found in the populations of the Sahara and Negev deserts (Policard & Collett 1952; Bar-Ziv & Goldberg 1974). Sand pneumoconiosis has been identified in samples of tissue associated with the mummy of Nakht-ankh in the Manchester Museum collection (Tapp 1979: 97–99) (see Plate 27). Initial microscopic examination identified the samples as lung tissue and demonstrated scarring and a proliferation of both fibrous and elastic tissue. Among the fibrous tissue were several aggregations of fine particles; examination under polarised light showed birefringence, indicating that the particles had a crystalline structure and were probably silica. This was confirmed by studies using analytical electron microscopy (AEM) (Curry *et al.* 1979).

Pneumoconiosis would have posed some chronic health issues for many persons in ancient Egypt and had a significant impact on their lives and well-being. Various treatments were available to alleviate some of the symptoms (Campbell 2008). These included expectorants to remove lung secretion, such as antimony for loosening a dry cough, and inhalation of bitumen poured over hot stones (P. Ebers 319, 323). The garden plant *Ammi*, now acknowledged as a respiratory vasodilator, was prescribed in the P. Ebers (319, 323) as a treatment for a cough.

Parasitic infections: the result of close contact with water and soil

Parasitic diseases have been the cause of considerable suffering in the populations of both ancient and modern Egypt, and would have posed a major health issue in pharaonic times. Worm infestations were already recognised as the most significant cause of these diseases; because of their size, some worms (e.g., the tapeworm, *Taenia* sp., and the guinea worm, *Dranculus medinensis* – with respective lengths of 200mm and 1m) could be observed and identified. Many of the terms used in hieroglyphs for parasitic conditions carry a worm determinative, and some case descriptions in the medical papyri strongly indicate worm infestations as the cause of disease.

The Manchester project on schistosomiasis (see below) indicated the presence of schistosomiasis in 70 per cent of the mummy tissue samples tested. However, a related study of ancient Egyptian pharmacy (see Chapter 5f and below) suggested that a viable remedy may have existed for this condition.

Many patients in ancient Egypt would have suffered from these diseases, their infections caused either by single or multiple parasites. Some of these conditions are described below.

Schistosomiasis

Schistosomiasis is a disease arising from the body's reaction to a parasitic infection caused by a trematode worm (see Chapter 2a, 6g). This parasite has a complex lifecycle that alternates between humans and snails that live on the banks of rivers. Infection occurs during contact with water infested with cercariae, the free-swimming form of the worm released by the snail. The cercariae infect the human host, mate in the portal vein and deposit eggs, which can be found in most of the internal organs but especially the urinary tract. The eggs ulcerate through the bladder, causing bleeding, and then pass into the urine. If an infected person urinates into water, the eggs hatch out and the cycle begins again.

Patients would have suffered from a variety of symptoms depending on the organs affected. Without effective treatment chronic conditions likely to develop and continue are abdominal pain; diarrhoea and blood in the faeces and urine (see Chapter 6g); irritation of the bladder causing frequent and painful urination; and wheezing, shortness of breath and a persistent cough. In advanced cases there can be narrowing of the rectum or colon, liver enlargement, liver scarring and bladder cancer (Fig. 6.1). The ancient Egyptians may have attempted to treat this disease with herbal therapies (see below) but undoubtedly it would have been a major cause of concern for many patients throughout the millennia.

A major international project initiated in the 1990s provided an unprecedented opportunity to study the epidemiology of this disease in Egypt over a 5000-year period spanning antiquity to the present day (Contis & David 1996). Schistosoma ova have been detected in Egyptian mummies (well characterised by

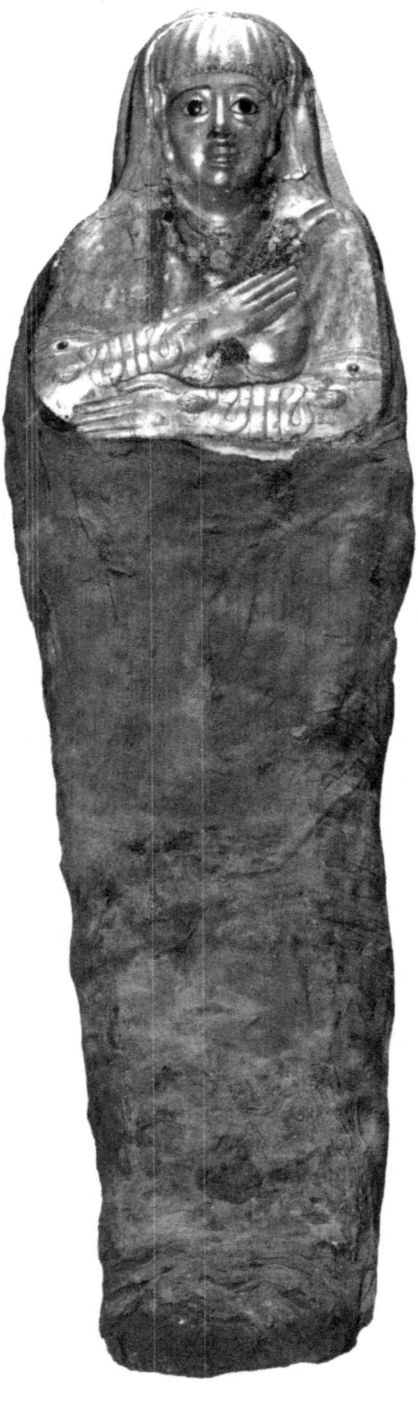

Figure 6.1. Mummy of a woman with a gilded cartonnage chest cover. Calcification of the bladder, a secondary pathological indication of schistosomiasis, was radiologically observed in this mummy, and immunological and molecular studies on a biopsy sample of the bladder tissue confirmed the presence of the disease. Roman Period. From Hawara, now in The Manchester Museum, 1766 (courtesy of The Manchester Museum, The University of Manchester).

their terminal spines), and have also been found in naturally mummified bodies excavated in Nubia. Currently, this chronic, debilitating disease continues to affect some 200–300 million people in over seventy countries, with the problem being exacerbated by the construction of river dams and irrigation schemes that provide additional breeding sites for the snails, an intermediary host in the parasite's lifecycle.

The aims of the Schistosomiasis Research Project, a ten-year programme set up in 1986 by Egypt and the United States of America, were to identify the contemporary epidemiological pattern of this disease in Egypt and to seek more effective methods to treat the disease and reduce its occurrence. In 1995 researchers at the University of Manchester were invited to undertake a parallel study focusing on the epidemiology of schistosomiasis in ancient Egypt in order to provide informative comparative data for the project (David 2008a: 7–8).

The development of a range of diagnostic techniques over many years has enabled researchers to identify schistosomiasis in mummified remains. Pioneering studies in palaeohistology undertaken by Ruffer (1910b) provided the first opportunity to identify this disease, allowing him to observe calcified schistosoma in the kidneys of two mummies. In 1980 researchers used the same techniques to identify the parasite in the mummy of Nakht (Millet *et al.* 1980). Radiology can demonstrate secondary pathological indications of schistosomiasis: for example, calcification of the bladder was observed in Mummy 1766 in the Manchester collection (David 1979: 34). Immunological techniques (ELISA) have also been used to confirm the presence of schistosome infection at the time of an individual's death (Deelder *et al.* 1990; Miller *et al.* 1993).

To achieve access to a sufficiently large number of samples for the Schistosomiasis Research Project, the Manchester researchers established the International Ancient Egyptian Tissue Bank (Lambert-Zazulak 2000), which acquired material from a variety of institutions, archaeological sites and chronological periods. Pioneering research was undertaken on these materials involving the first use of immunocytochemistry to detect disease in mummies (Rutherford 2008a). The results were confirmed by ELISA and DNA studies (Rutherford 2008b). For this investigation, the researchers revisited Mummy 1766 (in which schistosomiasis had already been observed – see above) to obtain a biopsy sample of bladder tissue. A 2000-year-old male schistosome was also discovered in this sample, and molecular studies undertaken on these remains produced the first identification of parasite DNA in a mummy (Rutherford 2008b).

Filariasis

Filariasis is an infection caused by a group of roundworms known as filarias. The adult worm, found in the body's lymphatic system, gives birth to larvae (microfilaria) rather than laying ova. During this stage of its lifecycle the parasite circulates in the blood but is not able to develop further unless it is ingested by blood-feeding insects, such as mosquitoes and black flies; it subsequently develops in the insect's gut and, when the host next bites an animal to obtain blood, it may transfer to a human host where it finally grows into an adult worm in the lymphatic system. However, the worms sometimes block the lymphatic system, causing fluid retention (oedema) in parts of the body. This can produce gross oedema (elephantiasis) characterised by severe swelling in the arms, legs, breasts and genitalia, and sometimes by a thickening of the skin.

Fragments of filarial worms were found in samples of scrotal skin taken from the Leeds Mummy, Nesyamun, as part of a multidisciplinary scientific investigation (David & Tapp 1992: 151–52). This demonstrated that he had suffered from filariasis, but it was not possible to identify any evidence of elephantiasis because mummification obscures any traces of oedema. However, a wall scene in the second portico of Hatshepsut's mortuary temple at Deir el-Bahri depicting the Queen of Punt may provide an iconographic example of filariasis (see Chapter 1c; Plate 8).

Strongyloidiasis

This disease is caused by a parasitic roundworm of the genus *Strongyloides*, which lives in the soil (see Chapter 6g). Larval forms of *Strongyloides* have been found in the mucosa and muscular intestinal wall from a mummy in the Manchester Museum collection (1777) (see Plate 28). The mummy belonged to Asru, a chantress in the Temple of Karnak who lived in the Late Period. The samples, taken from a mass of material found between the legs of the mummy, were examined both histologically and with transmission electron microscopy (TEM) (Curry *et al.* 1979; Tapp 1979).

Some individuals suffering from strongyloidiasis are asymptomatic or have generalised, non-specific conditions, but the disease can produce a variety of symptoms (see Chapter 6g). Asru probably suffered significantly from chronic strongyloidiasis (Tapp 1979: 99) and, although there is no confirmation that it caused her death, this cannot be ruled out. In antiquity such infections would sometimes have led to severe inflammation of the large intestines, and any subsequent spread to other parts of the body may have resulted in death.

Tapeworm (Taenia)

Tapeworms are flat, segmented worms that live in the intestines of certain animals. Their bodies essentially consist of packages of ova that are regularly shed into the environment to infect other organisms. Animals can become infected with these parasites when grazing contaminated pasture or drinking contaminated water. Eating undercooked meat from infected animals, especially pork and beef, is the main cause of tapeworm infection in humans.

These parasites can grow to considerable lengths (for example, the worm found in one modern patient exceeded 6m) and can cause a wide range of symptoms in humans, including nausea, weakness, abdominal pain, loss of appetite, diarrhoea and dizziness, although in many instances the patient is asymptomatic. However, an infection can occasionally produce a serious, life-threatening problem such as blockage of the biliary system.

Examples of *Taenia* infestation in mummies span the Pharaonic and Christian Periods. It was identified in a mummy from a Christian necropolis in El-Deir in the Kharga Oasis (Le Bailly *et al.* 2009) and also in the 20th Dynasty mummy of Nakht (ROM 1). Histological techniques and the use of electron microscopy enabled researchers engaged in a multidisciplinary study of this mummy to discover and identify numerous *Taenia* ova in the intestinal tract (Hart 1977; Millet *et al.* 1980). It is unclear whether pork or beef was the source of the tapeworm, but it is likely to have been the former as a small cyst of *Trichinella spiralis* was also found in the mummy, and this parasitic infestation is caused by eating undercooked pork. This discovery provides interesting historical evidence that pork was not, as some have claimed, universally prohibited in ancient Egypt, although it may have been eaten only at certain times of the year.

Guinea worm disease

Humans can become infected by the guinea worm (*Dracunculus medinensis*) as a result of drinking water that contains immature forms of the parasite. These develop in the person's stomach and subsequently burrow into the abdominal wall, where they mate before the male worm dies. The pregnant female worm then moves through the bodily tissues, usually reaching the feet or legs, where, after about a year, it causes irritation and ulcers and its ova are released into water in canals or pools. This contaminated water ultimately becomes the route by which the parasite is passed on to another person. The condition is usually asymptomatic until the worm attempts to break through the skin; then, at the site of this eruption, there is likely to be swelling, itching, burning and blistering, sometimes accompanied by fever, nausea and vomiting, diarrhoea and shortness of breath.

Although rare today, the disease is known to have existed in ancient Egypt. An interesting example is provided by the mummy of a young girl (1770) in the Manchester Museum collection (Isherwood *et al.* 1979; Tapp 1979). When a multidisciplinary investigation of the mummy was undertaken in 1979 radiography carried out before autopsy revealed a calcified nodule in the abdominal wall. This nodule was removed during autopsy and subjected to further radiographic scrutiny, which identified it as the calcified remains of a male guinea worm that had died in situ long before the girl's own demise. Calcium deposited in the worm ensured its natural preservation and also made it radiopaque, with the result that it was visible on the X-rays.

The autopsy revealed that the girl's legs had been amputated shortly before or at death. There has been speculation that they may have been badly ulcerated as a result of the guinea worm infection, and that amputation was perhaps undertaken in an unsuccessful attempt to save her life.

Ascariasis: roundworm infection

The roundworm *Ascaris* is a very common parasite found in tropical and sub-tropical countries. Immature forms of the worm are ingested through contaminated food, and then the larvae hatch in the small intestine before penetrating the intestinal wall and finally reaching the lungs. They continue to migrate along the airways and down the gullet, before again entering the intestine. Here, they mature into adults and lay ova that, on entering the soil, once again provide a source of infection.

When the worms are present in the lungs the disease can produce a cough, wheezing, chest pain and difficulty in breathing. If the intestine is affected there may be abdominal pain and distention, nausea, vomiting and diarrhoea. A heavy infestation can cause intestinal obstruction and constipation, and other complications include bowel inflammation, pneumonia and pancreatitis.

This infestation was found in intestinal tissue in a visceral package belonging to a mummy (PUM II) held by the Philadelphia Art Museum (USA) (Cockburn *et al.* 1980: 66).

Liver fluke infection (Fasciola hepatica)

Fasciola hepatica is a parasitic trematode that can affect the liver in humans and some animals. The condition is caused by eating contaminated watercress or raw or undercooked freshwater fish. Following ingestion, the immature forms of the parasite move from the intestines to the bile ducts in the liver where, over a period of four to six months, they develop into adult flukes and start to produce ova. Ultimately, they pass out into the intestines but some can remain in the bile ducts for twenty to thirty years, which can cause chronic inflammation of the bile duct. Other rare complications that result from heavy infections are stone formation, infections of the biliary system and bile duct cancer. Milder symptoms include abdominal pain, fever, nausea and vomiting, diarrhoea, hives, weakness, loss of appetite and weight loss.

Although this condition was probably common in ancient Egypt, it has rarely been recorded in palaeopathological material (Araujo *et al.* 2000). The partial remains of a fluke were tentatively identified in well-preserved liver tissue from a canopic jar associated with the 12th Dynasty mummy of Nakht-ankh in the Manchester Museum collection (Curry *et al.* 1979: 106). More recently, a study pioneering the use of discovery proteomics to identify disease in ancient Egyptian mummies has demonstrated the presence of proteins from a liver fluke in liver tissue dating from the Graeco-Roman Period (publication forthcoming).

Malaria

Malaria is another parasitic disease that may have been widespread in ancient Egypt (see Chapter 7b). The incidence of this condition would have increased during periods of climate change that resulted in a wetter environment, as this was likely to produce more swamps and a subsequent increase in mosquito populations.

Medical treatments

The medical papyri provide treatments for a wide and varied range of parasitic diseases associated with gastrointestinal and genitourinary conditions. Antihelminthics were prescribed to clear worms from the gastrointestinal tract. An interesting example, pelletierine, derived from the pomegranate, acts by paralysing tapeworms in the gastrointestinal tract; this was administered prior to purging with laxatives, and continued to be used as an effective treatment until sixty years ago (Campbell 2008: 229). There is one reference in the medical papyri (P. Ebers 265) to another antihelminthic, Balanites oil, which in the early 20th century was still regarded as a viable treatment for schistosomiasis (Campbell 2008: 229).

Laxatives played an important part in treating symptoms associated with gastrointestinal conditions. The ingredients, intended to ease defecation, included irritants such as castor oil and colocynth, bulk formers (whole grain, figs and fruit) and oils. Stomach demulcents included palatable ingredients such as barley water, honey and milk (Campbell 2008: 227).

Leg ulcers resulting from guinea worm infestation may have been treated with biocides such as antimony, malachite, copper and zinc; honey may also have been applied to these wounds. Coughs associated with some parasitic conditions would have been treated with expectorants or demulcents.

For some patients, this limited range of treatments would have provided some alleviation of their symptoms, but chronic parasitic infections always posed a major challenge to the general health and well-being of all sectors of Egyptian society.

(b) Individual social, domestic and occupational status: influence on health and disease

The impact of social status on the provision of healthcare

The extent to which social status affected an individual's health and access to medical treatment remains unclear. Some diseases arising from geographical and environmental conditions would have affected all levels of society (see Chapter 6a). In addition, there were some universal dietary issues. The gritty bread eaten by all classes was the main cause of tooth wear (see Chapter 2f), a problem that afflicted Egyptians throughout their history.

There is evidence that, at least to some extent, medical treatment was available and accessible to all social classes. For the upper echelons of society, the *swnw* provided medical treatment for the royal family, senior officials and administrators at the royal palaces (see Chapters 2 and 4e). In the towns built to house the families of the royal workmen there is archaeological, inscriptional and palaeopathological evidence that the state provided some level of healthcare (see Chapter 4a). A study has explored amputation and treatment for fractures in the skeletal remains belonging to the Old Kingdom pyramid-builders at Giza, and this has demonstrated that injury management was similar for both high officials and workers (Hussien *et al.* 2010).

At the Middle Kingdom town Kahun, built to accommodate the families of officials and workers at the adjacent pyramid site, the discovery of the famous Kahun Gynaecological Papyrus in the town's archive suggests that some centralised, state-organised social healthcare system existed within the community (see Chapters 4a, b, c). Again, in the New Kingdom, the state made a significant contribution to the families of the royal workforce at Deir el-Medina. Inscriptional sources relate that the king provided servants to grind the workers' corn, assist with the laundry and transport water to the site (Davis 1999: 40, 266). State medical assistance was made directly available to the Royal Gang through the appointment of designated workers to undertake medical duties for the workforce: they were allowed to take time off on a regular basis to prepare medicines and care for sick co-workers. In addition, provision was made to reimburse workers who lost daily payments because of sickness.

The state's involvement in medical care in these communities was undoubtedly intended to ensure that the royal workforce retained its fitness and was able to complete the king's tomb. Royal artisans were a specially favoured group, and there is no evidence that the use of child labour was the norm in ancient Egypt. However, at Tell el-Amarna there are indications that some of the hard labour was undertaken by a workforce of children and teenagers (see p. 99). Their welfare was disregarded, and they suffered from a growth delay of at least two years, probably as the result of nutritional deficiencies (Stevens & Dabbs 2018). Poor sanitation and general living conditions doubtless caused or exacerbated various health issues identified in their skeletal remains. The state seems to have considered this group to be disposable and replaceable, and their lowly social status clearly limited any opportunities to have access to a reasonable diet and medical treatment.

As well as receiving any state assistance, each family, whatever its status in society, was expected to fulfil a universal moral obligation to attend to its own sick, disabled and elderly members (Janssen & Janssen 2007: 220–37). In some cases, this would have involved provision of care over many years.

In many societies people affected by various kinds of disability are often at a disadvantage, encountering unequal and inadequate provision for their healthcare and employment. This appears to have been less of an issue in ancient Egypt, however, where there was some social acceptance of disability and attempts were made to address related difficulties (see Chapters 5d, 6e).

Public health, hygiene, and housing: their contribution to healthcare and well-being

Public health measures are aimed at protecting communities from the spread of disease and maintaining the health of the population. Essential aspects include the provision of adequate accommodation and an effective water supply for washing humans, animals, clothing and foodstuffs.

Domestic accommodation

Archaeological evidence indicates that the domestication of certain plants and animals probably first occurred in the ancient Near East and was subsequently established in Egypt by about 5000 BC, or possibly even as early as 8000 BC. This development obviously promoted interaction between humans and animals and led to increased disease transmission. Urban settlements, with crowded housing and a lack of sanitary provision, became very unhealthy living environments, where diseases such as tuberculosis, trachoma, malaria, parasitic infestations and possibly typhoid were commonplace. Other diseases, including influenza, pneumonia and tetanus, would also have flourished in this environment, although they usually do not leave indications in the palaeopathological record.

Among the material excavated at the workman's village at Tell el-Amarna were insect remains. As well as the human flea (*Pulex irritans*) and numerous pests of stored products, well-preserved specimens of the common bed bug (insects from the genus *Cimex*) have been discovered. The latter would have been more of an irritant than a disease vector to the occupants of the village, but provide the earliest record of an association between man and the bed bug ectoparasite (Panagiotakopulu & Buckland 1999).

Terraced houses with small rooms and little natural light were the mainstay of domestic architecture in ancient Egyptian cities, towns and villages. These are exemplified by the dwellings built for families of the royal workforce, although more spacious accommodation was provided at these sites for overseers and high officials (see Plate 29). Elsewhere, housing stock also included more salubrious detached villas for the elite and larger houses for senior priests (Thomas 2013, 2014), but generally living conditions in ancient Egypt were not conducive to health. The design of the buildings, their close proximity to neighbouring homes, a lack of proper sanitation and water sourced from the Nile, canals and wells all contributed to the problem.

The nature of the biblical plagues and the possible existence of bubonic plague in ancient Egypt remain speculative (see Chapter 7b). However, there were probably regular minor epidemics in the urban and rural communities, which may have included the unidentified 'Asiatic disease' (Györy 2010). There is little evidence of any attempt to use quarantine as a means of containing the spread of disease, although Amenhotep III (whose reign may have been a plague period) may have relocated his palace to the relatively isolated site of Malkata on the west bank of the river to try to find a disease-free environment (Habicht *et al.* 2021). His son Akhenaten may also have moved his capital city to Tell el-Amarna some years later for the same reason. The town of the royal necropolis workers, Deir el-Medina, was destroyed by fire during the reigns of these two kings and, although the cause may have been accidental, it was possibly an attempt to cleanse the place after an outbreak of disease (Habicht *et al.* 2021).

Nevertheless, despite the problems associated with domestic conditions, individual settlements were usually too small for density-dependent diseases to emerge and flourish. For example, a population of around 200,000 is required for smallpox to become established in a community (Lang 2013: 18–19) and, although a couple of instances of this disease have been tentatively identified in human remains, there is no extant evidence that this was a widespread highly infectious disease in ancient Egypt (see Chapter 7b). Similarly, poliomyelitis occurs in isolated palaeopathological and iconographic sources but is missing from the wider record (see Chapter 7b).

Personal hygiene

Personal hygiene was very important at all levels of Egyptian society. Herodotus (II, 79) claimed that, next to the Libyans, the Egyptians were the healthiest people in the world and provides detailed information about the hygienic practices of the priests. They had to undergo special rites and observe specific taboos in order to attain a level of physical purification that would permit them to enter a god's presence or to handle anything that had come into contact with the divine cult image (Herodotus II, 35, 37). Priests were obliged to shave their heads, and also the whole body every other day, to 'guard against the presence of lice, or anything else equally unpleasant, while they are about their religious duties'. They were also required to bathe in cold water twice a day and twice every night, performing their ablutions in the Sacred Lake attached to the temple.

This literary account is supported by evidence from scenes on stone blocks from Hatshepsut's Red Chapel at Karnak. These show a 'God's Wife' ('divine consort') undergoing purification before entering the temple for a special ceremony intended to achieve the ritual destruction of Egypt's enemies. The princess, standing in the Sacred Lake, was ritually bathed by her attendants with water from a jar: this rite made her an initiate of the temple and gave her a status equal to that of a priest (Ayad 2009: 93–94).

Priests were not required to remain celibate, but were expected to abstain from sexual intercourse during rotational periods of duty in the temple. An inscription in the Tomb of Idu at Saqqara (Strudwick 2005: 277) and Spell 21 in the Book of the Dead (Allen 1960: 151) refers to a requirement for sexual abstinence before entering sacred places; later Herodotus (II, 64) provided a statement on this:

> It was the Egyptians who first made it an offence against piety to have intercourse with women in temples, or to enter temples after intercourse without having previously washed … . The Egyptians are meticulous in their observance of this point, as indeed they are in everything else which concerns their religion.

Some Old Kingdom sources draw attention to an association between certain prohibited foodstuffs and the state of physical purity required to enter a sacred place (Strudwick 2005: 236, 277, 264; Teeter 2011: 34). Herodotus specifies that fish and beans were generally taboo for all priests, and other classical sources mention meat from cows, sheep and pigs, the flesh of pigeons or pelicans, shellfish, garlic, vegetables and salt.

However, it is unlikely that all these foods were forbidden to individual priests, especially since many items listed as components of the god's meals would eventually have provided the priests' daily rations at the completion of the rituals (see section below) (Teeter 2011: 33). Specific prohibitions probably applied only to the priesthoods of certain gods or temple localities: vegetables associated with a specific divine cult or meat from that temple's cult-animal would have been taboo for the cult's own priests and followers, but would have remained part of the dietary intake of priests in other districts.

As well as the specific information that Herodotus provides about practices associated with the elite, he also mentions hygienic measures that affected the well-being of the whole population. He attributed their good health to an unchanging climate and to the custom of purging oneself every month for three successive days to address the belief that all disease originated in food. Other comments he makes on personal cleanliness draw attention to the Egyptians' universal habit of using and scouring metal cups and continually laundering their linen clothes (II, 38).

Male circumcision, another important condition required to attain physical purity, is also mentioned by Herodotus (see Chapter 5a). In the Old and Middle Kingdoms circumcision may have been available only for royalty, the elite and initiates into the priesthood, perhaps mainly for boys between the ages of six and twelve years, although occasionally extended to adults (Filer

2001). From the Late Period onwards, in addition to its ritual significance, circumcision contributed generally to the Egyptian concept of physical purity and cleanliness.

Incidence of ill-health associated with particular occupations

Some occupations and workplaces were associated with particular health hazards. The conditions and circumstances of soldiers, agricultural workers and labourers at building and industrial sites are addressed in Chapter 6g. There would also have been health risks associated with some mummification procedures, such as the work of the 'cutters', who made the first incisions in the body and then removed the viscera (see Chapter 2e).

Dietary habits appear to have had a particularly deleterious impact on members of the priesthood and their families. Atherosclerosis is a degenerative disease involving a build-up of plaque that causes a narrowing and hardening of the arteries. The symptoms vary according to the site of the affected artery, but can include chest pain or angina; pain in the arm, leg or any site of an artery blockage; confusion if circulation to the brain is affected; muscle weakness in the legs from a lack of blood circulation; shortness of breath; and fatigue. The condition can induce strokes or heart attacks. It has been assumed that this condition, which is widespread in modern industrialised societies and linked to lifestyle factors such as a diet high in cholesterol, saturated fat and salt, is limited to modern times. However, analytical investigations of hundreds of mummies have shown that it occurred throughout ancient Egyptian history, and related particularly to the health of priests and their families.

One investigation (the Horus Study) used whole-body multislice computed tomography scanning to study fifty-two mummies in the Egyptian Museum, Cairo (Allam *et al.* 2011). This identified cardiovascular structures in forty-four mummies, of which twenty had either probable or definite atherosclerosis. These results covered a timespan of around 2000 years, from the Middle Kingdom to the Graeco-Roman Period, and included the earliest definite recorded case of the disease in a human – an unknown princess who lived between 1558 BC and 1550 BC.

A radiological investigation of twenty-four mummies in the Manchester Museum collection confirmed that the disease was present in three mummies belonging to individuals associated with temple worship – Asru and Perenbast, who were both 'Chantresses of Amun'; and Khary, a priest with the title of 'Divine Father of Amun' at the Temple of Karnak (Isherwood *et al.* 1979).

The Manchester team also carried out a multidisciplinary study on the 'Leeds Mummy', Nesyamun, in the collection of the Leeds City Art Gallery and Museum (David & Tapp 1992: 152). Histological examination of tissue samples removed from near the scrotum revealed well-developed plaques in the femoral blood vessels from the groin, again demonstrating the presence of atherosclerosis. According to inscriptions on the accompanying coffins, Nesyamun was a priest in the Temple of Amun at Karnak during the reign of Ramesses XI in the final years of the 20th Dynasty. His most important function was temple scribe: he held the titles of 'Scribe of the Sacred Bulls of Amun, Mut, and Khonsu', 'Scribe of the offerings made to all the gods of Upper and Lower Egypt' and 'Scribe of the accounts of the cattle of the estate of Amun'. His duties involved recording the quantity of corn offered to the sacred cattle kept in the temple enclosure to be slaughtered for the god's daily banquet and for temple festivals. Religious regulations governed the selection and slaughter of these animals, which, since they provided the god's food, had to be ritually pure. The process of selecting an animal and overseeing and performing the correct rites during slaughter and butchering were undertaken by a specialist priest (see Chapter 2d).

Whereas the diet of non-elite Egyptians consisted of bread, beer, pulses, vegetables, fruit and fish, with the rare addition of mutton, goat and pork, the lists of offerings inscribed on temple walls provide the main ingredients of the god's daily food intake. These were meat (especially beef – a luxury food mainly reserved for the elite), poultry, bread, cake, fruit, vegetables, honey, milk, wine and beer. The priests performing the rites known as the 'Reversion of Offerings' at the conclusion of the daily temple service subsequently removed the consecrated food from the god's altar and divided these offerings among themselves as part of the regular reimbursement for the performance of temple duties, finally taking the food home to their families, for whom it provided a regular staple diet.

Analytical studies on Egyptian mummies have demonstrated a high incidence of cardiovascular disease among the elite, particularly in the families of priests. Researchers in the Cardiovascular Group and Department of Dietetics at The University of Manchester set up a project with the aim of exploring whether this condition was linked to the special diet consumed by the priests and their families (David *et al.* 2010). This study confirmed that the ingredients of the god's daily food intake would have produced significant risk factors for atherosclerosis in priestly families. The total fat and saturated fat content of the food and the high intake of alcohol were particularly noticeable.

Evidence from ancient Egypt has shown that atherosclerosis is not an exclusively modern disease. It has enabled a comparison to be drawn between two distinctive diets that existed in parallel over a considerable timespan, making it possible to demonstrate that there is a causative dietary connection with this particular disease.

In addition, the Horus Study commented that, while the composition of the Egyptians' diet contributed to the development of atherosclerotic cardiovascular disease, it is also accepted that atherosclerosis emanates from a complex inter-play of genes and the environment. The research also recognised the important role of inflammation in both atherosclerosis and advancing age (Allam *et al.* 2009, 2011).

(c) The family unit: women and children

Apart from the royal family, the family unit (i.e., those who shared the same living accommodation) was small, usually consisting of parents, children and sometimes other close single relatives. A range of treatments and healthcare was available to meet the various general needs of individuals within the family unit, many of which are dealt with elsewhere in this volume.

Women and children, who were the main focus of the family, faced particular health concerns. There were the challenges associated with conception, childbirth and motherhood, while infants and young children were regarded as especially vulnerable to physical dangers. In both instances, these were addressed with special magical rituals and medical procedures designed to protect the recipients against disease or provide an effective cure.

Source material

Some 50 per cent of the population of ancient Egypt was female. However, although some studies have started to address women's role in society (Watterson 1991; Robins 1993), the subject has largely been ignored in the Egyptological literature of the past two centuries. This reflects the availability of ancient source material, which mainly records Egypt's male-dominated political and religious structure. It is assumed that women had a much lower rate of literacy and that most surviving documentation was written by men and expressed their world view, so that most information about women comes indirectly through these sources (Orriols-Llonch 2016: 194; Ollabarria 2022).

Women's own thoughts and opinions about their special needs and circumstances relating to reproductive health therefore remain inaccessible. However, all indications are that they were highly regarded members of society and played a key role within the family. Women's importance is reflected in the provision of medical treatment (Sullivan 1997): a significant proportion of the prescriptions in the medical papyri are devoted to issues relating to their health.

Children were central to the Egyptians' idea of family life, and childlessness was regarded as a great affliction that was addressed through prayers and medical treatment (Feucht 1995: 166–73). Fertility, conception and contraception, pregnancy, identifying the sex of the unborn and the treatment of neonates are all important sections in several documents including the Ebers, Carlsberg, London and Berlin Papyri and, most importantly, the Kahun Gynaecological Papyrus (see Chapter 4c; Ghalioungui *et al.* 1963; Bardinet 1995: 221–29, 437–43; Strouhal *et al.* 2014). However, the papyri are silent regarding normal childbirth, perhaps reflecting the fragmentary nature of surviving texts or because there was no need to record what was probably regarded as a natural process.

Parental roles in the creation of a child

The ancient Egyptians understood the connection between menstruation, conception and pregnancy (Sauneron 1962: 209; Feucht 2016: 205). Some cases in the medical papyri (e.g., P. Kahun 2 and P. Ebers 828, 829, 830) refer to bleeding but do not discuss the causes; however, it is likely that the majority were related to problems associated with menstruation.

Additionally, the Egyptians understood that parents played a dual role in the creation of a child (Feucht 2016: 204). According to some texts, the father was the creator of the child while the mother acted as the offspring's receptacle and nourisher in the womb (Sandmann 1938: 10 ff; Feucht 2001). They describe how the child was created in the father's heart and then passed via the semen into his testicles, before finally being transferred to the mother's womb. In another version of conception, both parents contributed equally to the child's creation, with the mother's milk forming the flesh and skin while the father's semen produced the bones (Feucht 2004: 38–40).

The dangers associated with pregnancy and childbirth

It was important to prevent or stop any bleeding during pregnancy, as it might indicate a miscarriage or premature birth. Attempts to do this employed magical rites as well as more practical solutions. The causes of bleeding were usually attributed to harmful powers, and magic was used to close the birth canal with a knot constructed from plant fibres, known as the 'Knot of Isis' (*tyet*).

An obscure example occurs in P. Kahun (17), but P. London (40, 41, 42) provides a clearer example: to attempt to stop or prevent bleeding during pregnancy, some type of tampon was inserted into either the vagina or the anus, which, it was believed, was connected in the belly with the woman's reproductive system. The magical incantations recited to accompany this procedure were regarded as particularly efficacious. In Case 40 in P. London the wording at the end of the incantation is to strengthen the egg, which implies re-attaching the foetus in the mother's uterus. Another incantation (Case 41) describes how Anubis, god of mummification, stopped a Nile flood for the goddess Tayet, likening this to staunching the flow of blood from a pregnant woman and thus preventing a miscarriage (Strouhal *et al.* 2014: 167).

Childbirth and its immediate aftermath could be fraught with difficulties. These would have had a profound impact on the family, with many men losing their wives and many older children growing up without their mothers. There would have been a high rate of infant mortality, with an estimated 20 to 50 per cent of babies dying in the first year of life, and perhaps fewer than 50 per cent of a mother's children surviving into adulthood (Fig. 6.2).

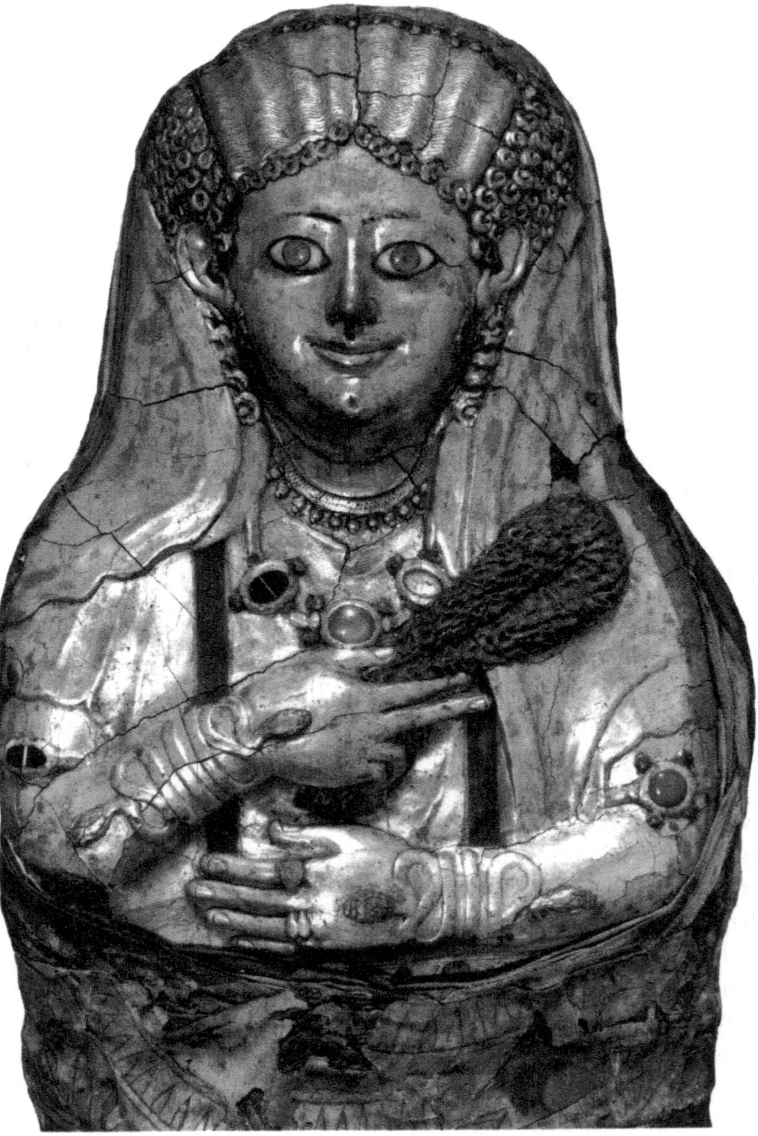

Figure 6.2. Mummy of a child in a gilded cartonnage outer casing. Age between three and four years, but lines of arrested growth in the upper limbs suggest previous illnesses. Dated to the Roman Period, when funerary preparation of child mummies was far more elaborate than in the pharaonic period. From Hawara, now in The Manchester Museum, 1769 (courtesy of The Manchester Museum, The University of Manchester).

The sources provide little information about those who attended the birth. There are no known medical titles for specialists in gynaecology or obstetrics as there were for some other disciplines, but it is likely that childbirth was supervised by older women in the community and by midwives (see Chapter 2d). Some attempt was made to alleviate and ease childbirth with magico/pharmaceutical treatments, and there were also remedies to expel the placenta: 'Remedy to cause the placenta of a woman to go down to its natural place: pin sawdust, put this in dregs [beer], smear a cloth pad and the woman sits on it' (P. Ebers 789).

Palaeopathological evidence

The ancient Egyptians would not have had sufficiently advanced diagnostic techniques to recognise some conditions and therefore these were not recorded in extant documentary sources. For example, they would not have been able to identify osteoporosis, which is detected by modern techniques such as dual energy X-ray absorptiometry (DEXA).

Now, however, palaeopathological studies are confirming that this disease did occur in Egypt (Zaki *et al.* 2009). An investigation of workers and elite officials engaged in the construction of the pyramids at Giza has shown a higher frequency of osteoporosis among elite women than female workers, perhaps because of the former's more sedentary lifestyle.

Another study of bone loss in female Nubian skeletons determined that osteoporosis occurred in younger age groups and related it to inadequate calcium intake and extended lactation (Dewey *et al.* 1969). Comparative histological studies on Nubian and Egyptian skeletal material found that earlier age onset of osteoporosis was more pronounced in the Nubian specimens. This has been attributed to nutritional differences, with Nubians depending on a grain diet (millet, barley and sorghum) low in calcium, iron and protein, while the Egyptian diet included more cereal (emmer wheat) and protein (Zaki *et al.* 2000).

Indeed, material relating to pregnancy and perinatal health has largely been derived from inscriptional and iconographic sources. Very little evidence of pregnancy and traumatic complications has survived in the osteological record (Sullivan 1997), and burials of pregnant women have rarely been identified. However, although their true potential has yet to be fully realised (David 2016: 182), palaeopathological studies on human remains now increasingly contribute new information about women's health in ancient Egypt.

The radiological investigation of a mummy in the Egyptian collection at the National Museum in Warsaw has led some researchers to conclude that this represents the only known example of a mummified pregnant woman and that these are the first radiological images of a foetus *in utero*. The report suggests that the woman died between the ages of twenty and thirty, and that the foetus's development was somewhere between the 26th and 30th weeks of the pregnancy

(Ejsmond *et al.* 2021). However, this interpretation has been disputed because of a lack of identification of foetal bones in the pelvic object; alternative proposals are that it may be a visceral package, condensed embalming materials or a calcified pelvic tumour (Saleem 2022).

Generally, palaeopathological evidence supports the conclusion that childbirth could be difficult and even life-threatening, and that these conditions occurred at all levels of society. For example, the mummies of Princesses Hehenit and Maatkare indicate that even royalty sometimes died in childbirth, the latter because of problems associated with a very narrow pelvis (see Chapter 2d).

Indeed, any woman with an abnormal pelvic structure faced the possibility of birth obstruction and consequent death in childbirth. This is apparent in several cases. In the *First Archaeological Survey of Nubia* Elliot Smith excavated the bodies of five Nubian women with extensively deformed pelves who had died as a result of childbirth (Derry 1935). The *Survey* also describes the condition of a Coptic female who died in childbirth as a result of sacroiliac joint dysfunction. Other deaths were caused by narrowing and obstruction of the birth canal (see Chapter 2d). The *First Archaeological Survey of Nubia* also describes a post-mortem on the mummified remains of a 4th century AD Coptic female infant from Kom el Ahmar that revealed a congenital defect of the uterus.

Burials of some foetuses have been found, indicating that the Egyptians considered them to be already viable individuals (Feucht 1995: 124–31; Feucht 2004: 45, note 71–72). Reports on the most famous examples – the two female foetuses found in the tomb of Tutankhamun – indicate the presence of multiple congenital afflictions, including Sprengel's deformity of the shoulder and other spinal conditions (Harrison *et al.* 1979), although these diagnoses have not been confirmed by more recent CT studies (Hawass & Saleem 2011).

Multiple births would also have posed difficulties during the pharaonic period. Iconographic evidence from a 5th Dynasty tomb belonging to Niankhkhnum and Khnunhotep at Saqqara may indicate that these two men (who both worked as palace manicurists) were identical twins (Evans & Woods 2016). However, it was probably rare for such individuals to live to adulthood, although better obstetrical practices may have offered more hope of survival in the Graeco-Roman Period.

Other gynaecological problems

The eminent obstetrician Augustus Granville performed the earliest true scientific autopsy of an Egyptian mummy, undertaken on a high-ranking woman, Irtyersenu, who lived during the 26th Dynasty. The mummy had been excavated from the Theban necropolis. Granville identified a mass around the right ovary as 'Ovarian dropsy' (cancer), and reported his findings to the Royal Society of London in 1825, concluding that this had caused the woman's death around the age of fifty. The body, subsequently known as the 'Granville Mummy', entered the Egyptian collections at the British Museum. More recent investigations, undertaken by a team of experts led by the museum's staff, have overturned Granville's original diagnosis, confirming instead that the mass was a benign cystadenoma and that tuberculosis was the probable cause of death (Donoghue *et al.* 2010).

Prolapse of the uterus was another condition recognised in ancient Egypt: palaeopathological examples have been found in the human remains of royal women associated with Mentuhotep II's burial at Deir el-Bahri and in some of the bodies excavated during the *First Archaeological Survey of Nubia*. A remedy 'To cause the uterus to leave its place' (P. Ebers 795) recommends fumigation as a treatment: 'Ibis of wax, place (it) on the coals and let the smoke enter her vagina'.

Problems with urination can be caused by many common infections, and symptoms include pain and burning when urinating, urinary urgency, a feeling of pressure in the urethra and lower back, and abdominal pain. P. Kahun 10 describes a disease of the urinary tract attributed to a disorder of the womb, and recommends drinking a mixture of medicinal herbs in beer, which would have a diuretic effect and could help by purging the urinary tract. Another case study partly preserved in P. Kahun 34 describes pain during urination, while P. Ebers 784 refers to pain on urinating and recommends a preparation of sea salt, sweet beer, honey and milk, which is to be poured into the rectum.

Nursing and childcare

It was customary for a mother to breastfeed her infant for a period of up to three years. The Egyptians may have recognised that this was the best and most reliable source of nourishment, and were perhaps aware that extended breastfeeding could delay the conception of a new baby.

However, this custom could cause chronic health problems for the mother. In pregnancy, and even more so with lactation, the maternal skeleton is eroded by the foetal demand for calcium, which, when compounded by a poor diet, can lead to abnormalities in the bone. Evidence of this was observed in a histological section of bone taken from a Nubian female of child-bearing age (Denton 2008: 80–82). This demonstrates an episodic removal, healing and subsequent removal of the bone that coincided with the woman's cycle of normal health interspersed with periods of pregnancy and lactation. A woman's general health could ultimately be undermined through several pregnancies and extended periods of lactation.

Another difficulty could arise when a mother did not have enough milk to breastfeed her child. Sometimes wet-nurses were employed for this task, on occasion becoming highly regarded members of the family unit (see Chapter 2d).

Studies of childhood in ancient Egypt (Janssen & Janssen 2007; Marshall 2022) show that mothers and their offspring faced continuing challenges. Pregnancy, birth, infancy and a child's early years were precarious stages of life, when every support and assistance was required. Sometimes pharmaceutical treatments could be prescribed for a variety of ailments and troubling conditions, but great reliance was also placed on magico-religious protection. Divinities such as Hathor, Taweret, Bes and Beset were especially powerful in this respect, while the possession of amulets was believed to ward off many evils (see Chapter 1a). Incantations were another powerful force available to women and children, and it was believed that the 'Spells for a Mother and Child' in P. Berlin 3027 offered them a special level of magical protection (Parkinson 1991: 58) (see Chapter 2d).

(d) Old age and health

Life expectancy

Some radiographic studies undertaken on the Royal Mummies have indicated an age-at-death of an individual ruler at variance with the inscriptional and historical data. This problem has been addressed by Wente (1980: 234–85), who suggests that a purely historical approach that ignores the radiological conclusions should be adopted. More recently, the approach to the demographic analyses of mummies and skeletal samples has been reviewed and it is now recognised that methods used to assign ages and sexes to skeletons are conditional upon the samples from which the methods are derived. So, for a more accurate determination, ageing and sexing are now undertaken in association with demographic studies (Konigsberg & Frankenberg 2013; Zakrzewski 2015).

Other inscriptional and palaeopathological sources provide evidence for the general population over 2000 years of pharaonic history. These indicate that, if people survived infancy, early childhood and occupational hazards, half the adult population probably lived into their thirties, with the average age-at-death for men in the late thirties and for women slightly younger (Masali & Chiarelli 1972). In addition, it is considered that some 90 per cent of the adult population probably did not live far beyond the age of fifty, although there were some notable exceptions (see below). Therefore, in ancient Egyptian terms, 'old age' is generally defined as the years covering the mid-thirties to the early fifties.

Attitudes towards old age

Unlike some other great ancient civilisations such as India and China, where the virtues of old age were praised, the Egyptians had a more ambivalent attitude. Some monumental inscriptions, prayers and funerary wishes express the hope for a good old age (*i3wt nfr*) with the wisdom and authority of advanced years without associated weakness (Frood 2010). Doubtless some older people acquired this wealth of experience and increased knowledge and wisdom that could be passed on to younger generations, but this is not generally emphasised or recognised even in the Wisdom Literature (Janssen & Janssen 2007: 139–43).

In fact, the Egyptians rarely praised the virtues of old age, but regarded it as a time of physical and mental decline. Indeed, extant literary accounts focus primarily on the various physical and mental problems that can come with old age. The most famous is in the Wisdom Instruction of Ptahhotep, preserved on three papyri and one wooden tablet, of which the earliest version dates to the Middle Kingdom. It was probably composed in the 6th Dynasty and contains thirty-seven maxims describing the basic values and mode of conduct required in Egyptian society. Ptahhotep, the vizier or king's first minister, sets out his advice to the young, commencing with an address to the king in which he describes the characteristic conditions of his own declining years. These include increasing weakness, weariness, loss of hearing and eyesight, inability to speak or breathe, memory loss, aches and pains, and mobility difficulties. In summary, he says: 'What age does to people is evil in everything, all taste is gone … ' (Lichtheim 1975: 63).

A similar picture of age-related physical decline is given in the fictional autobiography *The Story of Sinuhe*. Having fled to Syro-Palestine in his youth, Sinuhe describes the afflictions brought by advancing years, and yearns to regain his youthful faculties and return home to Egypt (Parkinson 1997).

However, the most serious conditions associated with old age do not appear to have affected everyone equally. Palaeopathological studies provide the most informative data for all classes, and for the elite there is also inscriptional evidence confirming that several kings (most notably Pepy II and Ramesses II) and some officials lived and retained their titles into old age, although the extent to which they were actually capable of performing their duties is not known (Hornung 1992).

Illnesses and afflictions associated with old age

The Egyptians defined old age in terms of increasing functional, physical and psychological incapacity rather than on the basis of an individual's chronological age. They would have understood and appreciated the current saying 'You're as old as you feel'. The range of problems they encountered in their declining years is represented in inscriptional, iconographic and palaeopathological sources.

Blindness was a significant problem that apparently affected all age groups (see Chapter 6e). Some evidence comes from palaeopathological material but, since the eyes are not usually well preserved in mummies, most is derived from inscriptional or iconographic sources. These sources show that trachoma, which

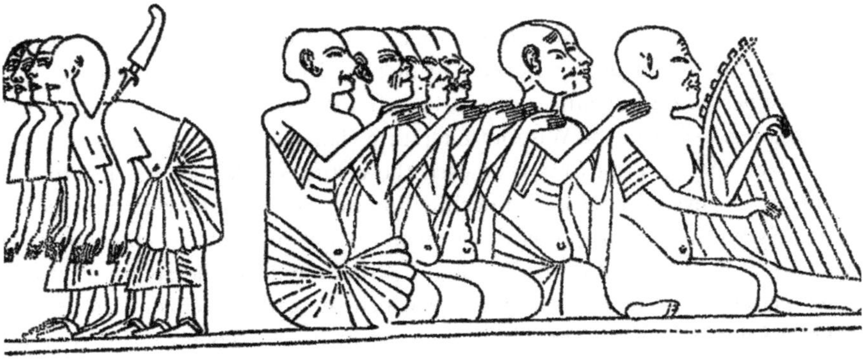

Figure 6.3. Representation of blindness in harpists, typically depicted with the artistic conventions of old age – baldness and rolls of bodily fat. A scene from the tomb of Meryra at Tell el-Amarna (Amarna tomb No. 4). Redrawn by K. N. White after Davies (1903: pl. 21) and Ghalioungui (1963: fig. 17).

is still prevalent today in Egypt and North Africa, was probably the commonest eye condition (Sandison 1967), but peripheral neuritis, cataracts, onchocerciasis ('river blindness') and possibly diabetes mellitus also occurred (David & Tapp 1992: 147). A tomb scene showing a harpist with a prominent, tortuous temporal artery may represent thrombosed ocular arteries, which are another cause of blindness (Jantzen 1968).

Deteriorating eyesight is often attributable to old age, a situation noted in inscriptions and perhaps represented in tomb wall scenes showing, for example, Paatenemheb (Jantzen 1968) and Nakht (Davies 1917): such scenes depict groups of musicians who provide entertainment at banquets and feature harpists who are shown with the artistic conventions of old age – baldness and rolls of bodily fat (Fig. 6.3). The harpist is often depicted as blindfolded or with his visible eye closed, which may indicate blindness (Fuchs 1964; Jantzen 1968). This perhaps implies that a special employment opportunity existed for the blind, but presumably considerable periods of musical training were required for these roles, and this perhaps favoured the employment of younger persons. However, once engaged on this career it is possible that such individuals continued to perform in their later years.

Loss of hearing is another affliction that would have come with old age, although there is also evidence that it could also be caused by various pathological conditions (see Chapter 6e).

Descriptions of old age include references to forgetfulness and intellectual impairment, but the medical papyri contain no allusions to any such malfunction in the elderly or in younger patients. Identification of cerebrovascular disease in tissue obtained from several mummies may indicate that some individuals suffered from 'strokes' (Ruffer 1911; Worth Estes 1993: 46).

Studies on skeletal and mummified remains have produced extensive evidence of degenerative diseases that often attend old age. These include osteoarthritis (associated with cartilage degeneration) in the spine, knees and hips (Gray 1966b, 1967, 1973; Dawson & Gray 1968: 41; Raven & Taconis 2005: 64) and osteoporosis. This condition is seen predominantly in women today, but a radiological survey of one museum collection has identified osteoporosis in equal numbers of male and female mummies (Raven & Taconis 2005: 64).

Spondylosis is another degenerative condition of the spine found in the palaeopathological record (Aufderheide & Rodríguez-Martin 1998: 96–97). This deterioration of the spine, mainly the result of ageing, can cause localised pain in the neck and upper, middle or lower back. Ankylosing spondylitis (a form of arthritis) has been reported in human remains (Aufderheide & Rodríguez-Martin 1998: 102–04); characterised by long-standing inflammation of areas of the body, especially the spine, it results in extreme fatigue, pain and stiffness in the spine, and swelling elsewhere caused by inflamed joints. It can develop before old age, but an existing condition will often deteriorate with advancing years.

Cancer and old age

The terms tumour and cancer are often used interchangeably, which can on occasion be misleading. A tumour is not necessarily a cancer, as the word tumour simply refers to a mass of tissue, and some of the wall scenes and references in the medical texts to swellings may represent a tumour. Some examples, however, may indicate a malignant tumour (cancer) that can proliferate rapidly and invade surrounding tissues, eventually spreading to other parts of the body via the bloodstream or lymphatic system.

Possible sources of evidence for cancer in ancient Egypt include human skeletal remains, mummified bodies, the medical papyri and artistic sources. As examples of the condition have rarely been found in animal fossils, non-human primates and early humans, the general lack of evidence in ancient remains may indicate that the condition was rare in antiquity. However, many cancers are associated with increasing age and it is therefore not as common in populations with a shorter life expectancy, as in ancient Egypt.

Another factor in the frequency of cancer is that unhealthy lifestyle choices such as particular dietary regimes, pollution, lack of exercise and smoking, which have caused a rapid global increase in cancer, are a relatively modern phenomenon (David & Zimmerman 2010). Genetic predisposition may increase a person's risk to cancer, and pathogens, particularly viruses, can also be a factor in the development of tumours (Turnbull & Hodgson 2005; Liao 2006). Schistosomiasis, for example, common in ancient Egypt, is now recognised as a potential cause of bladder cancer (Bedwani *et al.* 1998).

Palaeopathological evidence

Although the age-at-death for most Egyptians was considerably lower than in modern societies, the palaeopathological record shows the development of other degenerative diseases, including arthritis, osteoporosis and Paget's disease. On the basis that a lower incidence of cancer could be due to the population's shorter lifespan, it might be expected that bone tumours primarily associated with the young in modern times would be present in ancient societies, but these again are rare in antiquity.

Despite the long history of palaeopathological study of human remains globally and particularly in ancient Egypt, the direct evidence of cancer from human remains is still comparatively rare, although more recent studies are revealing further cases (Zink *et al.* 1999; Nerlich *et al.* 2006; Esche *et al.* 2010; Molto & Sheldrick 2018). This is despite the growing number of remains available for study and an increase in the number of bioarchaeologists. It has been suggested that the apparent absence of cancer in archaeological remains may be caused partly by issues of tissue preservation. However, earlier experimental studies on modern mummified tissue have demonstrated that mummification preserves the features of malignancy well (Zimmerman 1977). It is possible that methods of analysis of ancient specimens may be inadequate to detect initial changes within bone, so that the incidence of cancers in ancient Egypt might be not quite as rare as initially assumed (Kozieradzka-Ogunmakin 2015).

Today increasing scientific research on mummified remains facilitated through improved and more readily available imaging techniques, including computed tomography scanning and scanning electron microscopic imaging, is providing an additional dataset, which is increasingly able to detect cancer in the soft tissues of mummified bodies (Nerlich & Bianucci 2021) (see Plate 6). Additionally, aDNA techniques can assist with identifying tumour-related genes and proteomics may be able to detect certain protein combinations at higher levels, which may correlate with particular cancers. Such techniques, in combination with increased attention to detail by those conducting palaeopathological research, may result in an increase in the number of ancient individuals identified with cancer.

The incidence of cancer in contemporary ancient Greek society presents an interesting comparison. It is unclear whether Greece inherited any legacy of medical knowledge relating to cancer from Egypt. The Hippocratic Corpus (*c.* 400 AD) provides the earliest clear extant reference to cancer, and Greek texts generally describe a range of tumours and swellings and indicate that their physicians were aware of a difference between benign and malignant tumours. In fact, cancer was quite widely recorded and studied in classical Greece, although it is unclear whether this reflected a real increase in its incidence or – as is more likely – a greater awareness of the condition.

In the absence of surgical intervention, evidence of cancer should remain in all affected preserved specimens from ancient societies. Extant evidence from ancient Egypt and the supposedly low incidence of malignancy reported in some other early societies appear to indicate that cancer was less prevalent in pre-industrialised times than today. However, Greek literary sources suggest a wider prevalence, and many cases in these other contexts may simply remain undetected.

Iconographic and inscriptional evidence

Is there evidence for tumours in the artistic and textual record from ancient Egypt? Most scenes showing people depict the individual in idealised form, as youthful and fit. There are a few examples of individuals with swellings but, in most of these cases, it is difficult to categorically identify any specific disease.

The medical papyri describe certain pathological conditions that have been tentatively identified as cancer, although diagnosis is far from certain and some researchers have interpreted these conditions as merely swellings or growths, without suggesting a differential diagnosis. P. Ebers includes a series of prescriptions (857–77) that provides the most extensive description of swellings in the medical papyri. The manner in which this subsection is arranged and organised may preserve the main elements of an earlier, undiscovered 'Book of Tumours' (David & Zimmerman 2010).

One example is Case 813: 'Another [remedy] for one in whom there is eating (*wnmt*) on her uterus, in whose vagina ulcers appear … ' (translated Ghalioungui 1987: 207). Opinions differ as to the translation of *wnmt*, with Ebbell (1937: 111) suggesting cancer but Grapow *et al.* (1954–1973: IV 2) and Ghalioungui (1987: 207) remaining more cautious. Nunn (1996: 81) comments that 'eating' is a graphic description of advanced malignancy and wonders if this could be an example of uterine cancer. A more recent interpretation by Strouhal *et al.* (2014: 151–52) comments that the reference to ulcers could point to it being an ulcerative infection of the vaginal and uterine mucous membrane.

P. Ebers 873, 874 and 877 all refer to a swelling of Khonsu. Ebers 874 states:

> Instructions for a tumour of Khonsu. If you examine a large swelling of Khonsu on any part of a man and it is uneven, and it has made many swellings. Something has appeared in it like that which there is air … . Then you shall say concerning it: It is a swelling of Khonsu. You should not do anything against it. (translated Ghalioungui 1987: 249–50)

An explanation for these types of swelling is not forthcoming, as the description and hieroglyphs are not completely understood. It has been suggested that the condition may be leprosy, but leprosy does not appear to be attested in ancient Egypt at the time the Ebers Papyrus was compiled. The case could be an example of cancer, but bubonic plague and neurofibromatosis are other conditions that have been suggested (Nunn 1996: 75).

P. Edwin Smith 45 refers to round 'masses' on the chest:

> If you should examine a man for spherical masses on his chest, how you find [is]: they have spread on his chest, and, if you put your hand on his chest, on those masses [how] you find it [the chest] is very cool, there being no heat at all within it, and how your hands find it [is]: they not being (?) granular, neither can they make fluid, nor generate secretions of water, while they are ball-like to your hand. Then you are to say about him: 'One who has ball-like masses: a medical condition I will fight with'. (translated Sanchez & Meltzer 2012: 270–71)

The finding of 'no heat' in this case suggests that the ancient Egyptians recognised this condition as being different from an infection. Little treatment is offered, implying an insufficient understanding of the condition and a questionable prognosis. Various diagnoses have been suggested, including benign tumours such as neurofibromatosis (Sanchez & Meltzer 2012: 269–73).

Care of the elderly

Palaeopathological evidence indicates that some state provision existed to address the needs of the sick, disabled and elderly (see Chapters 2d, 6b, 6e). In addition, although 'pensions' were not universally available, the elderly in specific groups were given some support by the king or the state. For example, aged members of the royal workforce may have received a reduced monthly grain ration, while land allotments paid to soldiers during active service would have supported them as veterans in old age. Some high-status individuals, such as honorary priests and elite palace officials appointed by the king, enjoyed the privilege and benefit of a sinecure attached to their position (Janssen & Janssen 2007: 231–35). A legal text inscribed on the wall of a 19th Dynasty official, Samut, indicates that he bequeathed his property to Mut in return for a type of pension (Frood 2007: 89).

There was a moral expectation that each family would provide the primary medical care for its own members, although this is not stated in any extant legal document (McDowell 1998). A couple hoped that their children would care for them in old age, but those who were childless could resort to adoption, divorce or remarriage to beget an heir, or to polygamy or purchase of a slave (Janssen & Janssen 2007: 220–37). If none of these options were pursued, then the elderly had to rely on neighbours or distant relatives for assistance.

At all levels of society it was considered desirable to appoint someone as a 'Staff of Old Age' who could relieve an older person of some responsibilities. There were some historical periods when an elderly ruler or high official was able to devolve some duties to a deputy (his intended heir or successor) but still retain his own title and status, as is demonstrated in documents such as the *Instruction of Ptahhotep*, autobiographies such as that of Amenemhat and the installation of the 18th Dynasty vizier Useramun.

Combating old age

Ancient Egypt provides the earliest surviving evidence of a society that idealised youth and rigorously sought to combat or delay the ageing process. In life, Egyptians used a range of cosmetics to enhance their looks and promote a youthful appearance, which included deodorants, facial cosmetics and depilatory and skin cleansing creams, as well as treatments for greying hair and baldness.

Archaeological discoveries have provided some information about such cosmetics. For example, ointment jars containing cleansing cream were found in the burial of three queens of Tuthmosis III. Popular remedies to combat the symptoms of ageing are provided in the medical papyri, and include treatments for wrinkled skin, greying hair and baldness.

In his study of the Edwin Smith Papyrus, Breasted translates the title of a remedy on the verso of the document as 'Recipe for transforming an old man into a youth'. In alternative translations this is given as 'The Book of Passing Old Age as a Youth' or 'Beginning of the Book of Transforming an Old Man into a Youth'. The main ingredient in this recipe for treating wrinkled skin is the *hemayet* fruit. This word was not translated by Breasted, but more recently it has been rendered as 'bitter almonds' (Allen 2005: 113–15), an extract of which is mandelic acid, a product used today for skin care (Jacobs & Culbertson 2018).

P. Ebers contains recipes to treat greying hair (451–63) and to encourage hair growth on a bald head (464–74). Animal fats were a favourite ingredient in the latter, as seen in, for example, Ebers 465: 'Another [remedy] to cause hair to grow on a bald person: fat of lion, 1; fat of hippopotamus, 1; fat of crocodile, 1; fat of cat,1; fat of snake, 1; fat of ibex, 1; make as one thing, smear (or anoint) the head of the bald person with it' (translated Ghalioungui 1987).

The desire to retain youth continued beyond death. The body was mummified to preserve it for eternity, and there was generally no desire to reflect the reality of old age and sickness in religious art forms. It was customary for the elite to be depicted as young, vigorous and healthy in tomb wall reliefs and religious art, in the hope that they would continue in this form in the afterlife (see below).

However, physical conditions associated with old age are shown iconographically in some representations of servants and even the elite (Janssen & Janssen 2007: 151–61). Examples are found mainly in statuary, but some occur in tomb wall reliefs. The images almost exclusively depict men, although occasionally statues of elderly women servants have been identified. In all these figures physical signs of ageing are shown on their bodies rather than in facial features, and include male corpulence, pendulous breasts, postural difficulties and walking with a stick. Greying hair or baldness as typical signs of ageing are sometimes seen in depictions of servants, but baldness on an elite male represented a shaved head that indicated priestly status rather than loss of hair.

The Egyptian attitude to old age was inspired by the religious beliefs that underpinned and permeated almost all aspects of their society. A key feature was the general acceptance that, for those who had lived by society's rules, death did not represent personal annihilation but instead provided a means of attaining eternal life, where youth and physical perfection would ultimately be restored.

(e) Disability and deformity: an enlightened attitude?

Iconographic, inscriptional and palaeopathological sources

The palaeopathological record, medical papyri and funerary iconography provide an overview of disease and physical abnormalities found in Egypt (David 2017a). However, source material relating specifically to deformity and disability is incomplete and unreliable.

The interpretation of iconographic representations of deformity and disability in funerary art can be problematic. Religious art customarily represented the elite with idealised, perfect physical forms, whereas the non-elite would sometimes be depicted with physical abnormalities. This difference was derived from the concept that all the elements in religious scenes were expected to become functional once the priest had performed the 'Opening of the Mouth' ceremony. For this, the priest used a ritual adze to touch the mouth, hands and feet of all human representations in the wall scenes, and this was believed to imbue them with life and enable them to perform their duties throughout eternity. As a result of this magical intervention, the elite were expected to retain their youth and remain physically fit and active in the afterlife, and even the servants and workers shown with physical disabilities would be able to undertake any tasks required of them.

A departure from this tradition occurred during the Amarna Period when, from the middle of King Akhenaten's reign, iconographic sources show him and other members of the royal family, including Tutankhamun, with a distinctive physique. This is characterised by spindly legs, an enlarged skull, prominent lower jaw, well-developed breasts and wide hips. As Akhenaten's reign progressed, this art style became the normal way of representing all human figures. The identification of Akhenaten's mummy remains uncertain, so there is no firm palaeopathological evidence to confirm whether or not the iconographic sources present a true picture of his physique. However, the same unusual features occur in some iconographic images of Tutankhamun but are not visible in his mummy, which is firmly provenanced and identified. These unusual features may simply be characteristic of the art of this period – an attempt at realism directly related to contemporary religious innovations – or may indicate that he suffered from a specific medical condition (see Chapter 1c).

In general, however, traditional religious iconography records only a limited number of diseases and afflictions, and does not depict many of the conditions that would have been present in the elite population. The physical abnormalities most frequently represented in non-elite individuals (servants and workers) include dwarfism, kyphosis, blindness, poliomyelitis, clubfoot (talipes equinovarus), trauma, hernial swellings and genu recurvatum. Even in non-elite representations, however, some diseases and conditions are omitted, perhaps because they were difficult to depict or considered to be inappropriate as elements of tomb wall scenes. Some conditions, perhaps those regarded as especially dangerous, uncontrollable or capable of causing instability or destruction, may have been excluded through fear that they might introduce evil forces into the afterlife (Robinson 2017: 6).

Particular problems arise when interpreting funerary representations that may indicate either a specific medical condition or a stylistic convention used to depict a particular occupation (Fuchs 1964; Manniche 1978) (see 'Blindness' below).

Diseases and conditions omitted from funerary art are sometimes present in palaeopathological examples or described in the texts. These include parasitic diseases (although iconographic sources sometimes show secondary symptoms); scorpion or snake bites; diseases of the lungs, ears, nose, skin and cardiovascular systems; paralysis; joint pain; and dental and gynaecological problems.

The medical papyri do not record deformity or specific examples of disability, perhaps because many people with these conditions had a short lifespan and would not have sought treatment. In addition, some conditions, such as dwarfism, were seemingly regarded as a sign of 'otherness' or divine recognition, rather than a medical condition requiring treatment (see Chapter 5d). However, the texts prescribe some treatments for secondary conditions such as blindness, deafness, paralysis or joint pain that may have arisen as the result of underlying disabilities.

Palaeopathologists have access to a wide range of ancient Egyptian mummified and skeletal human remains for general disease studies. These also offer a rich resource for investigating deformity and disabilities, but much evidence is undoubtedly missing or is difficult to interpret. At best, this material represents an incomplete and sometimes nuanced perspective of the true situation.

Deformities and disabilities most often encountered

A single factor such as genetic inheritance, congenital abnormality, disease or general deterioration can be identified as the likely cause of some physical anomalies. In other cases there is more than one possible cause, or the condition can be the result of a combination of factors.

Genetic conditions

Egyptian iconographic and palaeopathological sources provide evidence of several conditions attributable to genetic factors. There are a few examples of osteogenesis imperfecta, a rare inherited bone disorder (Brothwell 1967; Dawson & Gray 1968: 13–14, 42; Gray 1969; Aufderheide & Rodríguez-Martin 1998: 365–66; Lowenstein 2009), and cleft palate, which is caused by arrested embryonic development (Aufderheide & Rodríguez-Martin 1998: 58). However, the condition most frequently encountered in the period spanning Predynastic to Roman times is achondroplasia (Dawson 1938; Kozma 2006). This commonest form of dwarfism is characterised by short limbs, a normal trunk, and a disproportionately large head (Dasen 1993: 9–11). Dwarfs were believed to possess powers of rebirth and regeneration, and their physical condition seems to have presented no barrier to employment at the highest levels (see Chapter 1c and below).

Congenital abnormalities

Recorded congenital abnormalities include several tentative identifications of clubfoot (see below); bone anomalies; spina bifida (where, during foetal development, the lower end of the spine fails to close around the spinal column) (Rabino Massa 1979; Molto 1989) and abnormal pelvic structures that led to complications in childbirth. Studies indicate that the two female foetuses found in Tutankhamun's tomb show multiple congenital conditions, including severe spinal conditions and Sprengel's deformity (see p. 180).

Some pathological causes of physical anomalies

Pathological causes of physical anomalies include acromegaly (a rare endocrine condition) (Worth Estes 1993: 443, n. 39; Brothwell 2002: 124, pl. 5.1C); gout (a metabolic disease) (Smith & Dawson 1924: 157; Nuki & Simkin 2006); spinal conditions including scoliosis and kyphosis; and cerebral palsy (see Chapter 2d).

Examples of spinal curvature are recorded in iconographic and palaeopathological sources. Pathological, congenital or degenerative factors can cause scoliosis (lateral curvature of the spine with rotation of the vertebrae) (Dawson & Gray 1968: 38–39; David 1979: 29; Worth Estes 1993: 44; Raven & Taconis 2005: 63) and kyphosis (forwards curvature of the upper spine) (Morse *et al.* 1964: Buikstra *et al.* 1993). Sometimes both conditions occur together, as in the mummy

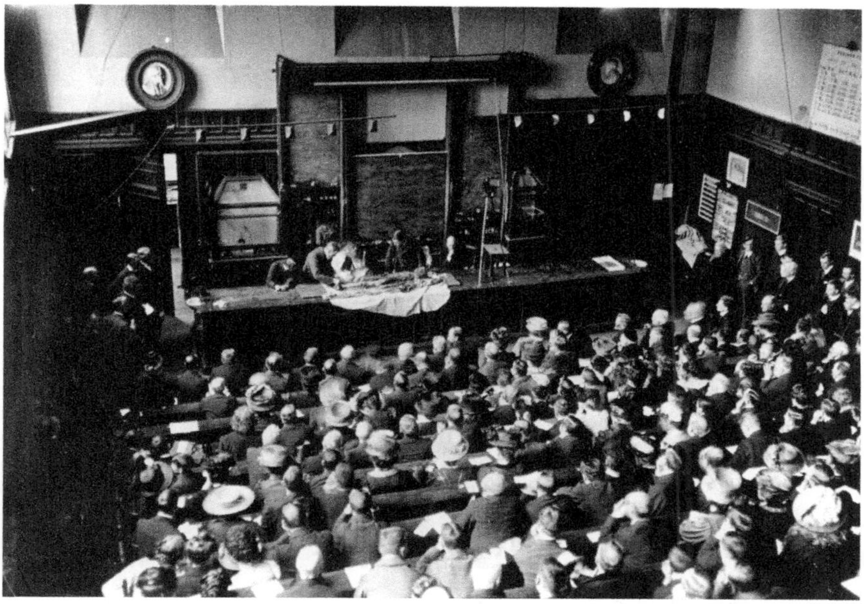

Figure 6.4. Dr Margaret Murray (centre) and her multidisciplinary team unwrap and autopsy the mummy of Nakht-ankh. This took place in front of an invited audience at The University of Manchester on 7 May 1908. More recent studies have demonstrated that Nakht-ankh suffered from several diseases (courtesy of The Manchester Museum, The University of Manchester).

of Khnum-nakht. First discovered by Dr Margaret Murray's interdisciplinary team when they unwrapped and autopsied the mummies of two brothers at Manchester Museum in 1908 (Murray 1910), this finding has been confirmed by further studies (David 1979) (Fig. 6.4). The condition would have greatly affected the quality of Khnum-nakht's life: the upper part of his body was bent towards the ground and he would have experienced great difficulty in walking.

Most evidence of deformity and disability found in human remains provides information about the presence of the condition and its effects upon the person when they were alive. This includes examples of amputation, where some but not all patients survived (Brothwell & Møller-Christensen 1963; David 1979: 83–89; Nerlich *et al.* 2000b; Dupras *et al.* 2008; Nerlich *et al.* 2010b; Finch *et al.* 2012; Finch 2012/2013).

The autopsy of the poorly preserved mummy of a young girl (1770 in the Manchester Museum collection) confirmed the findings of a preliminary radiological survey that showed that the lower parts of the legs were missing (David 1979: 83–89) (Fig. 6.5). The limbs may have been amputated shortly before death – the left one below the knee through the tibia, and the right one above

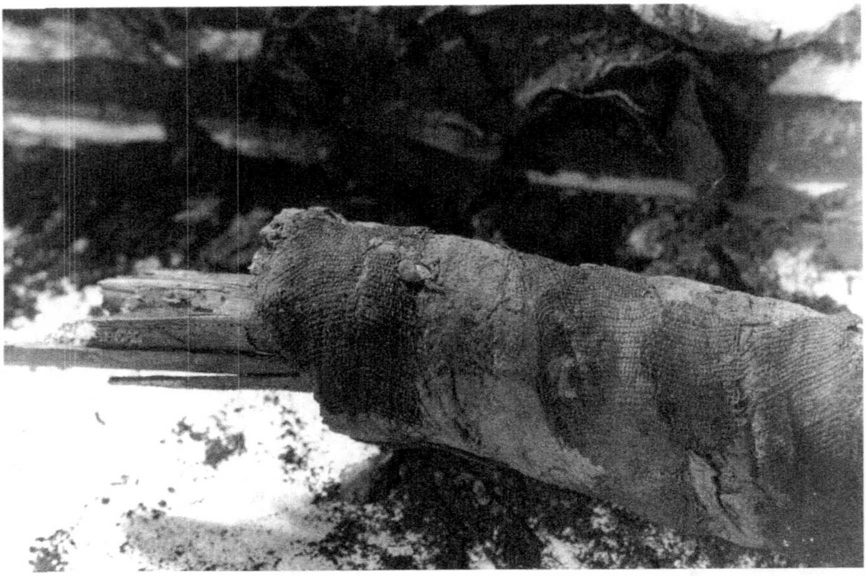

Figure 6.5. Right leg of a mummy (Manchester Museum 1770), revealed during the unwrapping of the mummy in 1975, showing amputation and prosthetic wooden limb inserted alongside bones (courtesy of The University of Manchester).

the knee through the femur. This was possibly an unsuccessful attempt to save the life of someone who, had she survived, would have been severely disabled.

Accidents and injuries

Deformities and disabilities were sometimes the result of accidents or injuries (see Chapter 4a). Fractures, wounds, dislocations and amputations could be the outcome of warfare (see Chapter 6g), interpersonal violence (see Chapter 6f), accidents (see Chapter 5c, 6g), legal punishments (see Chapter 6f) and medical intervention (see Chapters 5a, 5c).

These conditions are recorded in inscriptional, iconographic and palaeopathological sources. Some successful methods of treatment seem to have been available. For example, the Edwin Smith Papyrus (Breasted 1930; Sanchez & Meltzer 2012) describes trauma episodes, some perhaps acquired at building sites, and also wounds possibly sustained during battle. An equally high level of care and effective treatment was provided at the pyramid site for both men and women, regardless of their social status (Hussien *et al.* 2010). Treatments included joint manipulation to reduce fractures and dislocations and intravital amputations (see Chapters 5a, 5c).

Mental illness, intellectual impairment and malfunction

Mental illness or intellectual impairment and malfunction are generally ignored in ancient Near Eastern literature (Kellenberger 2013), and in most Egyptological studies it has been argued that, although Egyptian sources indicate that physicians treated symptoms characteristic of some conditions, they did not associate them with a particular disease or understand how they were caused (Worth Estes 1993: 107–08). Examples include references to seizures possibly associated with epilepsy and to psychic or mental symptoms perhaps indicative of severe psychiatric diseases such as schizophrenia (Ghalioungui 1963: 128–29). However, based on a new translation of the *Book of the Heart* (Papyrus Ebers, sections 854a–855z), Clayton (2022: 103) has suggested that sometimes when the Egyptians used the term *ib* (heart) they were describing a state of mind or being (cognitive and emotional states), rather than the clinical condition of the organ, and that this should be interpreted as a description of mental illness. This might then provide some insight into their ideas about the origins of mental illnesses. Emotional depression may also be recorded in a series of prayers inscribed in documents and on memorial stelae set up by the royal workmen in chapels at Deir el-Medina (Gunn 1916).

Hydrocephalus (an abnormal accumulation of fluid in parts of the brain) can be caused by genetic factors, infections, tumours or trauma. Rare pathological examples have been found from ancient Egypt and Nubia (Derry 1913; Aufderheide & Rodriguez-Martin 1998: 58) but they do not provide an accurate account. Hydrocephalus might have been much more widespread in the population, but this is not reflected in the palaeopathological record because few examples of the physical remains of children affected with hydrocephalus (from which they would have died at birth or in infancy) have been found.

Conditions where the cause cannot be precisely identified

Mummy (DUROM 1999.32) in the Oriental Museum, Durham provides a good example of a physical anomaly where the exact cause cannot be identified (Finch 2012/2013). The lower part of the left forearm was missing during the owner's lifetime. This may have been the result of genetic, congenital or developmental disorders, disease, trauma or surgical amputation. At the time of mummification, the missing limb was replaced with a prosthetic arm for use in the next life (Gray 1967).

Blindness can be the result of genetic inheritance, birth defects, accidents or eye disease (see Chapter 6d). Egyptian ophthalmologists were highly regarded in the ancient world, and some of their treatments are recorded in the Ebers Medical Papyrus (336–431). These include remedies for unidentified eye disease, trachoma, cloudiness and watering of the eyes, foreign bodies and eye injuries, inflammation, blood in the eye, and white spots on the eyes.

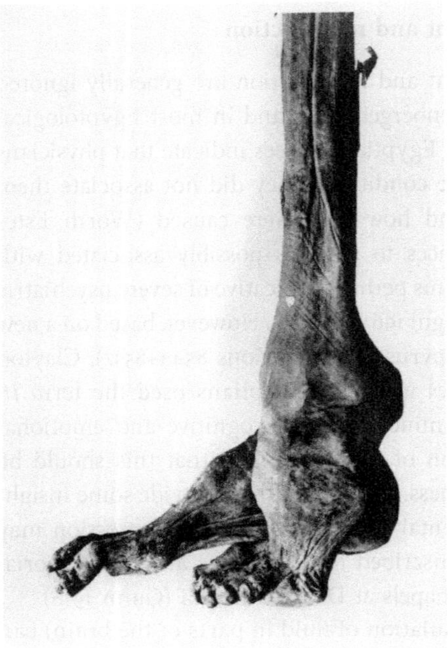

Figure 6.6. Deformed foot of the 19th Dynasty pharaoh Siptah. This has been attributed to either talipes equinovarus, inborn defect of the spine, cerebral palsy or poliomyelitis. Now in the Royal Mummies' Hall at the National Museum of Egyptian Civilization in Cairo, Egypt (Smith 1912: pl. 62).

The medical papyri also include prescriptions for deafness, another condition that can occur with advancing age or as the result of genetic inheritance, birth defects, accidents or disease arising from pathological conditions. Those recorded in mummified and skeletal remains include otitis media (infection of the middle ear), perforated ear drum (Benitez 1988) and mastoiditis (Smith & Wood Jones 1910: 284; Leek 1986: 191).

Walking difficulties can be the result of genetic factors, disease or accident. Sometimes the pathology indicates the most likely cause of a disability, but problems can arise when interpreting the evidence. For example, the initial anatomical examination of a mummy belonging to Khnum-nakht, carried out in Manchester in 1908, concluded that the left foot displayed a well-marked degree of congenital clubfoot (Murray 1910). In support of this it was remarked that the thickening of the skin and superficial tissues over the region of the cuboid were still quite evident. However, subsequent radiological investigations have shown no evidence of arthritis or secondary bone change in the foot, conditions that might be expected in a long-standing congenital deformity such as clubfoot. Consequently, the 'deformity' is now explained as the result of excessively tight bandaging of the foot when the embalmers wrapped the body after death (Brothwell 1967; David 1979: 29).

Other identifications of clubfoot in mummies have been controversial. The condition was diagnosed in the mummy of Tutankhamun (Hawass *et al.* 2010: 191), but disputed (Marchant 2013: 191–94), while the 'deformity' described in the original investigation of the 'Leeds Mummy', Nesyamun, was later recognised as evidence of tight bandaging of the foot (David & Tapp 1992: 109).

The body of the 19th Dynasty ruler Siptah provides the most famous example of a wrongly diagnosed case of congenital clubfoot in a mummy (Fig. 6.6). Discovered in the royal cache in the Tomb of Amenhotep II in 1898, the mummy was unwrapped in Cairo by Grafton Elliot Smith in 1905. He identified congenital clubfoot based on a shortening of the left leg and gross deformity of the ankle (Smith 1912: 71). Initially, this diagnosis was supported by Dzierzykray-Rogalski and Prominska (1994), but has been discarded in favour of theories that the king may have suffered from an inborn defect of the spine or a variety of cerebral palsy, brain damage at or before birth (Dodson 2016: 103) or a neuromuscular disease such as poliomyelitis (Harris & Weeks 1973).

So far, only rare examples of poliomyelitis have been tentatively identified in ancient Egypt. Palaeopathological evidence indicates that it may be present in a skeleton from Deshasha (Mitchell 1900; Harris & Wente 1980: 69), and an image on a funerary stela dating to the 18th Dynasty may also represent this condition. The scene shows the owner, Roma, a temple doorkeeper, with a grossly wasted and shortened right leg and a deformity of the foot. He may have contracted poliomyelitis in childhood and, if this occurred before growth of the leg bones was complete, the deformed foot would have compensated for walking on the shortened leg (Nunn 1996: 77; Jørgensen 1998: 118–19). Alternatively, this may depict a deformity caused by clubfoot, with associated wasting and shortening of the leg; however, the extreme shortening shown here is not usually associated with clubfoot. Another possibility is cerebral palsy, but poliomyelitis remains the most likely explanation.

More recently, the CT scan of a New Kingdom mummy in the Egyptian Museum in Cairo (coffin 4213) revealed shortening of the right leg and abnormalities of the foot that has been suggested as another example of poliomyelitis (Zaki *et al.* 2017).

Poliomyelitis has been considered a possible diagnosis in all these cases; however, this disease is very contagious and usually spreads widely throughout a population, but there is no evidence that this occurred here. So far, only a few examples have been tentatively identified as poliomyelitis, and this provides insufficient evidence to confirm that the disease was indeed present in ancient Egypt.

Life expectancy and old age

Estimates of life expectancy suggest that half the adult population probably reached only their mid-thirties while 90 per cent were unlikely to live much beyond the age of fifty. In this context, 'old age' was very unwelcome, being recognised as a time of life when deteriorating health and a range of debilitating conditions were likely to occur (Janssen & Janssen 2007) (see Chapter 6d).

Archaeological and inscriptional evidence contains references to rheumatism, arthritis, breathlessness, giddiness, baldness, deafness, failing eyesight, forgetfulness and senility. There is also palaeopathological evidence of osteoarthritis, ankylosing spondylitis, osteoporosis, peripheral vascular disease and aneurysm formation, and possibly diabetes mellitus.

Treatment and care of the sick, disabled and elderly

There was a remarkable degree of medical and social support for the sick, disabled and elderly. There is palaeopathological evidence that people lived with healed fractures, limb amputation and even severely incapacitating conditions such as cerebral palsy and paralysis (see Chapter 2d). Other examples include paraplegic patients found in a burial at Shurafa (Derry 1913) and amputees who were treated at Giza (Hussien *et al.* 2010) and elsewhere. The mummified remains of a 21st Dynasty priestess, Tabasety, revealed that although she had a relatively long life she was severely disabled due to a traumatic event early in her life, resulting in severe fractures to the pelvic region that never healed (Sousa 2019: 130–46). All these patients would have required either short- or long-term medical and nursing care and a high level of social support, which were probably provided either by individual families or by medical professionals at the temples or within the community.

It is evident that the Egyptians did not abandon or neglect those with long-term medical conditions. However, to what extent were they generally included in society (Jeffreys & Tait 2000)? Inscriptions and tomb wall scenes confirm that some people with disabilities or deformities were allowed to hold religious or public office, sometimes at a high level. In addition, special employment opportunities may have existed for people with particular conditions (see above and Chapter 5d).

Dwarfs (see Chapter 1c) often enjoyed particularly favourable employment opportunities (Dasen 1993; Kozma 2006). They often held privileged positions and were allocated specific responsibilities. Some took part in temple ceremonies or were employed and worked in royal and elite households, where they served as nurses, midwives and personal attendants. In particular, they looked after the master's clothing and jewellery – tasks that required dexterity and application. A depiction of a dwarf as a jeweller is in the Tomb of Mereruka at Saqqara (Duell 1938: plates 29–30, 32–33). They also sang, danced and played musical instruments to entertain the master's household. Other duties included the care of domestic pets and assisting with various activities on their employer's estate.

The remarkably successful career of Seneb demonstrates some of the opportunities that were available to dwarfs (see Chapter 1c). He held an important position at the Royal Court as 'Chief of all the Dwarfs of the Wardrobe' and was also a mortuary priest of the funerary cults of kings Khufu (*c.* 2589–2566 BC, 4th Dynasty) and Djedefra (*c.* 2566–2558 BC, 4th Dynasty). An inscription in his mastaba-tomb at Giza also attests to his wealthy status as the possessor of large flocks and herds.

It is likely that dwarfism was not regarded as a disease or deformity but as a normal if unusual human condition, perhaps an example of 'otherness' or even a divine manifestation that represented a blessing from the gods. It is noteworthy that Bes, a powerful apotropaic deity associated with fertility, marriage and the protection of women, displays many of the features of achondroplasia, and P. Leiden includes a so-called 'Spell of the Dwarf' to facilitate birth.

It is noteworthy that other contemporary societies had different attitudes to deformity (Laes 2017, see Chapter 7a). One example is the contrast between the perceptions and attitudes of the Egyptians and Greeks: while both regarded the human body as a reflection of their gods' own appearance, the Greeks believed that their deities possessed idealised, perfect bodies, and that any human departure from this was ungodlike and unacceptable. The Egyptian approach was more flexible: their religion did not stigmatise physical anomalies and their pantheon encompassed animal, hybrid and human representations.

In general, the Egyptians did not hope to find universal perfection in this world. No-one, including those with deformities and disabilities, expected to experience a trouble-free life; instead, everyone hoped to achieve an idealised state of perfection in the afterlife. This outlook may have promoted a general inclusivity and a willingness to find practical measures that would create a well-integrated society.

(f, i) Interpersonal violence

There is a wide array of images of violence, both collective and interpersonal, available throughout the timespan of ancient Egypt. As our observation of Egyptian scenes is divorced from their original time, it is necessary to try and distinguish images of violence from its practice (Bestock 2019: 268). Iconography highlights the violence of warfare, collective violence that was sanctioned and considered necessary. Such scenes often depict the binding and smiting of prisoners, demonstrating the continuation of violence after hostilities had ended. These pictorial representations are augmented by textual and archaeological sources. However, violence, and particularly the abuse that one could inflict on servants or subordinates, was condemned by the moral values of the day, as attested in Chapter 125 of The Book of the Dead, the Negative Confession: 'I have not caused pain … I have not caused harm to be done to a servant by his master … I have not inflicted pain on anyone' (Faulkner 1972: 29–34; Sales 2018).

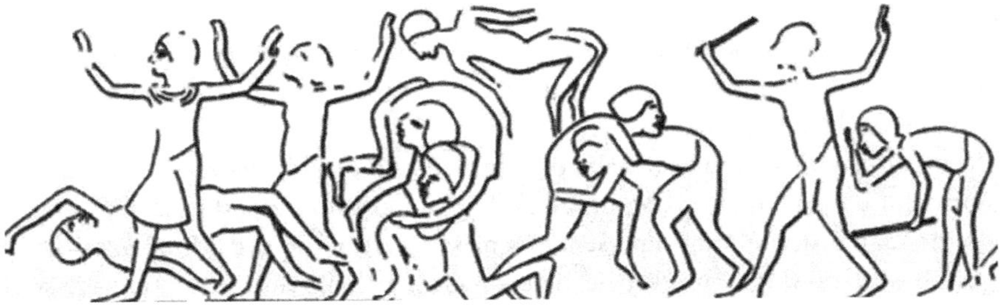

Figure 6.7. Wall-scene from the 18th Dynasty tomb of Meryra II at Tell el-Amarna (Amarna tomb No. 2) depicting wrestling, a sport that could result in parry fractures, in Nubia. Redrawn by K. N. White after Davies (1905: pl. 38) and Carroll (1988: fig. 2).

Injury patterns detectible in bioarchaeological studies provide tangible evidence and make a significant contribution to any evaluation of interpersonal violence. Analysis of wound location has been shown to be useful in distinguishing between accidental and violent injury. Fractures of the skull, face, ribs and hands, as well as multiple injuries, can signify interpersonal violence. Injuries to the cranium are a particularly useful indicator of violent conflict, and studies have linked the incidence of cranial trauma with the level of interpersonal violence in a population (e.g., Smith 1997; Walker 1997).

Parry fractures – injuries to forearms incurred while shielding oneself from a blow to the head – can be another indicator of this type of violence. Such injuries can be sustained in violent altercations but also in sporting activities such as stick fighting and wrestling, which were particularly popular in ancient Nubia (Carroll 1988) (Fig. 6.7). Care has to be taken not to interpret all forearm fractures as parry fractures, especially in the absence of cranio-facial injuries, as many of these injuries are likely to be the result of accidental falls. In addition, stress fractures resulting from repeated overuse and strain create fractures very similar in appearance, although these are usually accompanied by degenerative joint disease. Judd (2008) has suggested quantitative guidelines, including a range of measurements, that help to define the parry fracture configuration.

Importantly, skeletal injuries are estimated to represent no more than 40 per cent of all injuries acquired during assaults (Geldermalsen 1993; Matthew *et al.* 1996). Soft tissue injuries such as cuts, bruising and internal damage, sometimes fatal, are invisible in the bioarchaeological record, and so any assessment and interpretation of the levels of interpersonal violence will, as a consequence, always be an underestimate.

Many injuries that are described as being the result of interpersonal violence and warfare are consistent with those cases described in P. Edwin Smith. In this treatise treatments are rationally managed and the clinical approach to the challenges presented by these injuries is not too dissimilar from that practised today (Sanchez & Meltzer 2012: 5). Of the forty-eight cases in the papyrus, fourteen are head injuries, seven cervical injuries and one is an injury to the lower spine, all of which are typical of wounds sustained during violence. Other medical papyri recommend curative mixtures of herbal, animal and mineral products in the treatment of such injuries.

(f, ii) Law breaking

Information about crimes, criminal procedures and punishments meted out to law breakers is derived mainly from official records such as royal texts, decrees and court proceedings. No criminal law code, if one ever existed, has been preserved. Punishments, which were wide ranging, included loss of civil status, confiscation of property and belongings, hard labour, corporal punishment and death (Lorton 1977). Of these various sentences it is the after-effects of corporal punishment and hard labour that may have required medical treatment.

The main form of corporal punishment handed out by the courts was a beating, usually specified as 'one hundred blows with a stick'. A number of Old Kingdom tomb scenes show people being beaten, sometimes with sticks shaped to resemble a man's hand, often while tied to a post, such as the pillory scene depicted in the tomb of Mereruka at Saqqara (Kanawati *et al.* 2010: pl. 23) (Fig. 6.8). Certain scenes show the individual lying down being beaten on his back, and at a pillar, as in the mastaba of Khentika at Saqqara (James 1953: pl. 9) (Fig. 6.9). Many literary texts mention beatings by other individuals such as officials, tax collectors and schoolteachers, who frequently punished their subordinates without recourse to a court.

The medical papyri include several instances in which treatment is administered for the lacerations left by such beatings. P. Ebers 510 is 'a remedy to eliminate the weals following a beating', and recommends a mixture of 'honey; ox-bile; potter's clay; juice of *sꜣr*-plant; date-juice, cooked and bandaged therewith'.

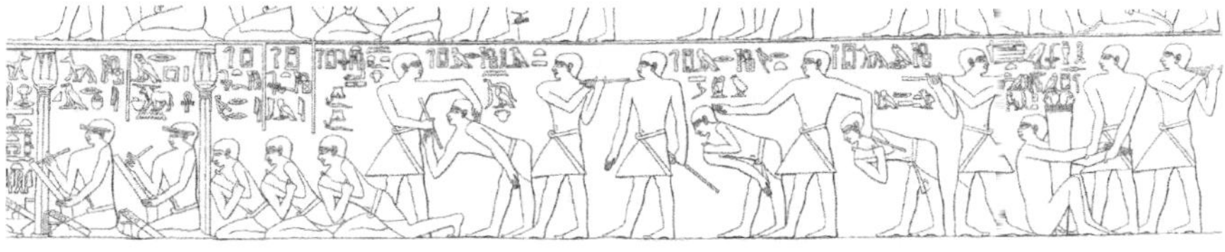

Figure 6.8. Punishment in ancient Egypt for non-payment of taxes. Scene from the 6th Dynasty mastaba tomb of Mereruka (chamber A4 west wall). Redrawn by K. N. White after Duell (1938: pl. 37).

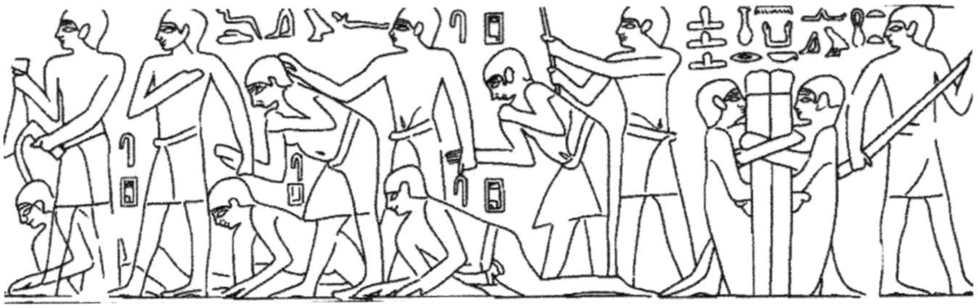

Figure 6.9. Corporal punishment being administered. Scene from the 6th Dynasty mastaba tomb of Khentika at Saqqara (room 1, north wall). Redrawn by K. N. White after James (1953: pl. 9).

While honey would be soothing and reduce infection, the action of some of the other constituents is less obvious. Similarly, P. Ebers 511–14 recommend various other medicaments to treat the lacerations. Case 514 advises a *ḥmꜣjt* plant placed on a cake dipped in honey and then swallowed. This remedy is quite unusual in that it is one of the few occasions that an oral medicine is prescribed, and in this instance probably intended as an analgesic preparation.

To the punishment of one hundred blows was sometimes added the sentence of 'five open wounds'. No details are provided as to what exactly this punishment entailed or to which part of the body the wounds were to be inflicted. The scenes depicting the beatings often show the miscreant being beaten on his back, so it is possible that the wounds may similarly have been inflicted on the upper torso.

A study of the skeletal remains of adult males from the South Tombs Cemetery at Tell el-Amarna by Dabbs and Zabecki (2015) may shed some light on this sentence. The scapulae of these individuals exhibited slot-type fractures, and the morphology of these wounds corresponds to sharp force trauma inflicted by spears or similar weapons (Bauer & Patzelt 2002). In all cases the injuries are healed, which indicates a period of time separating the punishment from the time of death. The hundred blows and five wounds punishment was not intended as a death sentence, as many beatings were followed by committal to a labour gang, often for an extended period of time. This is supported by the fact that injuries to the scapulae and the associated soft tissues are comparatively rapid to heal and the effects of such an injury on the ability to work would be less than those of injuries to other regions of the body (Scavenius & Sloth 1996). In addition, there is a thick envelope of muscle surrounding the scapula, which reduces the risk of unintentional damage to a vital organ.

The other main form of corporal punishment administered in ancient Egypt was mutilation, primarily amputation of the nose and ears. Additionally, amputations were carried out during warfare, where the hands and penises of the fallen enemy were removed. However, this was carried out to count numbers of enemies killed and to present these trophies to the king as evidence of success on the battlefield (see Chapter 5c).

Actual evidence for mutilation practices is limited and is mainly text-based, with most material coming from high-profile (often royal) contexts, which are unlikely to typify broader Egyptian society. The Turin Judicial Papyrus records corrupt royal judges being punished in this way, while the Nauri legal decree of Sety I threatens nose and ear mutilation for misappropriation offences. The fragmentary Karnak legal decree of Horemheb (*c.* 1323–1295 BC, 18th Dynasty) also mentions mutilation, albeit removing the nose only (Lorton 1977; Sperati 2009). Egyptian mutilation practices are also referred to by Diodorus Siculus (1, 78), who describes the severing of hands for theft and noses for adultery.

Transcripts of contemporary legal proceedings, such as the Tomb Robbery Papyri and various Deir el-Medina court disputes, frequently feature defendants and witnesses using the threat of mutilation as a deterrent in oaths: 'As Amun endures and as the Ruler endures, if I speak falsehood (replaceable by potentially any reprehensible action), may there be cut off my nose and ears, me being [banished] to Kush' (translated Loktionov 2017: 265).

Mutilation of the ears and nose usually leaves no trace on skeletal remains as the avulsed segment is composed of skin, cartilage and membrane mucosa, but not bone. It may, in some cases, be possible to detect mutilation on mummified remains, but it was mainly the elite of society who were mummified and as such they would have been unlikely to have suffered such an ignominy. Criminals and lawbreakers who were sentenced to such a punishment were very unlikely to have been mummified.

Amputated wounds would cause rapid blood loss and subsequent infection, and it is possible that fatalities may have occurred, particularly if multiple amputations were performed at the same time. However, the mutilation oaths and royal decrees imply that survival was expected because, as mentioned previously, the convicted persons were often then sentenced to hard labour in stone quarries and other similar settings.

From a medical perspective, there are indications that the ancient Egyptians had the surgical expertise to treat the aftermath of such wounds. Cases 11–14 of P. Edwin Smith describe treatments for various nasal fractures, while Case 23 is titled a 'slashing wound of the ear'. As discussed on p. 123, inflammation and infection were recognised and treated using agents such as fresh meat and honey. Cauterisation was advised to facilitate haemostasis, as attested in P. Ebers 872 and P. Edwin Smith 39, and it is possible that this may have been carried out immediately following amputation.

The ear and nose mutilations would have been a problem cosmetically and a mark of shame. The unfortunate individual who suffered such injuries would have not only experienced difficulties in social interaction but found the function of the particular sensory organs to be impaired. The visible portion of the outer ear, the auricle, collects sound waves and channels them into the ear canal, the external auditory meatus. Without the auricle the direction of the sound would be difficult to pinpoint, and there would also have been a degree of hearing loss and distortion. Similarly, cutting off an individual's nose will affect their breathing, which in turn impacts on their ability to smell. The front of the nose has two main functions: it guides airflow and filters out dust and other large particles. The loss of the nose would result in much more dust settling in the trachea and bronchi, almost certainly causing inflammation that could result in infection. Consequently, such mutilations would not only be a major disfigurement but would result in hearing and breathing difficulties. In addition, the unfortunate individual would be more prone to infection and his quality of life would be reduced.

(g) Occupational health: construction workers, agricultural labourers and fishermen

Task-related health issues have plagued individuals for as long as repetitive and hazardous actions have been carried out. The ancient Egyptians were no exception, as during their working lives they would have been subjected to a variety of occupational risks, many of which would have been detrimental to their health. For example, bites from insects and dangerous animals would have been a continual threat in the agricultural landscape where the majority of peasants worked. The back-breaking work in the numerous quarries and construction sites would have resulted in both acute and chronic injuries.

Workers employed in the various craft industries would have been subjected to specific occupational problems. The repetitive nature of their tasks and their habitual postures, together with poor ventilation and dust inhalation in their workplaces, would pose a variety of dangers. Metal workers were exposed to the glare of flames, which could disturb the management of body fluids, damage the cornea of the eye and cause respiratory difficulties. Glass blowers were prone to emphysema and circulatory complications from constantly blowing down tubes. Bakers were continually exposed to the heat and glare of the ovens as well as the risk of carbon monoxide poisoning (Halioua & Ziskind 2005). In addition, burns and traumatic injuries would have been a major concern in many of these ancient work places.

However, it was in agriculture and fishing that the majority of ancient Egyptians would have been employed and so, in these industries, was there any particular system of medical care available for the workers?

Agricultural workers

Many scenes tend to portray farming in the Nile valley in a favourable manner, but occupational hazards and environmental threats would have caused constant problems. This is well illustrated in the literature from ancient Egypt, both the *Satire on the Trades* and the later *Papyrus Lansing*.

The *Satire of the Trades*, also known as the *Instruction of Khety*, was a popular work composed during the Middle Kingdom that describes the advantages and superiority of a scribal profession and emphasises the hardships of other trades and professions. The text describes the impact of peasants' working conditions on their health:

> The fieldhand cries out forever. His voice is louder than the raven's. His fingers have become ulcerous with an excess of stench. He is tired out in Delta labour. He is well among lions but his experience is painful. The forced labour then is tripled. If he comes back from the marshes, he reaches his house worn out, for the forced labour has ruined him. (translated Simpson 2003: 431–37)

Papyrus Lansing: A Schoolbook is a 20th Dynasty anthology of texts also praising the profession of the scribe (Caminos 1954: 373–428; Lichtheim 1976: 168–78). The text similarly expresses the 'misfortunes' of the peasant, referring to the fields being waterlogged by the inundation, the ever-present menace of snakes in the fields and the harsh penalties incurred if the harvest was poor and the farmer was unable to fulfil his tax quota of grain. This situation would have been exacerbated by grain weevils and beetles, which can destroy significant amounts of stored cereals. In addition, locusts were probably common in the rich agricultural land bordering the Nile, and sudden plagues of these insects in ancient times no doubt caused considerable destruction of grains and other food crops, just as they do today (Panagiotakopulu 2004).

The farmer would have had to contend with bites from mosquitos, insects that would have been numerous in ancient Egypt. Conditions in pharaonic times would have been more favourable for mosquitos than today, due to the many more swamps along the Nile and the lack of sanitation in most of the ancient dwellings. Herodotus (II, 95) describes how the country was infested by swarms of mosquitos and how the population slept under nets to prevent their bites. Another deterrent, recommended in P. Ebers (845, 846), was the smearing of *behen* oil or bird fat, an early form of insecticide, on the skin.

The bite from a mosquito can result in malaria, which is caused by parasites of the genus *Plasmodium* (see Chapter 7b). The mosquito can also pass on filaria, which can block the lymphatic vessels, producing fluid retention. The gross oedema resulting, known as elephantiasis, is a condition marked by severe swelling in areas such as the arms, legs, breasts and genitals (as, for example, Nesyamun, see Chapter 6a) (David & Tapp 1992: 151–52; Kenawy & Abdel-Hamid 2015).

Other insects would similarly have tormented the population. Leishmaniasis is a disease caused by parasites of the genus *Leishmania* and the infection is transmitted to humans through the bites of female sandflies. Different species of the parasite can cause cutaneous ulceration and a more serious disorder that can damage internal organs (Zink *et al.* 2006).

Labouring in the fields in bare feet would have exposed the workers to infections and parasitic diseases such as strongyloidiasis, as noted above. This condition is caused by a roundworm that lives in the soil. Immature forms of the worm can invade the body through unprotected areas such as the feet, and then pass into the vascular system before reaching the lungs. The infection may cause respiratory, skin and digestive symptoms. It is difficult to determine whether strongyloidiasis is included within the medical papyri, as, although there are frequent mentions of parasitic worms, there is no obvious link with the strongyloides worm. However, it has been identified in the mummy of Asru (see Chapter 6a). Skin abrasions and wounds on the body would also have exposed workers to the risk of tetanus, caused by the bacterium *Clostridium tetani* (see Chapter 4f).

Many species of snakes roamed the fields and would have been a threat to farm workers. Common among them were vipers such as the sand and horned vipers, which inject a venom that acts cytotoxically on tissues and blood corpuscles. The bite of a cobra can lead to paralysis, internal bleeding and death (Strouhal 1997: 107). The priests of Serket had a special role in the treatment of venomous bites from scorpions and snakes (see Chapter 2a).

Farmers would have been vulnerable to attacks from domestic animals such as pigs and dogs, and such bites would have been quite likely to have turned septic, potentially resulting in a systemic infection. Both the Ebers and Hearst Papyri contain prescriptions for the treatment of animal bites, with the Hearst Papyrus (239–60) including specific remedies for the bites of crocodiles, lions, hippopotami and pigs. The Demotic Magical Papyrus of London and Leiden has an incantation aimed at dog bites, which was to be recited while applying crushed garlic to the wound (Griffith & Thompson 1904: Coll 19, 1–9). Garlic contains allicin which is a strong antibiotic and is released when the cloves of garlic are crushed.

Although the medical papyri include prescriptions for bites, wounds and other medical problems suffered by the agricultural workers, there is little indication of specific medical care being provided for them. It has been suggested that Methen, a 4th Dynasty official, also carried the title of *swnw grgt*, which has been translated as a physician who looked after the health of peasants who farmed the land of a master's estate (Halioua & Ziskind 2005: 119–20). Ghalioungui (1983: 71–73) thought this interpretation to be unlikely based on comments by scholars such as Spiegelberg, Grapow and

Godeckin. However, there is no consensus among these academics around an alternative translation.

Fishing

Fishing was pursued both for sport and as a livelihood. Economic fishing had a tradition going back to prehistoric times and scenes from all periods of ancient Egypt depict fishing in the shallow waters of the Nile, the marshes of the Delta and the deeper waters off the coast. Although many of these scenes portray fishing as both an idyllic pastime and occupation, the reality, particular for the fishermen who relied on fishing for their living, would have been more arduous and endangering.

Crocodiles, which inhabited the whole length of the Nile, posed a considerable threat to fishermen, who wore amulets for protection. The *cippi* of the Late Period were considered to confer protection against a range of dangerous animals, including the crocodile. The *Satire of the Trades* singles out the fisherman as being the worst of all occupations: 'I'll speak of the fisherman also, his is the worst of all jobs; he labours on the river mingling with crocodiles … ' (translated Lichtheim 1975: 184–92).

Crocodiles inflict serious injuries and sometimes death on their unfortunate victims. For the survivors, the wound may well bleed profusely and tissue damage could be extensive. Again, both the Ebers Papyrus (435) and the Hearst Papyrus (239) provide instructions to treat such a wound. Ebers 436 recommends: 'What one does for a bite-wound of a crocodile: If you examine a wound of a crocodile bite and you find his flesh open, its sides being separated; then you should bandage him with fresh meat the first day, like any human wound' (translated Ghalioungui 1987: 125).

The bandaging with fresh meat is fairly standard, but there is no mention of applying honey, which is used in many similar remedies. Honey would have been helpful, as such bites would be likely to become infected. Similarly, there is no reference to arresting haemorrhage, which would probably have been necessary following such a wound. Although not specifically mentioned in the papyri, it is likely that, in addition, invocations would have been addressed to the crocodile god, Sobek, by both the victim and the physician.

A particular hazard to fishermen as well as to boatmen and papyrus workers, who waded in the shallower waters of the Nile to cut papyrus plants, was urinary schistosomiasis (Kloos & David 2002; Ziskind 2009), a parasitic infection caused by trematode worms of the genus *Schistosoma* (see Chapters 2a, 6a). The main symptom of the disease is haematuria, and during Napoleon's campaign to Egypt and Syria (1798–1801) the comment was made that Egypt was the land of 'menstruating men'. The blood loss can lead to anaemia, loss of appetite and lowered resistance to other infections. It has often been suggested that the *aaa*

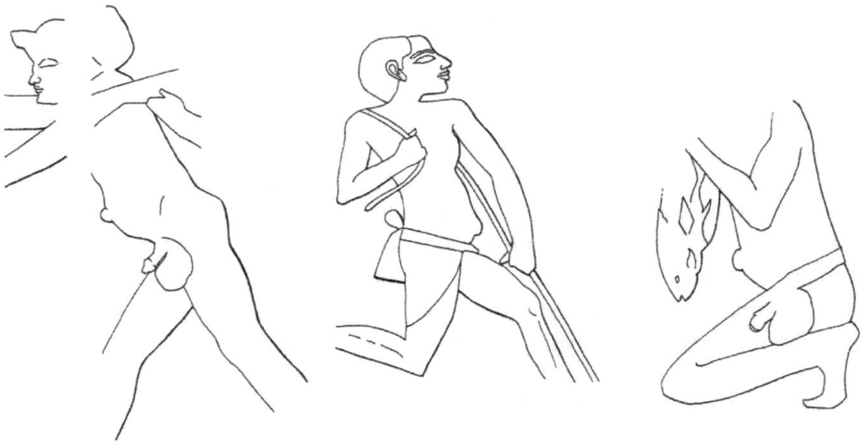

Figure 6.10. Examples of possible umbilical hernias from scenes in the 6th Dynasty mastaba tomb of Ptahhotep and the 5th Dynasty tomb of Mehu at Saqqara. Redrawn by K. N. White after Ghalioungui (1962: fig. 3) and Nunn (1996: 166).

disease, which is frequently mentioned in the medical papyri, is schistosomiasis, although many scholars dispute this. It would seem that this conclusion was the result of over-interpretation by early translators (Duke 2008). In hieroglyphs the word does have a discharging phallus as a determinative, although it is unlikely that the worm would have been visible to the naked eye.

Painted reliefs in the tombs of Ptahhotep and Mehu at Saqqara depict individuals suffering from abdominal distension and abnormalities of the navel, which could be associated with advanced schistosomiasis or might indicate an umbilical hernia (Ghalioungui 1962; Leca 1988: 216–17; Nunn 1996: 166) (Fig. 6.10). The Negative Confessions of Spell 125 of the *Book of the Dead* includes 'I have not waded in the water', which could indicate a recognition and avoidance of potential waterborne hazards such as schistosomiasis (Faulkner 1972: 29–34; Nunn 1996: 69).

7

Egypt's contribution to other ancient and modern medical systems

(a) Exchange of medical concepts and disease

Egypt's contribution to other medical systems: the political context

Ancient societies provided different types and levels of healthcare that often reflected a community's specific social and religious perceptions and beliefs. The individual experiences of medical practitioners and patients would have varied considerably, depending on the specific range of circumstances, opportunities and disadvantages present in the medical system of their own society. To place this into a historical context, it is first necessary to consider briefly the political and cultural ties that existed between Egypt and major neighbouring civilisations before comparing the extent and limitations of knowledge and expertise acquired by Egyptian medical practitioners over the millennia with the medical systems of Babylonia, Greece and Rome.

Throughout much of its history, ancient Egypt exerted considerable political, military and cultural influence over neighbouring lands, coming into contact with peoples living in Nubia, Asia Minor and around the Mediterranean. A two-way transmission occurred between Egypt and these regions that included an exchange of medical concepts and treatments. In addition, because they were internationally renowned for their knowledge and expertise, Egyptian physicians were invited to foreign courts to advise and practise their skills.

Sometimes Egypt's interaction with neighbouring lands resulted in the transference of disease, and there is some inscriptional evidence that certain diseases crossed political borders. Sources include Babylonian astronomical and other documents, letters in the Egyptian royal archive and occasional references in the medical papyri to treatments attributed to a foreign origin (see Chapter 7b). In addition, some Egyptian remedies contain pharmaceutical and other ingredients that were evidently imported from elsewhere.

Egypt's earliest recorded contacts were with Mesopotamia, where thousands of clay tablets preserve information about people's everyday lives. These include details of a medical system, first developed in Babylonian times, that continued for over two millennia. Egypt also had long-established links with the Aegean world, initially with the Minoan civilisation on Crete from at least the mid–late 3rd millennium BC (Kelder *et al.* 2018). At first, this involved irregular exchanges of precious objects and raw materials, but the development of greater ties from *c.* 2000 BC included the exchange of specialist craftsmen and ritual objects, diplomatic missions and a two-way transmission of medical knowledge. Contact between Egypt and the Minoans continued throughout the first part of the New Kingdom, but ceased sometime after the reign of Tuthmosis III, when Minoan culture went into decline. The power vacuum was filled by the Mycenaeans, who, moving out from southern Greece, established a base in the Aegean region.

Immigrants from various areas arrived in Egypt at different periods, but this process is particularly well recorded in the Late Period. Kings of the 26th Dynasty relied increasingly on Greek mercenaries to uphold their rule, and in the 6th century BC large numbers of immigrants from Ionia (on the coast of Asia Minor) settled in the Egyptian capital, Memphis. Between 664 and 610 BC other immigrants from the Ionian city of Miletus founded Naucratis as a Greek colony and trading post in the Egyptian Delta. This city (and the later foundations of Ptolemais and Antinoopolis in the Graeco-Roman Period) retained their exclusive Greek identity. However, there was also some degree of cultural and religious integration with the local Egyptian population (Lang 2013: 24), which may have been reflected in the medical provision in these communities (see below).

A final stage of immigration occurred when Egypt was conquered by the Greeks and then subsumed into the Roman empire. A significant number of immigrants now arrived in the country, bringing their own medical systems, which were mainly organised separately from and operated in parallel with native Egyptian medicine. However, there was undoubtedly some overlap, and some long-established Egyptian treatments now passed across to the Greek and Roman systems.

Transfer of medical knowledge

Over the millennia, although there was some transmission of concepts and practices, Egyptian medicine always retained a unique profile. This is particularly evident in societal attitudes towards deformity and disability and in the ways in which medical practitioners demonstrated respect for their patients regardless of the nature of the illness or its expected outcome. These important perspectives were probably inspired and underpinned by religious concepts and principles (see Chapters 5d, 6e).

It is well-evidenced that there was a continuing knowledge exchange between Egypt, Mesopotamia and Greece in which Egyptian medicine continued to be held in high regard. However, the true extent and impact of these exchanges remains unclear. This is partly due to the considerable variation in the level and availability of inscriptional, iconographic, archaeological and palaeopathological evidence for the study of each of these systems. In some instances, the source material – for example, human remains – are scarce or unobtainable. Sometimes, there are problems associated with the translation of inscriptions: whereas the ability to read and understand Greek and Latin was never lost, the cuneiform and Egyptian scripts have only been deciphered more recently. Even today some terms and ingredients in the prescriptions can pose difficulties for the translator.

Earliest contacts: Egypt and Mesopotamia

The medicine practised over the millennia in Mesopotamia is sometimes referred to as 'Babylonian medicine'. The subject is extensively explored by Geller (2010), but some key points of the system are discussed here to enable a comparison to be made with Egyptian medicine.

Sources

An abundance of inscriptional evidence survives from Mesopotamia. Cuneiform texts inscribed on thousands of clay tablets provide the closest to a complete account of everyday life in any ancient society. These include an extensive record of medical provision and treatment that contrasts with the much smaller number of Egyptian medical or magico-medical documents that have been identified, partly because papyrus (their most common writing material) was far less durable than clay.

The Mesopotamian literature provides a wealth of evidence relating to healing practices and practitioners. The oldest Babylonian medical texts date back to the Old Babylonian Period (the first half of the 2nd millennium BC), but most information is derived from three main types of medical literature. The *Diagnostic Handbook (Diagnostic and Prescriptive Series)* contains prognostic omens; vast numbers of prescriptions provide lists of mineral and botanical ingredients; and the therapeutic texts include a combination of recipes, lists of ingredients and incantations that were recited alongside medical rituals. These measures were intended to impress and hopefully to cure the patient.

The *Diagnostic Handbook* consists of a set of two tablets that contain medical omens and another thirty-eight tablets that provide explanatory advice on the diagnosis and prognostication of diseases (Scurlock 2018: 38–40). The physician (*āšipu*) reached a diagnosis on the basis of a personal examination of the patient, observing any physical signs and symptoms and noting the patient's response to his questions. A written version of the *Handbook*, edited by the physician Esagil-kin-apli, was already in use by the reign of the Babylonian king Adad-apla-idina

(1068–1047 BC). Plants or parts of plants, and some animal or mineral substances, formed the basis of more than a thousand medicines available in Mesopotamia (see above, Chapter 2f, i).

Demonic 'magic' and 'religion' were used alongside medical treatments. Magical recitations preserved in the texts include magical stories, threats and oaths, while religious elements included sacrifices and prayers to deities associated with magic and medicine (Scurlock 2018: 41–43).

Medical concepts

A crucial difference between early and later societies was the attribution of disease causation: the former assumed that external symptoms were caused by divine or demonic attack, whereas the latter explained symptoms as disease manifestations that originated in specific bodily organs, arising independently of any divine intervention.

The basis of both Egyptian and Mesopotamian medicine was the belief that divine intervention played an essential role in diagnosing and treating the sick, and this had a profound influence on their attitudes towards the nature and causes of disease, prognosis and therapeutic treatments (see Chapter 1b). However, records also show that both systems recognised that not all external symptoms were the result of divine/demonic attack.

Mesopotamian medicine, although essentially pragmatic and practical in its approach, was a complicated system that was probably derived from a theoretical background. It is likely that most of its procedures were based on philosophical theories that may have been taught as a component of medical training and practice, although literary treatises of this type have not yet been identified.

Medical practitioners

Babylonian procedures involved diagnosing and treating patients with a combination of skills provided by two separate sets of medical practitioners (Geller 2010: 43–44). The *āšipu*, primarily a priest and exorcist based at the temple, also functioned as a physician, visiting patients to diagnose illness and provide them with a prognosis. His treatments, based on the assumption that disease was the result of divine will or fate, employed magical means to cure the patient or provide protection against attacks by demons, enraged gods, witchcraft and evil omens.

The other practitioner, the *asû*, was not in conflict with the *āšipu* but was based in the community, perhaps working from his home or a small shop. He dealt mainly with afflictions attributable to natural circumstances – bites or environmental conditions, for example – and acted primarily as a pharmacist, who prepared and provided individually designed medicines for local patients.

He could identify the best sources of medicinal ingredients and had specialist knowledge of when they should be collected and how they should be stored. He also had extensive experience of how medicines should be prepared and administered.

Little is known about the educational routes employed in early societies to train and prepare medical practitioners for their careers. However, in common with Egyptian practice (see Chapter 3a), the Babylonian system probably provided some formal training, perhaps in specialised centres attached to the temples; instruction doubtless included copying and making commentaries on magico-medical texts. There is some indication that boys training to become *āšipu* (who usually came from priestly families) had to pass through a graded system of apprenticeships before they could practise medicine.

Egyptian and Mesopotamian sources provide little information about the lives or careers of individual medical practitioners: surviving names include the Egyptian healers Imhotep and Amenhotep, Son of Hapu; and Esagil-kin-apli, the editor of the Babylonian *Diagnostic Handbook*. In contrast, Graeco-Roman sources identify many famous physicians, including Hippocrates, Dioscorides, Erotian, Herophilus, Eristratus and Galen.

Treatments

The Egyptians generally relied on a combination of magico-religious and rationally based treatments that included basic surgery and some therapeutically viable pharmaceutical recipes (discussed in Chapter 5f). Most Mesopotamian treatments were based on pharmaceutical ingredients, but also involved animal sacrifices, prayers to deities and – with the emergence of astral medicine in the early 5th century BC (Geller 2010: 123) – the performance of healing rituals undertaken at propitious times during the zodiacal cycle.

Diagnosis of disease in Babylonian medicine relied on observation of various signs apparent in a patient's condition. The *Diagnostic Handbook* preserves details of how these were classified and expected to develop over the course of an illness. In some instances the signs and symptoms are listed and discussed systematically, from the head downwards.

The therapeutic texts are similarly organised and provide details of medications and treatments for specific conditions; these include salves, bandages, eye-drops, fumigants, enemas, urethral irrigations and tampons. The physicians apparently saw no contradiction in using these practical measures alongside the demonic magic and religious practices, which were believed to facilitate the patient's active participation in the healing process.

Attitudes towards ill-health and disability

In common with Egyptian medicine, Mesopotamian practice distinguished between the expected outcomes of specific conditions, identifying them as treatable, uncertain or incurable. Various perceptions of disability were recorded in cuneiform sources from the end of the 3rd millennium BC, and the same principles of assessment were applied to some of these conditions. For example, paralysis and epilepsy were identified and sometimes treated, but, despite a general commitment to recommend and pursue healing methods, some conditions, including cerebral palsy and hydrocephalus, were classified as incurable.

A birth anomaly was considered to be an evil omen: records state that, among the upper classes, priests were sometimes required to decide whether an infant should live or be thrown into a river (Kellenberger 2017: 51). There is no indication of how the non-elite dealt with this situation.

In contrast, the Egyptian attitude towards deformity and disability was very different (see Chapter 5d, 6e). Its religious and social systems offered inclusion and support and, not surprisingly, there is no evidence from pharaonic times that deformed infants were exposed to die, although documentary sources indicate that this occasionally occurred during the Graeco-Roman Period (West 1998; David 2017a: 84).

b) Egyptian healers invited to foreign lands, foreign diseases and drugs

Some earlier commentaries suggested that the content and format of Egyptian medicine underwent little change before the Persian invasion (e.g., Nunn 1996: 206). However, to accept this assessment one must largely ignore the interactions with and influences of Egypt's neighbours on her healing practices. This is particularly apparent for the Levant, where cultural communications are traceable from predynastic times and which increased markedly during the cosmopolitan New Kingdom. Reciprocal transmission of medical concepts and treatments is well attested, and the reputation of Egyptian medicine and the skills of Egyptian physicians were internationally renowned.

Exchange of medical personnel

An early illustration of foreign interaction in the medical sphere is revealed in a scene from the tomb of Nebamun (TT17), a scribe and royal physician during the reign of Amenhotep II. Nebamun is depicted receiving gifts from a Syrian prince who is considered to have travelled to Egypt to receive medical treatment (Säve-Söderbergh 1957 pl. 23; Shirley 2007) (Fig. 7.1).

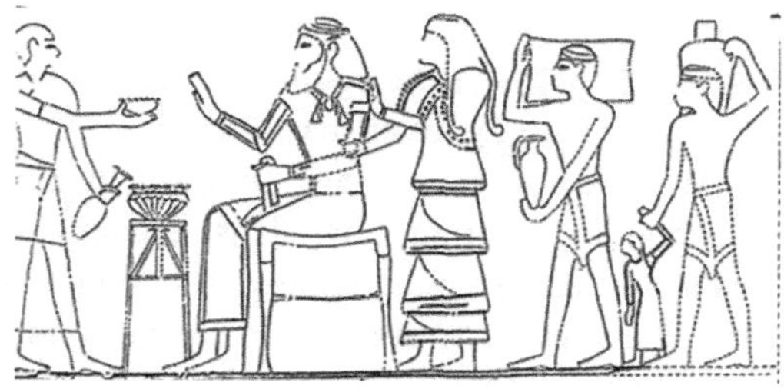

Figure 7.1. A scene of a Canaanite ruler bringing gifts to Nebamun, a royal physician. From the 18th Dynasty tomb of Nebamun at Thebes (TT17). Redrawn by K. N. White after Säve-Söderbergh (1957: pl. 23).

There is evidence of medical exchange preserved in the cuneiform letters from the diplomatic archive found at Tell el-Amarna (Moran 1992). Tushratta, King of Mitanni, sent, on loan, a statue of the goddess Ishtar of Nineveh to Egypt in the hope that the divine effigy would cure Amenhotep III of an illness. It is quite likely that royal medical staff accompanied the statue on its journey, providing opportunities for an exchange of knowledge and ideas with their Egyptian counterparts. An alternative suggestion is that the dispatch of the statue was associated with the solemnities of the marriage of Tushratta's daughter to Amenhotep (BM EA 23; see Plate 30).

The transfer of statues of healing gods and goddesses is well documented in the surviving diplomatic correspondence between Egypt and her eastern neighbours (Singer 2016). A further letter, probably sent during the reign of Akhenaten, documents an appeal by the ruler of Ugarit, Niqm-Adda, for palace attendants, and a request to include among the personnel a physician, as there were none in attendance at Ugarit at that time (BM EA 49).

A group of letters exchanged by Ramesses II with the Hittite court record more than one appeal to Egypt for medical help by the Hittites. Ramesses II sent drugs to Hattusili III, the ruler of the Hittite kingdom (Hatti), for the treatment of an eye condition, and Hattusili also requested an Egyptian physician to help his vassal Kurunta of Tarhuntas, even though there were already physicians in Kurunta's service. In a further letter Hatusili requested that an Egyptian physician prepare drugs to help his married sister conceive.

The Late Period/Ptolemaic Bentresh stela, although considered to be a propagandist work, refers back to the events of the reign of Ramesses II and again reflects the medical exchanges occurring at that time (see Plate 13). The stela includes details of a request by the prince of Bakhtan (perhaps to be identified with Bactria (Simpson 2003: 362)) for medical help to aid his ailing sister, and the subsequent sending of Thothemheb, a royal scribe from the House of Life. Although Thothemheb was unable to heal the princess, the later dispatch of a healing statue from Egypt was documented as effecting a cure.

Following the Persian invasion of Egypt, Udjahorresnet, a chief physician, was accorded a number of important positions by Cambyses, ruler of Persia, and further *swnw* served as court physicians in Persia during this period (see

Chapters 3b, 4e). This would probably have resulted in a transfer of medical knowledge between the countries. Medical astrology was known to have been introduced into Egypt at that time.

Alongside this exchange of medical personnel between Egypt and her neighbours, Egyptian physicians encountered new drugs and methods of treatment that were incorporated into Egyptian medical practice. This is attested in P. Ebers 422, a treatment for an eye condition, which states that an Asiatic communicated this preparation to a man from Byblos, where that particular drug was recommended. Among the compounds listed in P. Ebers 361, again a prescription for an eye disorder, is *prt-šni* fruit, which also is designated as originating from Byblos. P. Ebers 28, a remedy for the 'evacuation of the belly', has among its ingredients the *gngnt* plant, which is stated as being comparable to Cretan beans. Similarities have also been noticed between Egyptian medicine and that which originated from Assyria and Babylonia (Contenau 1938; Halioua & Ziskind 2005: 182; Geller 2010).

P. London incorporates seven incantations in foreign languages (27–33), transcribed into hieratic syllabic script. Six of these are in Northwest Semitic dialects, possible Phoenician or Aramaic. These cases are not in a separate group but fall within a series of typically Egyptian prescriptions, suggesting that they had been fully accepted and considered as legitimate remedies (Ritner 2000). The other case specifically mentions the language of Crete (Keftiu) and refers to treatment of the 'Asiatic disease', involving an incantation to be recited over yeast and various urines, presumably from different animals. A similar prescription appears in P. Hearst, although here the materials recommended are moringa-oil and scales from turtle shells.

Foreign diseases

The extensive links between Egypt and her neighbours would have enabled epidemics to readily cross the borders between the countries (David 2017a; Habicht *et al.* 2021). Transmission of diseases would have been aided by population movements, including the transfers of prisoners of war to Egypt during the military campaigns of the New Kingdom, the incursions of the Sea Peoples during the reign of Ramesses III and the use of foreign mercenaries in the Saite Period. Living conditions in Egypt, with overcrowded dwellings in the towns and cities, poor sanitation and unhygienic waste disposal, would have provided conditions conducive to the spread of disease (see Chapter 6b).

Biblical plagues

Ancient Egypt is often associated with the biblical plagues as recorded in the book of Exodus, in which God sent a series of ten plagues to force the Pharaoh to let the enslaved Israelites go free. Although it is possible that this account is simply fictional, a potential factual basis for it has been keenly debated, with suggestions including climatic and environmental events or a conglomerate memory of disconnected incidents at different times, merged to describe the Exodus. The sixth plague, characterised by boils that eventually formed ulcers on the skin, might be a symptom of an acute epidemic. The tenth plague, in which the first-born children and animals were massacred, has also been linked to an epidemic or plague.

The 'plague' (bubonic plague?)

One of the most devastating soft tissue infections is the 'plague', which has been responsible for several high-mortality epidemics throughout human history. The 'plague', usually considered to be bubonic plague, is caused by the bacterium *Yersinia pestis*, normally carried by rats and transferred to humans by the flea *Xenopsylla cheopis*, which commonly infests rats.

The origins and dispersal of epidemic diseases including the 'plague' have been the subject of much speculation. Most infections leave no specific trace upon bones and so it is to the mummified remains that attention has to be given. Although evidence of many diseases has been detected in mummified tissue, the only possible physical evidence of the 'plague' was noted by Ruffer (1910c). Bacilli similar to *Yersinia pestis* were detected in the lung and liver of a Ptolemaic mummy, but later investigators regarded this evidence as inconclusive.

Many modern researchers consider bubonic plague to have originated as a disease of Central Asiatic rodents. It is often suggested that it reached Egypt during the reign of Amenhotep III and that there may have been an earlier epidemic at the beginning of the New Kingdom (e.g., Aldred 1988: 149, 283; Kozloff 2006). However, Panagiotakopulu (2004) has suggested that bubonic plague was a disease endemic in the wild rodent population in Egypt and East Africa during pharaonic times and may have been present earlier.

Kozloff (2006) assembled a considerable body of circumstantial evidence to support the proposition that bubonic plague affected Egypt during the reign of Amenhotep III, such as the eight-year lapse in the written record and the unprecedented attention that Amenhotep gave to Sekhmet, the goddess of pestilence and war (see Plate 31). A frequent indicator of a fatal epidemic is mass or 'rushed' burials in which all age groups and both sexes are buried together. There are more examples of these multiple burials during Amenhotep III's reign than under any of his recent predecessors. In addition, the burial chambers were poorly decorated and the offering objects were of inferior quantity. There was also an unusually high number of married-couple burials, as though husband and wife died almost simultaneously.

Textual evidence

A rare mention of the plague being present in Egypt is found in an Amarna letter (EA II) sent from Burnaburiyaš, king of Babylon, to Akhenaten responding to the pharaoh's account that one of Amenhotep III's wives had died of the plague (Moran 1992). Another letter from the Amarna archive (EA 35), sent by the king of Alashiya (Crete), declares that he is able to send only a small quantity of copper as a gift, as the plague had afflicted the country and killed all the copper-workers.

There is other textual evidence to indicate that a plague existed in Western Asia and the Mediterranean at that time. The Hittite plague prayers of Mursili II (*c.* 1330–1295 BC), the ruler of the Hittites, describe an epidemic that killed his father, Suppiluliuma II, and his brother, Arnuwanda II, the subsequent ruler. According to this source the plague was passed on by Egyptian prisoners captured at a battle at Amka in Lebanon, and the epidemic then continued to afflict Hatti for some twenty years (Pritchard 1955: 394–96; Kuhrt 1995: 275–76).

It is difficult to identify a particular plague-like disease from references in the medical papyri, as they merely list signs and symptoms rather than specifying a particular ailment, and many of the cases could refer to a variety of different conditions. P. Ebers (873, 874) makes reference to a 'swelling of Khons' and one of the possible interpretations for this condition is bubonic plague. Similarly, in P. Hearst (XI, 12–15) and P. London (15, 8–10) there is a reference to the 'Asiatic Disease', perhaps bubonic plague. From Hittite sources it is known that there was an Asiatic plague roughly contemporary with the compilation of the Ramesside London Papyrus. During Egyptian–Hittite hostilities at the beginning of the 19th Dynasty, Egyptian prisoners captured in Syria are said to have brought a devastating plague into the Hittite camp (Ritner 2000: 111). If it was present, therefore, among Egypt's neighbours and trading partners, then it is more than likely that it would have spread to Egypt.

The first eight incantations on the verso of P. Edwin Smith are aimed at confronting an annual epidemic known as the 'pestilence of the year' (see verso, spell 6). Many of the incantations identify either the wind or the breath of Sekhmet as responsible for the pestilence, although the sixth spell identifies the swallowing of a fly as a cause of disease. The incantations are addressed not only to benign deities to protect, heal and overcome the disease but also to Sekhmet in the hope of placating her.

It was generally believed that epidemics were caused by hostile divinities or powers. These powers were not only gods but could be dead and living persons, even animals, and it was not the power or divinity who caused the problem but their agents, the so-called 'disease demons' (see p. 6).

The incomplete text the *Admonitions of Ipuwer* is preserved in P. Leiden I 344 recto and dated to the 19th Dynasty, although thought to be a copy of an older work (Parkinson 2002: 204–16, 308–09; Tobin 2003: 188–210). The document is a vivid account of upheaval, chaos and societal disintegration, and is sometimes cited as referring to possible epidemics at the end of the Old Kingdom. There is considerable debate, however, over whether the text is a historical account of actual events or a literary work contrasting order with chaos.

Future research may be able to provide a definitive answer as to whether the plague was present in ancient Egypt. The tooth's dental pulp as a preserved source of bacterial DNA has enabled investigators to demonstrate the presence of *Yersinia pestis* in samples from 300-year-old specimens found at archaeological sites in France (Drancourt *et al.* 1998; Barbieri *et al.* 2017). By using the technique of proteomics, *Yersinia pestis* was detected in proteins in the pulp, and it may be possible to apply such a technique to human remains from ancient Egypt.

Other epidemic diseases

There is some evidence for other infectious and epidemic diseases that may have been transmitted to Egypt from her neighbours. Among these is typhoid, which may have been the cause of the Plague of Athens (*c.* 430–426 BC), where it is estimated to have killed one-third of the population of the city (Papagrigorakis *et al.* 2006, *contra* Shapiro *et al.* 2006). In addition, there are indications that leprosy, malaria, poliomyelitis and smallpox may have afflicted the ancient Egyptians.

Leprosy

Leprosy, a chronic infectious disease caused by *Mycobacterium leprae*, is acquired by close personal contact over a long period and is thought to have originated in Asia (Monot *et al.* 2005). There is little indication of the disease in Egypt during the Dynastic Period, and perhaps the earliest evidence is to be found in four skulls excavated at the Dakhleh Oasis that have been dated to the Ptolemaic Period (Dzierzykray-Rogalski 1980). aDNA evidence of *M. leprae* has been found in a mummified individual from Abusir, also dating to the Ptolemaic Period (Neukamm *et al.* 2020). However, due to the stigma attached to leprosy, it is likely that victims were isolated from the community and did not have access to traditional burials and mummification, and so it is possible that there may be further, perhaps earlier, examples yet to be unearthed.

P. Ebers 874 and 877 discuss treatment for a swelling or tumour of Khonsu and this has rather tenuously been linked to leprosy by some researchers. However, as with many discussions relating to the medical papyri, particularly those where there are translational difficulties, this is not certain, and other suggestions have been put forward, including cancer, bubonic plague and neurofibromatosis.

Malaria

Malaria is a disease caused by parasites of the genus *Plasmodium* and the infection is transmitted to humans through the bites of infected female

Anopheles mosquitoes, which pass the parasites from their saliva into the human bloodstream. The deadliest form of malaria is caused by *Plasmodium falciparium*, although several other species of the parasite exist. Malaria causes symptoms that typically include fever, tiredness, vomiting and headaches, and in severe cases can cause seizures, coma and even death (Nerlich *et al.* 2008).

There are no references in the medical papyri that can be likened to the characteristic three- or four-day fever, although Spell 6 on the verso of P. Edwin Smith is an incantation for someone who has swallowed an insect. The later *Hippocratic Corpus* does describe the undulating fever typical of plasmodial infection.

Although there are no gross pathological changes to be found in mummies and skeletal remains to indicate that these individuals had suffered from malaria during life, recent analysis of skeletal remains at the North Tombs Cemetery at Tell el-Amarna has demonstrated specific areas of porosity and periostitis, indicative of malaria. These features have been observed in a high proportion of individuals, which could suggest that the disease was endemic among the Amarna residents (Dabbs & Rose 2015). Other factors also suggest that some form of epidemic disease affected the population of Tell el-Amarna, including high numbers of postweaning and sub-adult skeletons, the patterning and organisation of the cemeteries and the literary evidence from the Amarna letters (Dabbs & Zabecki 2014).

A specialised parasite-F test looking for antigens produced by species of *Plasmodium* has been able to identify malaria in mummies from many periods in ancient Egypt (Miller *et al.* 1994; Rabino Massa *et al.* 2000). However, Nerlich and his co-workers (2008) suggested that because less than 40 per cent of all the samples in these studies tested positive for the *P. falciparum* histidine-rich protein-2 antigen there are doubts about the specificity of the tests. More recently, aDNA investigations have detected the presence of species of *Plasmodium* in a number of mummy samples, dating from the New Kingdom until the Late Period, and such studies have suggested that malaria may not have been that uncommon in pharaonic times (Nerlich *et al.* 2008; Hawass *et al.* 2010; Khairat *et al.* 2013).

Poliomyelitis

The poliovirus produces a mild clinical condition in most individuals, but in a few cases it invades the central nervous system and can result in a degree of muscle paralysis. A diagnosis of poliomyelitis has been suggested in only a few instances from ancient Egypt (see Chapter 6e). However, because of the sporadic appearance of these cases and the absence of similar deformities in other mummies, the presence of poliomyelitis is not proven. There is no evidence for poliomyelitis epidemics in Egypt and such contagions were unknown in the world before the 20th century AD.

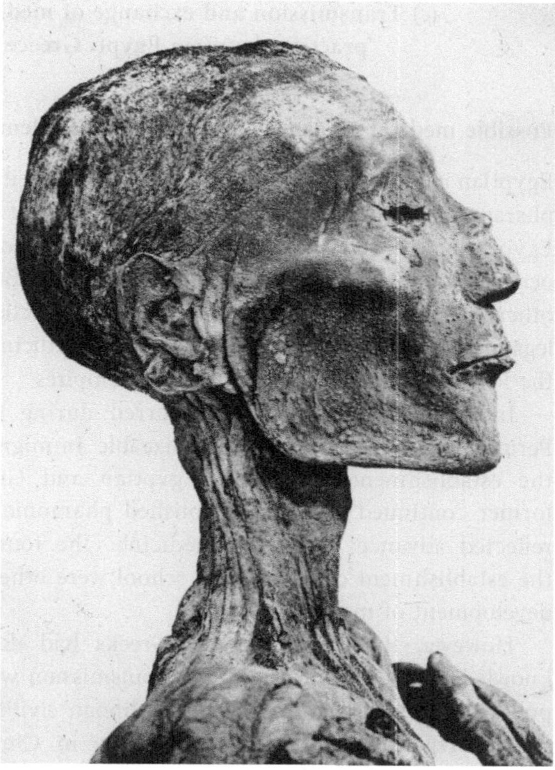

Figure 7.2. Ramesses V's mummified head. The lesions on his face suggest that he suffered from smallpox. Found in the second cache of mummies in the tomb of Amenhotep II in the Valley of the Kings by Victor Loret. Now in the Royal Mummies' Hall at the National Museum of Egyptian Civilization in Cairo, Egypt (Smith 1912: pl. 56).

Smallpox

Smallpox, caused by the variola virus, results in a high fever and characteristic rash, and kills up to about one-third of those infected, although today the disease has been eradicated from the world. Its origin is uncertain, but it is suggested it may have come from East Asia or Africa. The infection does not leave any trace on the skeleton but pustules can be detected on the soft tissues (see Plate 32).

Although nothing in the extant medical papyri can be related to smallpox, the earliest evidence of lesions resembling those of smallpox was found on the faces of three mummies dating from the 18th and 20th Dynasties, one of whom was Ramesses V (Strouhal 1996) (Fig. 7.2). Using electron microscopy, a corpuscle of the virus was detected in the skin of Ramesses, and an immuno-precipitation test further confirmed the diagnosis of smallpox. In addition, the evidence of poor-quality mummification carried out on the body of Ramesses as well as historical evidence from Turin Papyrus 1923 relating to unusual burial arrangements and possibly anti-epidemic precautions could imply that an epidemic of smallpox occurred at that time.

(c) Transmission and exchange of medical concepts and practices between Egypt, Greece and Rome

Possible medical transmissions before the Ptolemaic Period

Egyptian medicine has traditionally been studied either as an important aspect of pharaonic culture or, later, from the perspective of Greek medicine practised in Egypt during the Graeco-Roman Period (Jouanna 2012). Significant developments occurred in Greek medicine from the 5th century BC, when the Hippocratic and other systems gave rise to new concepts and practices. The transmission of this legacy formed the basis of many aspects of medicine that continued throughout the Ptolemaic (Hellenistic) and Roman Empires.

In Egypt, major changes occurred during the Ptolemaic and Roman Periods, when the arrival of a sizeable immigrant population resulted in the establishment of parallel Egyptian and Greek medical systems. The former continued the long-established pharaonic traditions, while the latter reflected advances in Greek medicine. The foundation of Alexandria and the establishment of its medical school were other key factors in the further development of medical science.

However, the Egyptians and Greeks had doubtless exchanged medical knowledge at a much earlier date. Transmission would have occurred through political and trading links with the Minoan civilisation (see above). The main sources regarding disease and medicine in Crete are archaeological items (including inscribed tablets from the palace archives at Knossos and Pylos) and skeletal remains (Kelder *et al.* 2018). This contrasts with Egypt, where evidence from inscriptions and mummies provides a more comprehensive picture of healthcare in that society. Nevertheless, there are clear similarities between the two systems: for example, physicians were attached to the palaces to care for elite patients, while priest–healers employed in temples or sanctuaries probably served the whole society, and magico-religious practitioners, 'wise women' and midwives provided treatments for urban and village communities.

There were also similarities between medical practices in Crete and Egypt. In some cases, where the cause was attributed to the displeasure of deities or spirits, the Minoans used spells and incantations to exorcise ill-health. However, practical healing procedures were also employed; these addressed conditions arising from observable causes such as trauma, often resulting from accidents or misuse of weapons or tools. In these instances, pragmatic measures might be applied: Minoan physicians probably possessed a basic knowledge of surface anatomy and were apparently competent to perform both therapeutic and ritual (trepanation) surgery. Herbal medicine also made a major contribution: a *materia medica*, largely derived from native plants and others imported from the eastern Mediterranean, was available to both palace physicians and community healers.

When the Mycenaean civilisation replaced the Minoan they inherited their medical traditions, and a further two-way transmission with Egypt may have then occurred as a result of the trading and cultural interactions that continued until the end of the 12th century BC.

Later, the settlers in Greek cities established in Egypt from the 26th Dynasty onwards may have been accompanied by their own physicians/healers. However, they may also have consulted the local Egyptian physicians, and this perhaps resulted in a two-way transmission of medical knowledge long before the Ptolemaic Period provided a more obvious opportunity for such exchanges.

Source material

As mentioned above (Chapter 7a), there is a great discrepancy in the quantity, quality, type and accessibility of the source material relating to these different systems, which makes it difficult to compare their similarities and differences. This incongruity (evident when considering Egypt and Mesopotamia, see Chapter 7a) is also apparent when a comparison of Egyptian and Graeco-Roman medicine is attempted, since whereas there is an extensive Greek and Roman philosophical/medicinal literature, only very limited Egyptian documentation has survived.

The *Hippocratic Corpus*, which includes some seventy disparate treatises, is the principal primary source for early Greek medicine (Craik 2018). These anonymous texts are attributed to Hippocrates, a highly regarded physician and writer; he was born on the island of Kos in *c.* 460 BC and founded a medical school there, but also lived for some time in Thessaly. The style and content of these texts indicate that they were probably written by different authors, and perhaps even drawn from different periods. Nevertheless, Hippocrates was traditionally regarded as the 'father of medicine' and the descendant of Asclepius, the god of medicine.

One papyrus, *Anonymous Londinensis*, which dates from the 2nd century AD, is probably based on an earlier history of medicine. It gives the names of twenty-four physicians including Hippocrates, and also some – including Plato – who are otherwise known only from their philosophical works.

Medical knowledge is also embedded in non-medical literature. For example, a discussion of the effects of battle wounds in Homer's epic tale *The Iliad* is a primary source for Greek anatomy and physiology. Owing to a complex, overlapping association between philosophers and physicians, medical material is found in the works of some philosophers such as Aristotle and Plato and in fragmentary texts of other pre-Socratic individuals who studied the nature of the body. Furthermore, inscriptions on stelae give praise and thanks to physicians for helping local communities.

Even after the changes introduced in the 5th century BC, Greek medicine retained a belief in divine intervention to cure the sick. Miraculous cures are recorded in the temples of Asclepius, and many votive offerings associated with these temples have been discovered. In contrast, the Roman system, which drew substantially on Greek medical practice, prioritised 'rational', observational diagnosis and treatment over magico-religious methods (Stok 2018).

Additional source material includes quantities of surgical instruments that enabled surgeons to undertake a variety of procedures. Although generally patients were treated at home, the Romans were the first to introduce hospitals (*valetudinaria*) in the 1st and 2nd centuries AD, exclusively for the treatment of slaves and soldiers (Bliquez 2018).

Medical concepts

To a greater or lesser degree, Mesopotamian, Egyptian and Graeco-Roman medicine each possessed a combination of magico-religious practices and pragmatic treatments. For example, they all included pharmaceutical therapies: these were a predominant treatment in Babylonian medicine, and some passed into Graeco-Roman pharmacology (Geller 2010: 114–17); however, the extent of this transmission remains uncertain.

A basic difference between the earlier systems and Graeco-Roman medicine (as exemplified by the Hippocratic tradition) is the level of divine intervention that each attributed to the causation, treatment and healing of disease. Whereas deities played a central role in Egyptian and Mesopotamian medicine, the Greeks and Romans, although mindful of the gods' involvement in healing, recognised that environmental, dietary and physical factors generally caused ill-health, and thus pragmatic methods were often sought to treat a wide variety of illnesses. However, although some scholars believe that the Hippocratic system was an entirely scientific approach, at first it probably involved a complementary mixture of magico-religious elements and pragmatic treatments; over time, the latter gradually became predominant, although divine intervention always retained some significance.

Aelius Galenus (commonly Anglicised to Galen), a Greek physician born in Pergamum, pursued his career in Rome (Johnston 2018), as did many other Greek physicians. Renowned as a physician, surgeon and philosopher, he was one of the greatest contributors to ancient medicine, and his developments in anatomy, pathology, pharmacology and neurology continued to permeate Western medicine for over a thousand years. Galen's work owed much to the tradition of Hippocrates, the earlier Greek physician who, according to Galen, had developed medicine into a science in the 5th century BC.

A basic tenet of Hippocratic medicine was the assumption that an individual's health or diseases were the result of a balance or imbalance in four bodily humours: blood, phlegm, yellow bile and black bile. It was believed that gender, social class, geographical location, living conditions and diet were also significant factors in a person's well-being. In addition, an individual's mind was thought to have an impact on the causation or development of a disease. These principles were taught and practised at Hippocrates' school of medicine at Kos.

Erotian, a lexicographer who lived in the reign of the Roman emperor Nero, later classified the contents of the Hippocratic Corpus under several main headings. These dealt with anatomy, physiology and pathology, and the basic theories of medical practice that underpinned the therapies (practical measures classified as 'surgical' or 'dietary') discussed in other sections.

Treatments

Surgery

Surgery did not feature in Mesopotamian medicine, and the extent of its use in pharaonic Egypt remains uncertain (see Chapter 5a). However, surgical procedures were developed and practised in Ptolemaic Alexandria – where, in the newly established medical school, dissections were performed on living criminals (Stok 2018) (see Chapter 3a and below) – and they made an increasingly significant contribution during the Roman Empire.

Large numbers of surgical instruments, mainly from Roman times, are known from both archaeological and literary contexts (Bliquez 2018). Evidence from the Asclepeion at Epidaurus (350 BC) indicates that surgery had become an important method of treatment. For example, lists inscribed on three marble boards give details relating to some seventy patients accommodated at the temple: these include their names, medical conditions, case histories and cures. Surgical procedures may have been facilitated by 'dream therapy', which was available in healing centres; this was possibly used to induce a hypnotic trance in patients.

Pharmacy

Pharmaceutical treatments were an important element of Greek and Roman medicine. For example, Dioscorides is a major pharmacological source for the early Roman Empire (see Chapter 2f, i, p. 53).

Healing sanctuaries

There is evidence that, in later times, sanatoria were developed as integral features of some religious shrines in Greece and elsewhere. Healing sanctuaries, which were associated with various deities, combined a temple for the worship of the resident god with a centre where medical advice, prognosis and treatment were provided. Here, the sacred water that patients drank or bathed in was a key feature of these sanctuaries and believed to possess medicinal properties (Edelstein & Edelstein 1945). The cult centres also accommodated the practice of incubation: the supplicant would make a donation to the temple and then undergo 'dream therapy' in a small dark chamber within the complex. While the patients were in this induced state it was believed that the deity, thought to reside in the sanctuary, could reach them through dreams and provide them with care or prescribe treatments that the priests would deliver (see Chapter 3c).

The most significant Greek shrines were dedicated to the Greek god of medicine, Asclepius, who, during the Ptolemaic Period, came to be identified with an Egyptian, Imhotep (see Chapters 2b, 3c, 4e). Mythological sources identify Asclepius' father as the god Apollo, regarded as a renowned healer or founder of medicine. Various places in Greece claimed to be Asclepius' birthplace, but the origins of his cult remain obscure; it may have incorporated several earlier healing traditions, although it seems to have emerged in parallel with the development of Hippocratic medicine.

The conquests of Alexander the Great and his successors, followed by the expansion of the Roman Empire, facilitated the spread of this healing cult, which went on to become one of the most popular and widespread in the ancient world (Caldwell 2018). Over 700 cult centres have been identified to date, including the three largest sanctuaries at Pergamum, Epidaurus and on the island of Kos (Jackson 1990) (see Plate 33), in addition to Messene, Corinth, Gortys and Alipheira (Curnow 2012/2013: 67–83). Cult centres and healing sanctuaries were established in Egypt for Imhotep and Amenhotep, Son of Hapu, under the Ptolemaic Dynasty (see Chapter 3c), and there is also evidence that the cult of Asclepius travelled as far as the regions known today as Spain, Turkey and Britain.

Archaeological evidence provides further information about the likely purpose and function of these cult centres. It indicates that Pergamum, Kos and Epidaurus each incorporated a self-contained unit where healing procedures were carried out away from the main complex; however, at other sites this facility was included in the main sanctuary area. In some instances, where archaeology cannot identify the exact purpose or use of a building, ancient literary sources are able to provide useful additional or confirmatory information. The evidence generally indicates that the special rooms that accommodated incubation were always an important feature of Asclepius' sanctuaries (see Plate 8). This central and popular healing practice was probably one of the main reasons for the cult's unequalled success.

Similar cult centres associated with various other healing deities were established at various sites in Egypt. These were located either within or adjacent to temples, and offered incubation and total or partial immersion in water as treatments for patients who sought cures for physical or mental ailments (see Chapter 3c).

Although the concept of healing cult centres seems to have been introduced to Egypt from Greece, where they flourished from the 5th century BC, there is some evidence that incubation was probably practised much earlier in Egypt, from at least the end of the New Kingdom (*c.* 1000 BC), as a feature of the shrine of the local goddess, Meretseger, at Deir el-Medina (Sadek 1988; Bruyère

1929, 1930). In addition, Quirke (1992: 136) discusses the 19th Dynasty stela of Qenherkhepeshef (BM EA 278) discovered at Thebes as a possible indication of incubation. However, the water supply system for bathing the sick, introduced in the Graeco-Roman Period, may represent the key innovation that the Greeks and Romans, with their specialist knowledge of hydraulic engineering, contributed to the concept of the healing sanctuary in Egypt (pers. comm. K. N. White). The most completely preserved sanatorium in Egypt can be seen in the precinct of the Temple of Isis-Hathor at Denderah; archaeological and inscriptional evidence indicates that some other temples acted as similar centres of healing at this period (see Chapter 3c).

The cults of some of these deities also travelled widely outside Egypt during the Roman Empire. The cult of Isis was particularly successful in this respect and continued to exert considerable influence even after the arrival of Christianity. A good example of this development is the Temple of Isis in the city of Savaria (modern Szombathely, Hungary), which was one of the goddess's largest cult centres during the Roman Empire. Excavations were started here in 1955 and continued from 2001 onwards under the directorship of Ottó Soszrarits (see Plate 34). This work has revealed the extensive remains of the site, confirming that it functioned both as a divine sanctuary for the goddess and as a centre where patients could undergo medical therapies. It featured a sophisticated water supply system, separate from the urban provision that served Savaria (Sosztarits 2013). This arrangement was considered necessary on religious grounds, since it was required that all water in general use at the temple should come from a 'pure' source. A completely independent drainage network incorporated a well and made use of trapped rainwater that fell within the sacred precinct. However, Nile water, transported at considerable expense from Egypt, was used for the libations offered to deities in all the regular temple rituals at these shrines.

The mythology of pharaonic Egypt, linking Isis to the annual Nile inundation and the renewal of fertility, was based on a belief in the spiritual power of water. The main celebration of the cult of Osiris and Isis in Egypt marked the annual Nile flood. This association with water was continued and celebrated in Roman times with a major annual festival, the Navigium Isidis or Isidis Navigium (Giunio 2013), marked by a procession of priests and cult adherents who, dressed in distinctive costumes and carrying sacred emblems, transported a model ship from the Isis temple to the sea or a local river.

Since there was now no direct physical connection between the Nile and the Isis celebrations in cult centres outside Egypt, the Navigium Isidis celebrated the goddess in a new role as 'Mistress of the Seas' and 'Protector of Seafarers and Rulers and Peoples of the Roman Empire'. The festival was held on March 5; this differed from the annual Osirian celebration in Egypt, but appropriately coincided with the ending of winter storms in the Mediterranean, which allowed seaborne trade to resume, including the transport of grain shipments from Egypt to Rome.

Attitudes towards ill-health and disability

A greater emphasis on 'pragmatic' as opposed to 'magical' treatments in Greek and Roman medicine inspired various developments in the delivery of treatment; in Roman times these included significant advances in robust and interventional methods of surgery. The Greeks believed that all their gods (except the disabled Hephaestus) were physically perfect, and that the design of the human body was based on this flawless image (see Chapter 6e). These beliefs underpinned the often harsh attitudes that they adopted towards those who had deformities or disabilities (Rose 2017: 139–53) (see Chapters 5d and 6e). This attitude continued under the Romans, although the Stoics (who argued that misfortune should be accepted without complaint) offered an alternative view – namely, that the ideal of a perfect, beautiful and healthy body should be replaced with the belief that virtue was the highest good (Gevaert 2017: 213–21).

Immigration to Egypt in the Graeco-Roman Period: the impact on medical concepts, provision and practices

The interchange of ideas about medical concepts and practice that took place between Egypt and Greece facilitated the transmission of aspects of pharaonic medicine into classical, medieval and even later traditions. As summarised above, opportunities for this knowledge transfer would have arisen either from general interaction between the two medical systems over the millennia or the more direct contact between the Egyptian and Greek communities that followed the foundation of trading centres such as Naucratis and the later conquest of Egypt by Alexander the Great in 332 BC, and the country's subsequent colonisation under Ptolemaic and Roman rulers.

In this context, Alexandria, founded by Alexander the Great on the north-west coast of the Nile Delta, played a key role. It soon became a leading Hellenistic city with its own medical school where a cosmopolitan group of physicians and scientists congregated to innovate, practise and develop new ideas and techniques. The medical school was ultimately significant in the transmission of medical knowledge to Europe and the Middle East.

New opportunities now arose for foreigners to settle on crown land in Egypt and cultivate it in exchange for a commitment to military service in the Ptolemaic and Roman Periods. These settlements became established in several areas: the Fayoum, where there was new land reclamation, became particularly popular. The settlers were not homogeneous – they belonged to various ethnic groups and came from different homelands, but most shared a Greek outlook and followed

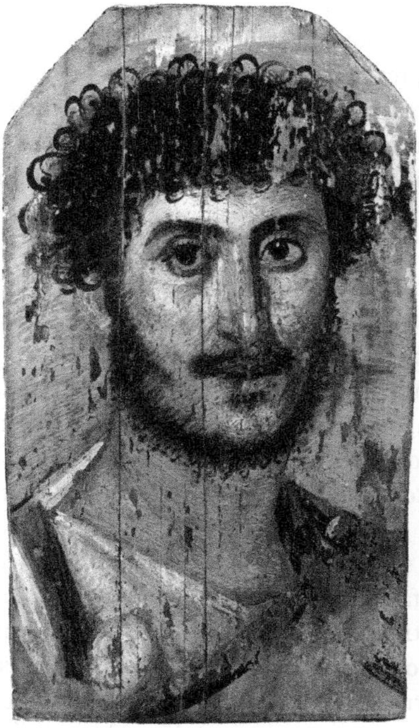

Figure 7.3. Painted wooden panel portrait of a young man, originally placed over the face of a mummy. Mummification was one of the Egyptian practices that some immigrants adopted during the Roman Period. From Hawara, now in The Manchester Museum, 2263 (courtesy of The Manchester Museum, The University of Manchester).

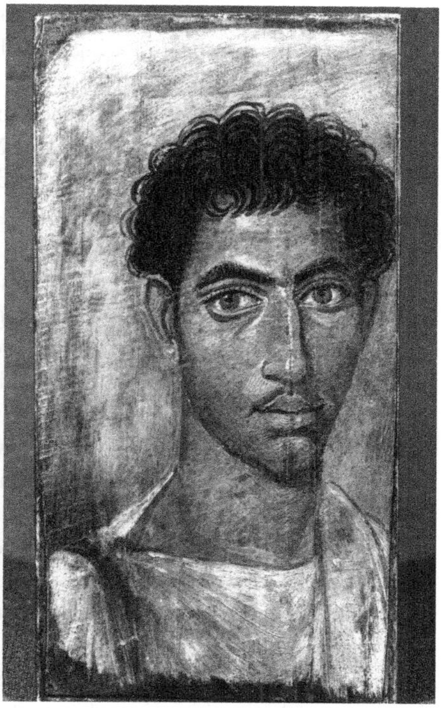

Figure 7.4. Painted wooden panel portrait of a young man, originally placed over the face of a mummy. Unlike the stylised facial representations seen on coffins of the pharaonic period, these portraits from Roman Egypt appear to depict individual people. From Hawara, now in The Manchester Museum, 10306 (courtesy of The Manchester Museum, The University of Manchester).

Greek values and beliefs. At least superficially, the indigenous and immigrant communities developed parallel but separate lives. For example, separate and distinctive Egyptian and Greek legal and educational systems were introduced, although archaeological and iconographic evidence from contemporary tombs and temples indicates that there was some degree of hybridisation in the art forms, and in some religious beliefs and customs.

Some immigrants did adopt Egyptian religious beliefs and funerary practices, particularly mummification (Fig. 7.3). Panel portraits, incorporated into some Roman Period mummies, and possibly representing realistic likenesses of their owners, show that people in these communities displayed a wide variety of facial and physical features (Fig. 7.4). Mummies of the Graeco-Roman Period held today in museum collections worldwide provide valuable opportunities for studies on diet, therapeutic treatments and the incidence of disease prevalent in that era (David 1979).

Lang's (2013) study of medicine in Ptolemaic times discusses the impact that climate, geography, demography, agriculture, botany, biological inheritance and magico-religious beliefs would have had on disease incidence and medical practice. The new immigrants would have brought their own experience, knowledge and attitudes regarding medical care and treatment. As they adapted mentally and physically to their new environment, they would have encountered fresh challenges while gradually learning to live alongside the resident Egyptian population.

The two communities generally faced similar health issues. These included problems exacerbated by environmental factors including seasonal epidemics, respiratory diseases and animal bites or stings, in particular those of scorpions and snakes. People from both societies would have suffered from eye diseases, gynaecological conditions and dangers surrounding childbirth. Mummy studies have shown that a wide range of parasitic infestations occurred throughout Egypt (Chapter 6a). These included malaria, a particular problem for communities in the Delta and Fayoum, where lakes and canals provided abundant breeding grounds for mosquitoes, the vector of this disease.

Degenerative osteoarthritis is often observed in Egyptian remains from pharaonic times onwards, and there is palaeopathological evidence that skeletal malformation, disease and deterioration occurred among both the indigenous and the immigrant populations (Fig. 7.5).

Dietary deficiencies and mild nutritional stress, with associated enteric diseases such as typhoid and dysentery, also existed in pharaonic times, as well as viral and bacterial infections, including tuberculosis. The immigrant population would have had to cope with dietary changes and diseases caused by local bacteria, viruses and parasites (Lang 2013: 2–19). There is no evidence, however, that the immigrants brought any major plagues with them, or that they succumbed to these illnesses on arrival in Egypt.

Tooth wear and to a lesser extent periodontal disease, mainly attributable to the diet, were fairly commonplace in pharaonic Egypt. However, evidence from mummy studies has demonstrated that these conditions decreased during the Graeco-Roman Period, while the rate of caries increased. The changing incidence of these conditions would have been the result of dietary changes partly introduced by the immigrants.

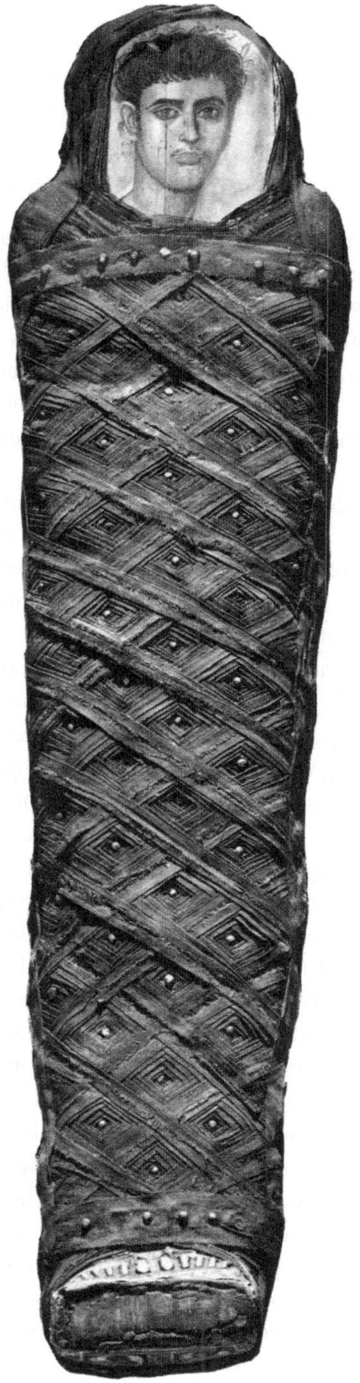

Figure 7.5. Mummy of an adolescent male enclosed in diagonal bandaging interspersed with gilded studs; a cartonnage piece covers the feet. The panel portrait shows a boy wearing a gilded laurel wreath. Inside the elaborate casing, the body is poorly preserved. Unusually in a young person, there are early osteoarthritic changes present in the knee joints. Roman Period. From Hawara, now in The Manchester Museum, 1768 (courtesy of The Manchester Museum, The University of Manchester).

The indigenous and immigrant communities therefore encountered the same basic health and lifestyle challenges, and despite retaining two separate medical systems there was probably some overlap and exchange of ideas and treatments (Marganne 1993; Lang 2013: 41).

The central role of Alexandria in Greek medicine

Although Alexandria was built on an earlier Egyptian settlement, it remained essentially Greek in character and developed into a leading city of the Hellenistic world. Nevertheless, its population included significant numbers of Egyptian and Jewish residents, as well as residents of mixed background, the result of marriages between non-elite Greeks and native-born Egyptians.

The city acquired a wealth of notable buildings. These included the Pharos, the famous lighthouse completed in 280–279 BC, which was regarded as one of the wonders of the ancient world. There was also a renowned library at Alexandria, which contained many scrolls (estimates range from 30,000 to as many as 900,000) (Bagnall 2002; Ryholt & Barjamovic 2019). The library's collections included numerous volumes describing the practices and procedures of ancient Greek medicine, many of which were later adopted by the Romans. Outstanding philologists were engaged by the library to edit these texts. Members of an associated research institute, the Museion, were appointed by the king and undertook scientific research, for which they were rewarded with generous salaries. However, these institutions were not bases for the practice of Alexandrian medicine, although some famous physicians may have had connections with the library and Museion. Alexandria's international reputation as a centre for medical research and experimentation had been established by elite sects who mainly followed the principles of Greek medicine, although some concepts and drug ingredients were perhaps adopted from the parallel Egyptian system. The latter continued to be used by the non-elite population of Alexandria and indigenous communities throughout the country.

Famous members of the Alexandrian sects included Herophilus of Chalcedon, a mid-3rd-century BC physician who was acknowledged as the first medical teacher in Alexandria (Stok 2018) (see Chapter 3a). Herophilus discovered that the nervous system is connected to motion and sensation, and distinguished between different types of pulse. With his contemporary, Erasistratus of Chios, he carried out research relating to the venous and nervous systems.

According to Aulus Cornelius Celsus, writing in the 1st century AD (Scarborough 1976), both these men, with authorisation from the Ptolemaic rulers, practised dissection and vivisection on criminals supplied by the prisons (Stok 2018: 360). This grisly resource offered a unique opportunity to examine the structure of internal organs and their disposition and functions within the body. However, human dissection and vivisection, although unique, were temporary features of the medical and scientific research carried out at Alexandria. There is no evidence that any animal dissection or vivisection was ever undertaken, or that invasive internal surgery on humans or animals ever played any part in indigenous Egyptian medicine.

It could be possible that public opinion was more receptive to the concept of human dissection and vivisection because of the ancient Egyptian custom of mummifying the dead (von Staden 1989: 29). However, this seems unlikely, as there was no correlation between the aims and techniques employed in these procedures (Lang 2013: 253). For example, mummification, based on religious beliefs and carried out to restore the body in preparation for the next life, utilised very limited and specific invasive procedures. On the other hand, human dissection and vivisection were carried out for purely investigative and scientific reasons, and usually involved full autopsy or extensive dismemberment of the corpse.

Evidence for transmission and exchange of medical concepts from Egypt to the Graeco-Roman tradition

Circumstances during the Graeco-Roman Period provide a unique opportunity to examine how Egyptian and Greek medicine functioned in tandem. Important questions remain, however, regarding the extent to which medicine was considered to be part of an individual's ethnocultural identity (Lang 2013: 42–43). As for a patient's choice, did they seek medical advice and treatment exclusively within their own community, or did they sometimes consult medical practitioners in the alternative system? (Lang 2013: 125–33).

More generally, researchers have questioned the true extent to which Egyptian medicine may have influenced Greek and subsequently Roman traditions. Some classical literary sources indicate that Egyptian medicine and its practitioners were held in high esteem. For example, Homer (4, 227–323) recounted that the gifts Menelaus and Helen brought back from Egypt included drugs to treat a variety of conditions; he also states that the Egyptian physicians were 'the wisest of men'. This seems to acknowledge the superiority of pharaonic medicine over Greek and all other systems. Theophrastes (371–*c.* 287 BC), in his *History of Plants* (9.15), reiterates Homer's opinion of Egyptian physicians and claims that Egypt produced more medicinal plants than any area other than Greece. The biography of Plato in Diogenes Laertius' *Lives of the Philosophers* (3rd century AD) praises the skills of Egyptian priest-physicians and uses Homer's comments to support this claim.

Herodotus (II, 84) described Egypt as 'full of doctors' and commented that they were specialists in different branches of medicine (III, 1). This contrasted with the Greek system, where the practitioners were generalists in both theory and practice. He also emphasised that Egyptian physicians were highly regarded and in great demand among the elite of foreign lands. He discussed the good health enjoyed by the Egyptian population, which he attributed to an even climate and a beneficial diet. Another author, Isocrates (436–338 BC), in his work *Busiris* (*Isocrates*, vol. 3, 21–22), attributed the Egyptians' good health and longevity to the use of safe and effective drugs, while the 1st-century BC account of Diodorus Siculus (1, 821–22) also comments on the Egyptians' beneficial diet, along with their methods of administering medical treatment in accordance with a written code compiled by a group of foremost physicians.

It has been argued (Jouanna 2012) that there was a change in attitude once the Greeks moved towards an increasingly pragmatic approach to medicine in the 5th century BC. Rather than attributing the origins of medicine to the Egyptians, Greek writers now claimed that distinction for themselves. They stated that it was Asclepius, inheriting this knowledge from his divine father Apollo, who founded medical science, which was carried forward by his descendants, ultimately becoming the basis of the Hippocratic tradition. Jouanna (2012) comments that histories of medicine by Greek authors between Hippocrates (5th century BC) and Galen (2nd century BC) do not acknowledge any major transmission from Egyptian medicine. However, in his *Natural History* (7, 114), Pliny the Elder (AD 23–79) states that the Egyptians claimed to have discovered medicine, while Clement of Alexandria linked its foundation to Egypt, with a subsequent transmission to the Greeks.

In addition to the literary affirmations, researchers have identified several medical concepts and techniques that may have been transmitted from Egypt to Greece, including the presence of Egyptian mineral and herbal ingredients in the Hippocratic pharmacopeia. Evidence of the direct influence Egypt had on Greek medicine is exemplified by the very similar gynaecological tests found in some Egyptian medical papyri (notably P. Carlsberg and P. Kahun) and the Hippocratic source *On Sterile Women* (chapter 214) (Iversen 1939). Other researchers have considered whether the pathogenic agent (*wẖdw*) mentioned in Egyptian sources was the origin of a Cnidian concept (later replaced by the Hippocratic doctrine of humours) that corrupt nutriment residues not evacuated from the body were a major cause of disease (Steuer & Saunders 1959; Bardinet 1995) – a view that continued into Victorian England.

Other important discoveries may have been transmitted from Egypt to Greece. For example, records show that it was the Egyptians who first developed an anatomical and medical vocabulary, and pharaonic sources also contain the earliest extant references to anatomical observations, experiments in surgery and pharmacy and the use of splints, bandages and compresses.

Breasted's commentary (1930) claimed that the Edwin Smith Papyrus provides evidence that the Egyptian physicians made some significant objective and scientific advances, although these discoveries are usually attributed to the Greeks many centuries later. This viewpoint has been discussed in detail by Ghalioungui (1963: 58–66) and reviewed more recently by Sanchez & Meltzer (2012: 1–7).

The Edwin Smith Papyrus, a didactic trauma treatise that demonstrates a detailed anatomical knowledge, contains in the first section forty-eight clinical observations of surgical procedures relating to the head, neck and parts of the thorax (Breasted 1930: 5–7; see Chapter 1c, 5c). The ancient author discusses these in relation to the organs affected, starting from the head and working downwards – a sequence still used in medicine today. The papyrus also mentions the concept of 'syndromes' (defined by Ghalioungui (1963: 116) as 'collections of manifestations forming recurrent and distinctive clinical pictures'). Again, this very significant advance is usually attributed to the Greeks. Furthermore, the author of this papyrus describes traumatic hemiplegia and a squint, probably indicating that Egyptian physicians already understood the relationship between the nervous system and voluntary movements, and they appear to have been aware that the side and localisation of the paralysis depended on the situation of the nervous lesion. Ghalioungui (1963: 61) goes on to contrast this with Hippocrates' comments about the brain 1000 years later, and it was not until the 4th century BC that the Alexandrian physicians Erasistratus and Herophilus definitively formulated the anatomical relationship between the peripheral nerves and the central nervous system.

In general, the Egyptian medical papyri show that there was a well-established routine procedure involving careful observation of the patient and ongoing analysis of the symptoms, followed by a recommended treatment. Much later, these are identified as important stages in the Hippocratic method. Other Hippocratic treatments foreshadowed in the Edwin Smith Papyrus include instructions to deal with the fracture of a clavicle (Case 35) and a treatment to reduce dislocations of the jaw (Case 25). Used later in the 1st century BC by a Cypriot physician, Apollonius of Kitium, this technique was ultimately transmitted through Islamic medicine to Europe and is still practised today (Forshaw 2020).

The Egyptians may also have been the first to understand the circulation of the blood. As indicated in P. Edwin Smith and P. Ebers, they also seem to have identified the link between the heart and pulsation. For example, P. Ebers 854(a) states that a patient's pulse could be taken by a priest of Sekhmet, a physician, or a *s3w* (amulet man/magician).

In conclusion, it is likely that Egyptian physicians achieved some significant discoveries centuries ahead of the Greeks, but this is not fully recognised because Egyptian records are so much more limited in number and scope than the sources available for Greek medicine.

(d) Egypt's contribution to later medical systems

Medicine in the later Classical and Islamic periods

The development of Classical and Islamic medicine

'Classical medicine', which incorporated elements of Roman, Greek and earlier traditions (including pharaonic medicine), was widely practised throughout the later years of the Roman Empire. As previously discussed (Chapter 7c), the famous medical school at Alexandria acted as a specific route for the transmission of ancient knowledge to other areas of the Roman Empire (Cilliers 2018: 1017). Many of the early traditions were absorbed into Islamic medicine and ultimately, through Greek, Latin and Arabic manuscripts, significant ideas and practices were transmitted from the ancient sources into medieval and later European medicine. Here they continued to develop over many centuries to become the basis of 'Western' medicine, with some concepts even continuing down to the present day.

Transmission of Classical medicine: the historical and political background

The preservation and transmission of Classical medicine occurred within the context of the political circumstances dominating the later years of the Roman Empire. The Empire was now divided into an eastern, Greek-speaking sphere ruled from Constantinople, and a western, Latin–Germanic section still governed from Rome. During the 4th to 7th centuries AD (*c.* AD 300–650) the western empire disintegrated, marking the onset of the Dark Ages. This dissolution was characterised by economic difficulties, epidemics, civil wars and incursions by pagan and Christian Germanic tribes (Cilliers 2018: 1013). Rome was sacked on several occasions and the last western Roman emperor was deposed in AD 476.

However, North Africa (the Roman province of Africa Proconsularis), which was now part of the eastern Roman Empire, was spared the ravages suffered in other areas of the Roman world. Led during the 4th and 5th centuries AD by Carthage and other cities, the area continued to enjoy relatively stable conditions and even survived subsequent conquest by Germanic Vandals. The Roman Emperor Justinian then reconquered North Africa and once again brought it under Christian Byzantine rule. Throughout this period, an integrated system of medical theory and practice, largely based on Greek medicine, continued to flourish there, following a theoretical and philosophical approach and incorporating some practical measures adopted from local indigenous healing traditions.

Routes of transmission through North Africa and northern Italy

Relatively stable political conditions enabled North Africa to play a key role in preserving and transmitting Classical medicine. Medical schools, vital to preserving and transmitting this knowledge, were established at Carthage, at

Ravenna in northern Italy and elsewhere. They had links with the great medical institution at Alexandria in Egypt, and their scholars were able to access the great works of Classical medicine held in the Alexandria collections.

When political conditions in North Africa eventually deteriorated, fleeing refugees probably transported Classical medical expertise and documentation to Spain and Italy. In particular, Ravenna now emerged as a leading centre where medical texts were copied, translated and categorised (Sigerist 1958: 135); eventually this knowledge was carried forward to monasteries in France, before finally reaching northern Europe during the 6th to 8th centuries AD (Cilliers 2018: 1030).

An important step in the transmission of Classical knowledge was the translation of medical texts from Greek into Latin. Earlier in the Roman Empire, physicians and philosophers of diverse ethnic backgrounds had possessed a good knowledge of Greek, but by the 3rd century AD this was no longer true, and it became necessary to produce manuscripts in Latin to make medical science more widely available (Cilliers 2018: 2017). North African centres played a vital part in this process, also producing works by their own renowned medical writers, several of whom continued to be popular down to medieval times.

Transmission of ancient medical knowledge to Islamic (Arab) medicine

In the 7th century AD the Arab invasions swept away the remnants of the Roman/Byzantine empires in North Africa and the Middle East, and introduced a new religion, Islam, which established new ideas and customs across the region. This represented a major transition in political and religious power, but seemingly did not involve a complete break with pre-Islamic culture, particularly Graeco-Roman and Byzantine precedents.

As the Muslim conquests continued across Asia and Africa, 'Islamic medicine' became the predominant system of treatment in these areas. It assimilated diverse concepts and practices from Graeco-Roman, Christian and pre-Islamic sources, including magical and mystical beliefs. Later directives dealt with the correct treatment of patients and the organisation of employment and financial relief for the needy (Katz 2005; Gaumer 2017: 410).

Medical literature written in Arabic now not only preserved knowledge from earlier Classical sources but ultimately provided an additional route for its transmission to Europe, often through Latin translations, where it continued to have a major impact on Western medicine until at least the 17th century AD.

The wider influence of ancient Egyptian medicine

The limitations of Egyptian source material

The wealth of evidence relating to disease and medical treatments in Greek, Roman and Islamic societies (Brothwell and Sandison 1967; Dols 1984; Bagnall

1993; Scheidel 2001) is mainly derived from documents written in Greek, Latin and Arabic. Knowledge of these languages has continued uninterrupted from ancient to modern times. In contrast, extant source material for pharaonic medicine is very limited and for centuries the key to translating and understanding the Egyptian scripts, in which these manuscripts were written, was lost. Even after Champollion deciphered hieroglyphs and opened the language for future study, obscurity still surrounded the meanings of some words found in the medical papyri. Nevertheless, there is arguably sufficient evidence to indicate that Egyptian pharaonic medicine provided the basis for 'Western' medicine.

Some significant advances and contributions from pharaonic medicine

A key stage in this inheritance was the extent to which transmission occurred between Egyptian and Greek medicine (see above). Despite some fundamental differences between the two systems, and although available evidence is limited, there is a convincing case that the Greeks did inherit some very significant discoveries and practical treatments from the Egyptians. In this context it is interesting to speculate whether Naucratis, the city established for the Greeks in Egypt in the 26th Dynasty, played any part in the transmission from Egypt to Greek medicine. For example, did the Greek physicians practising pre-Hippocratic medicine in Naucratis gain new knowledge from their Egyptian counterparts that eventually contributed to the 'pragmatic' approach that evolved in Greek medicine in the 5th century BC (pers. comm. K. W. White)?

The pharmaceutical and surgical traditions

Pharmaceutical therapies and surgery were the commonest methods of practical treatment in ancient medicine. Inscriptional, iconographic and palaeopathological evidence has shown that the Egyptians performed a limited range of surgical procedures. These seem to have been successful in some cases and were an advance on the sole reliance on pharmaceutical treatments observed in Mesopotamian medicine.

Egyptian experimentation provided a basis for developments in surgical techniques and instruments in Graeco-Roman medicine (Bliquez 2018). The Alexandrian medical school played a key role in the development of surgery: new knowledge and skills acquired through autopsies and vivisection contributed to surgical advances under the Roman Empire, and in turn influenced Islamic and early European medicine.

Based on extensive inscriptional evidence from Classical sources, modern scholarship has generally credited the Greeks with initiating a pharmaceutical tradition that was continued under the Romans (Scarborough 2018). However, although no extant *Egyptian Herbal* has yet been discovered, the Egyptian medical literature gives some idea of the richness of their pharmacopeia, providing the earliest recorded applications of some well-known drugs. These occur later in Classical writings and in Hebrew, Syriac, Persian and Arabic sources. Efficacious drugs mentioned in these sources may have been discovered independently and do not provide conclusive evidence of borrowing from Egypt. However, it is the distinctive recipes with unexpected and fanciful ingredients (for example, hedgehog spines to treat alopecia and skinned mice for childhood illnesses) that are found in both Egyptian and later sources that provide a clearer indication of transmission (Harris 1987: 115). A multidisciplinary study at Manchester has confirmed that the Egyptians were using therapeutic and reproducible pharmaceutical treatments nearly 2000 years before Hippocrates (David 2010; see Chapter 5f).

Provision of care for the sick and infirm

Egypt produced trained physicians, including specialists in a variety of fields, from at least as early as the Old Kingdom. This need to train and employ professional health workers was recognised and developed in all the later medical systems.

Sanatoria established in Egypt provided dedicated accommodation where the sick could stay while receiving healing treatments. Contemporary centres were also established elsewhere in the Hellenistic world. Although the concept of dream therapy may have existed in Egypt before this date, the idea of 'hospitals' as locations where a variety of complementary medical treatments were offered in parallel is probably Greek in origin. This concept, later expanded and developed during Roman times, eventually became a key feature of Islamic medicine.

The Egyptians demonstrated an inclusive and caring attitude towards sickness, deformity and disability that may have been influenced by their underlying religious beliefs and practices (Garland 2010; David 2017; Gevaert 2017). This approach was not evident in contemporary societies where different religious and ethical standards prevailed (discussed in Chapters 5d and 6e), and the Egyptian perspective was reflected and repeated only much later, when new beliefs and attitudes were introduced with the arrival of Christianity and Islam.

Egypt's legacy to European and modern 'Western' medicine

Overall, the evidence suggests that the legacy of ancient Egyptian medicine can be traced via Classical and Islamic traditions through to medieval and later practices in Europe, with some aspects still surviving today in modern 'Western' medicine (Stannard 1999; David 2012/2013).

Sometimes a specific medical observation in the texts indicates that the Egyptians achieved a particular pioneering breakthrough thousands of years ago. There is also evidence that some of their concepts, knowledge and overall approach towards particular treatments have influenced modern attitudes. For example, some of the medicinal ingredients identified in ancient Egyptian remedies were probably transmitted through later sources (see above) and eventually incorporated into the *materia medica* of Europe in medieval, Renaissance and later times; some even continue in use today, often in a synthesised form.

In ancient Egypt some type and level of medical care and treatment appears to have been available to everyone, regardless of wealth or status. Specific guidelines defined and protected the relationship between healthcare providers and their patients, and there was an enlightened attitude towards deformity and disabling physical and mental health issues. Healers provided some level of treatment for all their patients, regardless of the severity of their condition; even for the terminally ill, appropriate palliative care was offered. It is perhaps this centrality and importance of the patient's role that should be regarded as the Egyptians' most significant and enduring legacy to the modern world.

Bibliography

Adler, C. J., Dobney, K., Weyrich, L. S., Kaidonis, J., Walker, A. W., Haak, W., Bradshaw, C. J., Townsend, G., Sołtysiak, A., Alt, K. W., Parkhill, J. & Cooper, A. (2013). 'Sequencing ancient calcified dental plaque shows changes in oral microbiota with dietary shifts of the Neolithic and Industrial revolutions.' *Nature Genetics* 45(4): 450–55.

Al Sadhan, R. & Alma, K. (1999). 'Miswak (chewing stick): a cultural and scientific heritage.' *Saudi Dental Journal* 11(2): 80–88.

Aldred, C. (1988). *Akhenaten: King of Egypt*. London, New York: Thames and Hudson.

Aldred, C. & Sandison, A. T. (1962). 'The Pharaoh Akhenaten: a problem in Egyptology and pathology.' *Bulletin of the History of Medicine* 36: 293–316.

Allam, A. H., Thompson, R. C., Wann, L. S., Miyamoto, M. I. & Thompson, G. S. (2009). 'Computed tomographic assessment of atherosclerosis in ancient Egyptian mummies.' *Journal of the American Medical Association* 302(19): 2091–94.

Allam, A. H., Thompson, R. C., Wann, L. S., Miyamoto, M. I., Nur El-Din, Ael-H., El-Maksoud, G. A., Al-Tohamy Soliman, M., Badr, I., El-Rahman Amer, H. A., Sutherland, M. L., Sutherland, J. D. S. & Thomas, G. S. (2011). 'Atherosclerosis in ancient Egyptian mummies: the Horus Study.' *Journal of the American College of Cardiology: Cardiovascular Imaging* 4(4): 315–27.

Allen, J. (2005). *The Art of Medicine in Ancient Egypt*. New York, New Haven, CT: Metropolitan Museum of New York & Yale University Press.

Allen, T. G. (1960). *The Egyptian Book of the Dead: Documents in the Oriental Institute Museum at the University of Chicago*. Oriental Institute Publications 82. Chicago, IL: University of Chicago Press.

Anderson, S. R. (1997). 'The eye and its diseases in ancient Egypt.' *Acta Ophthalmologica Scandinavica* 75: 338–44.

Anthes, R. (1928). *Die Felseninschriften von Hatnub, nach den Aufnahmen Georg Möllers*. Leipzig: J. C. Hinrichs.

Araujo, R., Reinhard, K. & Ferreira, L. F. (2000). 'The role of mummy studies in paleoparasitology.' *Chungara Revista de Antropología Chilena* 32: 111–17.

Argilés, M., Sabi, M. & Marqués-Caiyo, M. S. (2021). 'Antibacterial analysis of the minerals used for ocular remedies in ancient Egypt.' In R. Dinarès Solà, M. F. Georges & M. R. Guasch-Jané (eds), *Pharmacy and Medicine in Ancient Egypt: Proceedings of the Conference Held in Barcelona*, Egyptology 34. Oxford: Archaeopress.

Armitage, P. L. & Clutton-Brock, J. (1981). 'A radiological and historical investigation into the mummification of cats from ancient Egypt.' *Journal of Archaeological Science* 8: 185–96.

Assmann, J. (1996). *Das Grab des Amenemope (TT41)*. Theben 03. Mainz: Philipp von Zabern.

--- (2003). *The Mind of Egypt: History and Meaning in the Time of the Pharaohs*. Cambridge, MA: Harvard University Press.

Aufderheide, A. C. & Rodríguez-Martín, C. (1998). *The Cambridge Encyclopedia of Human Paleopathology*. Cambridge: Cambridge University Press.

Aufrère, S. (2021). 'Egypt.' In M. Beretta (ed.), *A Cultural History of Chemistry Volume*, vol. 1. *In Antiquity*. London: Bloomsbury Academy, 53–63.

Austin, A. (2014). *Contending with Illness in Ancient Egypt: A Textual and Osteological Study of Healthcare at Deir el Medina*. Los Angeles: UCLA Electronic Theses and Dissertations.

--- (2017). 'The cost of a commute: a multidisciplinary approach to osteoarthritis in New Kingdom Egypt.' *International Journal of Osteoarchaeology* 27(4): 537–50.

--- (2022). 'Dental health and dentistry in ancient Egypt: possible evidence for dental filling and extraction at Deir el-Medina.' *International Journal of Paleopathology* 38: 95–106.

Ayad, M. (2009). *God's Wife, God's Servant: The God's Wife of Amun (c. 740–525 BC)*. London: Routledge.

Baadsvik, E. L., Weiger, M., Froidevaux, R., Rösler, M. B., Brunner, D. O., Öhrström, L., Rühli, F. J., Eppenberger, P. & Pruessmann, K. P. (2021). 'High-resolution MRI of mummified tissues using advanced short-T2 methodology and hardware.' *Magnetic Resonance in Medicine* 85(3): 1481–92.

Badawy, A. (1978). *The Tomb of Nyhetep-Ptah at Giza and the Tomb of Ankhmahor at Saqqara*. Berkeley, CA: University of California Press.

Bagnall, R. S. (1993). *Egypt in Late Antiquity*. Princeton, NJ: Princeton University Press.

--- (2002). 'Alexandria: Library of Dreams.' *Proceedings of the American Philosophical Society* 146(4): 348–62.

Le Bailly, M., Mouze, S., Chaves da Rocha, G. & Heim, J.-L. (2009). 'Identification of Taenia sp. in a mummy from a Christian Necropolis in El-Deir, Oasis of Kharga.' *Journal of Parasitology Research* 96(1): 213–15.

Baines, J. (1987). 'Practical religion and piety.' *Journal of Egyptian Archaeology* 73: 79–83.

Baines, J. & Lacovara, P. (2002). 'Burial and the dead in ancient Egyptian society: respect, formalism, neglect.' *Journal of Social Archaeology* 2: 5–36.

Baines, J. & Málek, J. (1980). *Atlas of Ancient Egypt*. Oxford: Phaidon Press Ltd.

Balabanova, S., Parsche, F. & Pirsig, W. (1992). 'First identification of drugs in Egyptian mummies.' *Naturwissenschaften* 79: 358.

Barbieri, R., Mekni, R., Levasseur, A., Chabrière, E., Signoli, M., Tzortzis, S., Aboudharam, G. & Drancourt, M. (2017). 'Paleoproteomics of the dental pulp: the plague paradigm.' *PLoS One* Jul 26;12(7): e0180552. doi: 10.1371/journal.pone.0180552.

Bardinet, T. (1995). *Les Papyrus Médicaux de l'Égypte Pharaonique*. Lyon: Fayard.

Bar-Ziv, J. & Goldberg, G. M. (1974). 'Simple siliceous pneumoconiosis in Negev Beduins.' *Archives of Environmental and Occupational Health* 29(3): 121.

Bastian, L. A. & Piscitelli, J. T. (1997). 'Is this patient pregnant? Can you reliably rule in or rule out early pregnancy by clinical examination?' *Journal of the American Medical Association* 278(7): 586–91.

Bauer, M. & Patzelt, D. (2002). 'Intracranial stab injuries: case report and case study.' *Forensic Science International* 129: 122–27.

Bay, N. S. & Bay, B. H. (2010). 'Greek anatomist Herophilus: the father of anatomy.' *Anatomy and Cell Biology* 43(4): 280–83.

Beck, S. (2018). *Exorcism, illness and demons in an ancient Near Eastern context: the Egyptian magical Papyrus Leiden I 343 + 345*, Palma 18. Leiden: Sidestone Press.

Becker, M. J. & Turfa, J. M. (2017). *The Etruscans and the History of Dentistry: The Golden Smile through the Ages*. London, New York: Routledge.

Bedwani, R., Renganathan, E., El Kwhsky, F., Braga, C., Abu Seif, H. H., Abul Azm, T., Zaki, A., Franceschi, S., Boffetta, P. & La Vecchia, C. (1998). 'Schistosomiasis and the risk of bladder cancer in Alexandria, Egypt.' *British Journal of Cancer* 77(7): 1186–89.

Benitez, J. T. (1988). 'Otopathology of Egyptian mummy PUM II: final report.' *Journal of Laryngology and Otology* 102: 458–90.

Bertol, E., Fineschi, V., Karch, S. B., Mari, F. & Riezzo, I. (2004). 'Nymphaea cults in ancient Egypt and the New World: a lesson in empirical pharmacology.' *Journal of the Royal Society of Medicine* 97(2): 84–85.

Bestock, L. (2019). *Violence and Power in Ancient Egypt: Image and Ideology before the New Kingdom*. London, New York: Routledge.

Bietak, M. (2012). 'The archaeology of the "Gold of Valour".' *Egyptian Archaeology* 42: 32–33.

Blackman, A. M. (1925). 'Oracles in Ancient Egypt.' *Journal of Egyptian Archaeology* 11: 249–53.

Blackman, A. M. & Davies, W. V. (1988). *The Story of King Kheops and the magicians: transcribed from Papyrus Westcar (Berlin Papyrus 3033)*. Reading: J. V. Books.

Bleiburg, E., Barbash, Y. & Bruno, L. (eds) (2013). *Soulful creatures: animal mummies in ancient Egypt*. New York: D. Giles Ltd.

Bliquez, L. J. (1996). 'Prosthetics in classical antiquity: Greek, Etruscan and Roman prosthetics. II.' In W. Haase (ed.), *Rise & Decline of the Roman World*, II. Berlin: Walter de Gruyter, 2662–76.

--- (2018). 'Greco-Roman surgical instruments: the tools of the trade.' In P. T. Keyser & J. Scarborough (eds), *Science and Medicine in the Classical World*. Oxford: Oxford University Press, 555–92.

Blomstedt, P. (2014a). 'Cataract surgery in ancient Egypt.' *Journal of Cataract and Refractive Surgery* 40: 485–89.

--- (2014b). 'Orthopedic surgery in ancient Egypt.' *Acta Orthopaedica* 85(6): 670–76.

Blustein, Y., Stern, N. & Kottek, S. S. (1987). 'A case of prosthetic dentistry in ancient Egypt.' *Bulletin of the History of Dentistry* 35(2): 120–24.

Borghouts, J. F. (1978). *Ancient Egyptian Magical Texts. Religious Texts*, Translation Series: NISABA, vol. 9. Leiden: E. J. Brill.

--- (1982). 'Divine intervention in ancient Egypt and its manifestation.' In R. J. Demarée & J. Janssen (eds), *Gleanings from Deir el-Medina*. Leiden: Nederlands Instituut Voor Het Nabije Oosten, 1–70.

--- (1994). 'Magical practices among the villagers.' In L. Lesko (ed.), *Pharaoh's Workers: The Villagers of Deir el Medina*. Ithaca, NY: Cornell University Press, 119–30.

Bourriau, J. (1988). *Pharaohs and Mortals: Egyptian Art in the Middle Kingdom*. Cambridge: Cambridge University Press.

Bos, G. (1993). 'The miswak, an aspect of dental care in Islam.' *Medical History* 37: 69–79.

BP (1973). *British Pharmacopoeia*. Her Majesty's Stationery Office.

BPC (1973). *The British Pharmaceutical Codex*. The Pharmaceutical Press.

Braverman, I. M., Redford, D. B. & Mackowiak, P. A. (2009). 'Akhenaten and the strange physiques of Egypt's 18th Dynasty.' *Annals of Internal Medicine* 150: 556–60.

Breasted, J. H. (1906 [this edition 2001]). *Ancient Records of Egypt*, 5 vols. Champaign: University of Illinois Press.

--- (1930 [reissued 1991 with a foreword by T. A. Holland]). *The Edwin Smith Surgical Papyrus: Hieroglyphic Transliteration, Translation and Commentary*, VI. 2 vols. Chicago, IL: University of Chicago Press.

Brewer, D. G. (2001). 'Animal husbandry.' In D. B. Redford (ed.), *The Oxford Encyclopedia of Ancient Egypt*, vol. 1. Oxford: Oxford University Press, 89–94.

Brewer, D. G., Redford, D. B. & Redford, S. (1992). *Domestic Plants and Animals: The Ancient Egyptian Origins*. Warminster: Aris & Phillips.

Brier, B. (2023). 'Warrior Tutankhamun: fragile pharaoh no more.' *Ancient Egypt* 23(2): 14–21.

Brothwell, D. R. (1967). 'Major congenital anomalies of the skeleton: Evidence from earlier populations.' In D. Brothwell & A. T. Sandison (eds), *Diseases in Antiquity*. Springfield, IL: C. C. Thomas, 423–43.

--- (2002). *Digging up Bones*. Rev. ed. Ithaca, NY: Cornell University Press.

Brothwell, D. R. & Møller-Christensen, V. (1963). 'A possible case of amputation, dated to c. 2000 BC.' *Man* 63: 192–94.

Brothwell, D. & Sandison, A. T. (eds) (1967). *Disease in Antiquity: A survey of diseases, injuries and surgery of early populations*. Springfield, IL: C. C. Thomas.

Brown, N. R. (2017). '"Come my staff, I lean upon you": the use of staves for the divine transformation of the deceased in ancient Egypt.' *Journal of the American Research Center in Egypt* 53: 189–201.

Brunton, G. (1947). 'The oracle of Kom el-Wist.' *Annales du Service des Antiquités de l'Égypte* 47: 293.

Bruyère, B. (1929, 1930). Mertseger à Deir el-Medineh, I & II. Cairo: *Mémoires publiés par les membres de l'Institut Français d'Archéologie Orientale* I: 58/1 & II: 58/2.

--- (1959). La Tombe No. 1 de Sen-Nedjem à Deir el-Médineh. Tome LXXXVIII. Cairo: *Mémoires publiés par les membres de l'Institut Français d'Archéologie Orientale* 88.

Budge, E. A. Wallace. (1902). 'The Nile: notes for travellers in Egypt.' London: Harrison & Sons.

Buikstra, J. E., Baker, B. J. & Cook, D. C. (1993). 'What diseases plagued the ancient Egyptians? A century of controversy considered.' In W. V. Davies & R. Walker (eds), *Biological Anthropology and the Study of Ancient Egypt*. London: British Museum Press, 24–53.

Burridge, A. L. (1993). 'Akhenaten: a new perspective: evidence of a genetic disorder in the royal family of 18th Dynasty Egypt.' *Journal of the Society for the Study of Egyptian Antiquities* 23: 63–74.

Burzacott, J. (2017). '"A remarkable wooden toe": Swiss Egyptologists study 3000-year-old prosthesis.' *Nile Magazine* 9 (August–September): 6–8.

Caldwell, L. (2018). 'Roman medical sects: the Asclepiadeans, the Methodists, and the Pneumatists.' In P. T. Keyser & J. Scarborough (eds), *Science and Medicine in the Classical World*. Oxford: Oxford University Press, 637–54.

Caminos, R. A. (1954). *Late Egyptian Miscellanies*, Brown Egyptological Studies 1. London: Oxford University Press.

Campbell, J. M. (2008). 'Pharmacy in ancient Egypt.' In R. David (ed.), *Egyptian Mummies and Modern Science*. Oxford: Oxford University Press, 216–36.

Campbell, J. M., Campbell, J. R. & David, A. R. (2010). 'Do the formulations of ancient Egyptian prescriptions stand up to pharmaceutical scrutiny?' In J. Cockitt & R. David (eds), *Pharmacy and Medicine in Ancient Egypt: Proceedings of the conferences held in Cairo (2007) and Manchester (2008)*. Oxford: Archaeopress, 15–19.

Campbell, J. M. & David, A. R. (2010). 'The application of archaeobotany, phytogeography and pharmacognosy to confirm the pharmacopoeia of ancient Egypt 1850–1200 BC.' In J. Cockitt & R. David (eds), *Pharmacy and Medicine in Ancient Egypt: Proceedings of the conferences held in Cairo (2007) and Manchester (2008)*. Oxford: Archaeopress, 20–29.

Capart, J. (1907). *Une rue de tombeaux à Saqqarah*. Brussels: Vromant & Cie.

Carroll, S. T. (1988). 'Wrestling in ancient Nubia.' *Journal of Sport History* 15(2): 121–37.

Casini, E. (2018). 'Rethinking the multifaceted aspects of mandrake in ancient Egypt.' *Egitto e Vicino Oriente* 41: 101–16.

Cassar, P. (1974). 'Surgical instruments on a tomb slab in Roman Malta.' *Medical History* 18: 89–92.

Celsus, Aulus Cornelius (translated W. G. Spencer, 1938). *De Medicina*, Loeb Classical Library. Cambridge, MA: Harvard University Press.

Černý, J. (1927). 'Le culte d'Amenophis Ier chez les ouvriers de la nécropole thébaine.' *Bulletin de l'Institut Français d'Archéologie Orientale* 27: 159–203.

Černý, J. & Gardiner, A. H. (1957). *Hieratic Ostraca*. Oxford: Griffith Institute.

Červiček, P. (1986). *Rock Pictures of Upper Egypt and Nubia*, Annali dell'Istituto Universitario Orientale di Napoli, Supplemento n. 46, fasc. 1. Rome: Herder.

Chamberlain, A. (2006). *Demography in Archaeology.* Cambridge: Cambridge University Press.

Charpentier, G. (1981). *Recueil de Matériaux Épigraphiques Relatifs à la Botanique de l'Egypte Antique.* Paris: Trismégiste.

Chassinat, É. (1921). *Un Papyrus Médical Copte, Mémoires publiés par les membres de l'Istitutut Français d'Archéologie Orientale* 32. Le Caire: L'Institut Français d'Archéologie Orientale du Caire.

Chitgopkar, S. D. & Khan, M. (2005). 'Painless reduction of anterior shoulder dislocation by Kocher's method.' *Injury* 36(10): 1182–84.

Chohayeb, A. A. (1991). 'The dental heritage of ancient Egypt.' *Bulletin of the History of Dentistry* 39(2): 65–69.

Christenson, B. (2006). 'Queen of Punt.' *Clinical Infectious Diseases* 42(9): 1344–45.

Cilliers, L. (2018). 'Medical writings in the late Roman West.' In P. T. Keyser & J. Scarborough (eds), *Science and Medicine in the Classical World.* Oxford: Oxford University Press: 1013–34.

Clayton, J. (2022). *Mental Illnesses in the Ancient Egyptian "Book of the Heart".* Wallasey: Abercromby Press.

Clement of Alexandria (translated A. Roberts & J. Donaldson). 'Stromata part VI.' In P. Kirby, *Early Christian Writings* (accessed 20 April, 2021) <html://www.earlychristianwritings.com/text/clement-stromata-book6.html>.

Cockburn, A., Barraco, R. A., Peck, W. H. & Reyman, T. A. (1980). 'A classic mummy: PUM II.' In A. and E. Cockburn (eds), *Mummies, Disease and Ancient Cultures.* Cambridge: Cambridge University Press, 52–70.

Cockitt, J. & David, R. (eds) (2010). *Pharmacy and Medicine in Ancient Egypt: Proceedings of the conferences held in Cairo (2007) and Manchester (2008).* Oxford: Archaeopress.

Cole, D. (1986). 'Obstetrics for women in ancient Egypt.' *Discussions in Egyptology* 5: 27–33.

Collier, M. (2016). 'The sting of the scorpion.' In C. Price, R. Forshaw, A. Chamberlain & P. Nicholson (eds), *Mummies, Magic and Medicine in Ancient Egypt: Multidisciplinary essays for Rosalie David.* Manchester: Manchester University Press, 102–14.

Collier, M. & Quirke, S. (eds) (2004). *The UCL Lahun Papyri: Religious, Literary, Legal, Mathematical & Medical.* Oxford: Archaeopress.

Contenau, G. (1938). *La Médecine en Assyrie et en Babylonie.* Paris: Maloine.

Contis, G. & David, A. R. (1996). 'The epidemiology of Bilharzia in ancient Egypt: 5000 years of schistosomiasis.' *Parasitology Today* 12(7): 253–55.

Corthals, A., Koller, A., Martin, D. W., Rieger, R., Chen, E. I., Bernaski, M., Recagno, G. & Davalos, L. M. (2012). 'Detecting the immune system response of a 500-year-old Inca mummy.' *PLoS One* 7(7): e41244.

Counsell, D. (2006). 'Intoxicants in Ancient Egypt: The Application of Modern Forensic Analytical Techniques to Ancient Artefacts and Mummified Remains in the Evaluation of Drug Use by an Ancient Society; a Historical and Scientific Investigation.' Unpublished PhD thesis, University of Manchester, Faculty of Life Sciences.

--- (2008). 'Intoxicants in ancient Egypt? Opium, nymphea, coca and tobacco.' In R. David (ed.), *Egyptian Mummies and Modern Science*. Cambridge: Cambridge University Press, 195–215.

Craik, E. (2018). 'Hippocrates and early Greek medicine.' In P. T. Keyser & J. Scarborough (eds), *Science and Medicine in the Classical World*. Oxford: Oxford University Press, 215–34.

Crevecoeur, I., Dias-Meirinho, M. H., Zazzo, A., Antoine, D. & Bon, F. (2021). 'New insights on interpersonal violence in the Late Pleistocene based on the Nile valley cemetery of Jebel Sahaba.' *Scientific Reports* 11, 9991.

Curnow, T. (2012/2013). 'The Cult of Asclepius: its origins and early development.' In R. David (ed.), *Bulletin of the John Rylands University Library of Manchester*, vol. 89 supplement: *Ancient Medical and Healing Systems: Their Legacy to Western Medicine*. Manchester: Manchester University Press, 676–84.

Curry, A., Anfield, C. & Tapp, E. (1979). 'Electron microscopy of the Manchester Mummies.' In A. R. David (ed.), *The Manchester Museum Mummy Project: Multidisciplinary Research on Ancient Egyptian Mummified Remains*. Manchester: Manchester Museum, 103–11.

Dabbs, G. R. & Rose, J. C. (2015). 'The presence of malaria among the non-royal of the North Tombs Cemetery.' *Horizon* 16: 7.

Dabbs, G. R., Rose, J. C. & Zabecki, M. (2015). 'The bioarchaeology of Akhetaten: unexpected results from a capital city.' In S. Ikram, J. Kaiser & R. Walker (eds), *Egyptian Bioarchaeology: Humans, Animals, and the Environment*. Leiden: Sidestone Press, 43–52.

Dabbs, G. R. & Zabecki, M. (2014). 'Abandoned memories: a cemetery of forgotten souls?' In B. W. Porter & A. T. Boutin (eds), *Remembering the Dead in the Ancient Near East*. Boulder, CO: University Press of Colorado, 236–38.

--- (2015). 'Slot-type fractures of the scapula at New Kingdom Tell El-Amarna, Egypt.' *International Journal of Paleopathology* 11: 12–22.

Dasen, V. (1993). *Dwarfs in Ancient Egypt and Greece*. Oxford, New York: Clarendon Press.

Daumas, F. (1957). 'Le sanatorium de Dendera.' *Bulletin de l'Institut Français d'Archéologie Orientale* 56: 35–57.

David, A. R. (ed.) (1979). *The Manchester Museum Mummy Project. Multidisciplinary Research on Ancient Egyptian Mummified Remains*. Manchester: Manchester Museum.

--- (1996). *The Pyramid Builders of Ancient Egypt: A Modern Investigation of Pharaoh's Workforce*. London: Routledge & Kegan Paul.

--- (2002). *Religion & Magic in Ancient Egypt*. Harmondsworth: Penguin Books.

--- (ed.) (2008a). *Egyptian Mummies and Modern Science*. Cambridge: Cambridge University Press.

--- (2008b). 'The ancient Egyptian medical system.' In R. David (ed.), *Egyptian Mummies and Modern Science*. Cambridge: Cambridge University Press, 181–94.

--- (2010). 'The "Pharmacy in Ancient Egypt Project" at the KNH Centre for Biomedical Egyptology.' In J. Cockitt & R. David (eds), *Pharmacy and Medicine in Ancient Egypt: Proceedings of the conferences held in Cairo (2007) and Manchester (2008)*. Oxford: Archaeopress, 1–5.

--- (2012/2013). 'Introduction: ancient medical and healing systems: their legacy to Western medicine.' In R. David (ed.), *Bulletin of the John Rylands University Library of Manchester*, vol. 89 supplement*: Ancient Medical and Healing Systems: Their Legacy to Western Medicine.* Manchester: Manchester University Press, 7–24.

--- (2016). 'Understanding the lives of ancient Egyptian women: the contribution of physical anthropology.' In S. L. Budin & J. MacIntosh Turfa (eds), *Women in Antiquity*. London, New York: Routledge, 181–93.

--- (2017a). 'Illness from afar: epidemics and their aftermath.' In P. P. Creasman & R. H. Wilkinson (eds), *Pharaoh's Land and Beyond: Ancient Egypt and Its Neighbours*. Oxford: Oxford University Press, 271–85.

--- (2017b). 'Egyptian medicine and disabilities: from pharaonic to Greco-Roman Egypt.' In C. Laes, *Disability in Antiquity*. London, New York: Routledge, 75–89.

David, A. R. & Tapp, E. (1992). *The Mummy's Tale: the Scientific and Medical Investigation of Natsef-Amun, Priest in the Temple at Karnak*. London: Michael O'Mara Books Limited.

David, A. R. & Zimmerman, M. R. (2010). 'Cancer: an old disease, a new disease or something in between?' *Nature Reviews Cancer* 10(10): 728–33.

David, A. R., Kershaw, A. & Heagerty, A. (2010). 'Atherosclerosis and diet in ancient Egypt.' *Lancet* February 27; 375 (9716): 718–19.

David, R. & Murphy, E. (2021). *The Life and Times of Takabuti in Ancient Egypt: Investigating the Belfast Mummy*. Liverpool: Liverpool University Press.

Davies, N. de G. (1903). *The rock tombs of El Amarna: Part I. The Tomb of Meryra*, Archaeological Survey of Egypt 13, EEF. London: Kegan Paul, Trench, Trübner & Co., Bernard Quaritch.

--- (1905). *The rock tombs of El Amarna: Part II. The Tombs of Panehesy and Meryra II*, Archaeological Survey of Egypt 14, EEF. London: Kegan Paul, Trench, Trübner & Co., Bernard Quaritch.

--- (1917). *The Tomb of Nakht*. New York: The Metropolitan Museum of Art.

--- (1927). *Two Ramesside Tombs at Thebes*. New York: Metropolitan Museum of Art.

Davies, S. (2006). *The Sacred Animal Necropolis at North Saqqara: the Mother of Apis and Baboon Catacombs: The Archaeological Report*. London: Egypt Exploration Society.

Davies, W. V. & Friedman, R. (1998). *Egypt*. British Museum Press, London.

Davis, B. G. (1999). *Who's Who at Deir el-Medina: A Prosopographical Study of the Royal Workmen's Community*, Egyptologische Uitgaven 13. Leiden: Nederlands Instituut Voor Het Nabije Oostenleiden.

Dawson, W. & Gray, P. H. K. (1968). *Catalogue of Egyptian Antiquities in the British Museum. I, Mummies and Human Remains*. Oxford: British Museum Press.

Dawson, W. R. (1938). 'Pygmies and dwarfs in ancient Egypt.' *Journal of Egyptian Archaeology* 24: 185–89.

Deelder, A. M., Miller, R. L., De Jonge, N. & Krijger, F. W. (1990). 'Detection of schistosome antigen in mummies.' *Lancet* 335(8691): 724–25.

Demarchi, B., Boano, R., Ceron, A., Bello, F. D., Favero-Longo, S. E., Fiddyment, S., Marochetti, E. F., Mangiapane, G. L., Mattonai, M., Pennacini, C., Ribechini, E., Woolley, J., Zilberstein, G. & Righetti, P. G. (2020). 'Never boring: non-invasive palaeoproteomics of mummified human skin.' *Journal of Archaeological Science* 119: https://doi.org/10.1016/j.jas.2020.105145.

Denton, J. (2008). 'Slices of mummy: a histologist's perspective.' In R. David (ed.), *Egyptian Mummies and Modern Science*. Cambridge: Cambridge University Press, 71–82.

Denton, J. (2016). 'Slices of a mummy: a thin perspective.' In C. Price, R. Forshaw, A. Chamberlain & P. Nicholson (eds), *Mummies, Magic and Medicine in Ancient Egypt: Multidisciplinary Essays for Rosalie David*. Manchester: Manchester University Press, 276–85.

Derchain, P. (1965). *Le Papyrus Salt 825 (B.M. 10051)*, 2 vols. Brussels: Palais des Académies.

Derry, D. E. (1909). 'Anatomical Report.' In *Archaeological Survey of Nubia*, Bulletin 2. Cairo: National Printing Department.

--- (1913). 'A case of hydrocephalus in an Egyptian of the Roman Period.' *Journal of Anatomy and Physiology* 47: 436–58.

--- (1935). 'Note on five pelves of women of the Eleventh Dynasty in Egypt.' *Journal of Obstetrics and Gynaecology of the British Empire* 42(3): 490–95.

Descriptions de l'Égypte (1809). Publié par les orders de sa Majesté l'Émpereur Napoléon le Grand, Imprimerie Impériale, Paris.

Dewey, J. R., Bartley M. H. Jr. & Armelagos, G. J. (1969). 'Rates of femoral cortical bone loss in two Nubian populations.' *Clinical Orthopaedics and Related Research* 65: 61–66.

Di Cicco, C. O. (2005). 'Queen of Punt Syndrome [abstract].' Programme and abstracts of the 14th Congress of the European Academy of Dermatology and Venereology (London), *Journal of the European Academy of Dermatology and Venereology* 19 (Suppl. 2): 1–412.

Dioscorides, Pedanius (translated T. A. Osbaldeston & R. P. Wood, 2000). *De Materia Medica: Being an herbal with many other medicinal materials: written in Greek in the first century of the common era: a new indexed version in modern English*. Johannesburg: IBIDIS.

Dodson, A. (2016). *Poisoned Legacy: The Fall of the Nineteenth Egyptian Dynasty*. Cairo: The American University in Cairo Press.

Dodson, A. & Hilton, D. (2004). *The Complete Royal Families of Ancient Egypt*. Cairo: The American University of Cairo Press.

Dols, M. W. (1984). *Medieval Islamic Medicine: Ibn Ridwan's treatise "On the prevention of bodily ills in Egypt"*. Berkeley: California University Press.

Donoghue, H. D., Lee, O. Y.-C., Minnikin, D., Besra, G. S., Taylor, J. H. & Spigelman, M. (2010). 'Tuberculosis in Dr Granville's mummy: a molecular re-examination of the earliest known Egyptian mummy to be scientifically examined and given a medical diagnosis.' *Proceedings of the Royal Society of London. Series B, Biological Sciences* 277: 51–56.

Drancourt, M., Aboudharam, G., Signoli, M., Dutour, O. & Raoult, D. (1998). 'Detection of 400-year-old Yersinia pestis DNA in human dental pulp: an approach to the diagnosis of ancient septicemia.' *Proceedings of the National Academy of Sciences of the United States of America* 95: 12637–40.

Duell, P. (ed.) (1938). *The Mastaba of Mereruka / by the Sakkarah Expedition*, vol. 1, Oriental Institute Publications 31. Chicago, IL: University of Chicago Press.

Duke, L. (2008). 'Schistosomaisis in ancient Egypt: The "AAA" debate.' *The Proceedings of the 17th Annual History of Medicine Days, Faculty of Medicine, University of Calgary, March 7th and 8th, 2008 in the Health Sciences Centre, Calgary.* Alberta: University of Calgary, 77–83.

Dunlop, R. H. & Williams, D. J. (1996). *Veterinary Medicine: An Illustrated History.* St Louis, Baltimore, Boston: Mosby.

Dupras, T., Mathews, S., De Meyer, M., Peeters, C. & Vanthuyne, B. (2008). 'Just cut it off: amputation in ancient Egypt.' *Paleopathological Association 35th Meeting.* Abstracts: 6.

Dupras, T. L., Williams, L. J., De Meyer, M., Peeters, C., Depraetere, D., Vanthuyne, B. & Willems, H. (2010). 'Evidence of amputation as medical treatment in ancient Egypt.' *International Journal of Osteoarchaeology* 20: 405–23.

Dzierzykray-Rogalski, T. (1980). 'Paleopathology of the Ptolemaic inhabitants Dakhleh Oasis (Egypt).' *Journal of Human Evolution* 9(1): 71–74.

Dzierzykray-Rogalski, T. & Prominska, E. (1994). 'A further report on Pharaoh Siptah's handicap (XIXth Egyptian Dynasty).' *HOMO – Journal of Comparative Human Biology* 45 (Supplement): S45.

Ebbell, B. (1937). *The Ebers Papyrus.* London: Oxford University Press.

Ebeid, N. I. (1999). *Egyptian Medicine in the Days of the Pharaohs.* Cairo: General Egyptian Book Organisation.

Ebers, G. M. & Stern, L. C. (1875). *Papyros Ebers, das hermetische Buch über die Arzeneimittel der alten Ägypter in hieratischer Schrift.* Leipzig: Englemann.

Edel, E. (1976). *Ägyptische Ärzte und ägyptische Medizin am hethitischen Königshof: neue Funde von Keilschriftbriefen Ramses' II aus Boğazköy.* Opladen: Westdeutscher Verlag.

Edelstein, E. J. & Edelstein, L. (1945). *Asclepius: A Collection and Interpretation of the Testimonies*, 2 vols. Baltimore, MD: Williams & Wilkins.

Ejsmond, W., Ożarek-Szilke, M., Jaworski, M., Szilke, S. & Jaroszewska, K. (2021). 'A pregnant ancient Egyptian mummy from the 1st century BC.' *Journal of Archaeological Science* 132 (August): 10.1016/j.jas.2021.105371.

Elhabashy, S. & Abdelgawad, E. M. (2019). 'The history of nursing profession in ancient Egyptian society.' *International Journal of Africa Nursing Sciences* 11: 1–7.

Emboden, W. (1978). 'The sacred narcotic lily of the Nile: Nymphea caerulea.' *Economic Botany* 32: 558–64.

--- (1979). *Narcotic Plants: Hallucinogens, Stimulants, Inebriants and Hypnotics, their Origins and Uses.* London: Studio Vista.

--- (1981). 'Transcultural use of narcotic water lilies in ancient Egyptian and Maya drug ritual.' *Journal of Ethnopharmacology* 3(1): 39–83.

--- (1989). 'The sacred journey in dynastic Egypt: Shamanistic trance in the context of the narcotic water lily and the mandrake.' *Journal of Psychoactive Drugs* 21(1): 61–75.

Emery, W. B. (1958). *Great Tombs of the First Dynasty*, III. London: Egypt Exploration Society.

Erman, A. (1901). *Zaubersprüche für Mutter und Kind: aus dem Papyrus 3027 des Berliner Museums*. Berlin: Königliche Akademie der Wissenschaften.

Esche, E., Mummert, A., Robinson, J. & Armelagos, G. J. (2010). 'Cancer in Egypt and Nubia.' *Anthropologie (1962–)* 48(2): 133–40.

Eshraghian, A. & Loeys, B. (2012). 'Loeys-Dietz syndrome: a possible solution for Akhenaten's and his family's mystery syndrome.' *South African Medical Journal* 102(8): 661–64.

Evans, L. & Woods, A. (2016). 'Further evidence that Niankhkhnum and Khnumhotep were twins.' *Journal of Egyptian Archaeology* 102: 55–72.

Evershed, R. P. & Clark, K. (2021). 'Trends in use of organic balms in Egyptian mummification revealed through biomolecular analysis.' In D. H. Shin & R. Bianucci (eds), *The Handbook of Mummy Studies: New Frontiers in Scientific and Cultural Perspectives*. Singapore: Springer, 653–715.

Faulkner, R. O. (1969). *The Ancient Egyptian Pyramid Texts*. Oxford: Clarendon Press.

--- (1972). *The Ancient Egyptian Book of the Dead*. London: British Museum Press.

Favry, N. (2016). 'The transmission of offices in the Middle Kingdom.' In G. L. Miniaci & W. Grajetzki (eds), *The World of Middle Kingdom Egypt (2000–1550 BC)* II, MKS 2. London: Golden House Publications, 117–31.

Feucht, E. (1995). *Das Kind in alten Ägypten*. Frankfurt, New York: Campus Verlag.

--- (2001). 'Birth.' In D. B. Redford (ed.), *The Oxford Encylopedia of Ancient Egypt*, 1. Oxford: Oxford University Press, 192–93.

--- (2004). 'Der Weg ins Leben.' In V. Dasen (ed.), *Naissance et Petite Enfance dans l'Antiquité*. Fribourg, Göttingen: OBO 203, 33–53.

--- (2016). 'Motherhood in pharaonic Egypt.' In S. L. Budin and J. MacIntosh Turfa (eds), *Women in Antiquity*. London, New York: Routledge, 204–17.

Filer, J. (1995). *Disease*. London: British Museum Press.

--- (2001). 'Hygiene.' In D. B. Redford (ed.), *The Oxford Encylopedia of Ancient Egypt*, I. Oxford: Oxford University Press, 133–36.

Finch, J. (2011). 'The ancient origins of prosthetic medicine.' *Lancet* 377(9765): 548–49.

--- (2012/2013). 'The Durham Mummy: deformity and the concept of perfection in the ancient world.' In R. David (ed.), *Bulletin of the John Rylands University Library of Manchester*, vol. 89 supplement: *Ancient Medical and Healing Systems: Their Legacy to Western Medicine*. Manchester: Manchester University Press, 111–32.

--- (2018). 'The complex aspects of experimental archaeology: the design of working models of two ancient Egyptian great toe prostheses.' In J. Draycott (ed.), *Prostheses in Antiquity (Medicine & the Body in Antiquity)*. London, New York: Routledge, 29–48.

Finch, J. L., Heath, G. H., David, A. R. & Kulkarni, J. (2012). 'Biomechanical assessment of two artificial big toe restorations from ancient Egypt and their significance to the history of prosthetics.' *Journal of Prosthetics and Orthotics* 24(4): 181–91.

Fischer-Elfert, H. W. (2004). *Science in Ancient Egypt*. Sächische Akademie der Wissenshaften zu Leipzig. Papyrus Turin No. "54003" (accessed September 30, 2022) <https://sae.saw-leipzig.de/de/dokumente/papyrus-turin-provv-861>.

Forman, W. & Quirke, S. (1996). *Hieroglyphs and the Afterlife*. London: British Museum.

Forshaw, R. J. (2009a). 'Dental health and disease in ancient Egypt.' *British Dental Journal* 206(8): 421–24.

--- (2009b). 'The practice of dentistry in ancient Egypt.' *British Dental Journal* 206(9): 479–84.

--- (2013). 'Hesyre the first recorded physician and dental surgeon in history.' *Bulletin of the John Rylands University Library of Manchester*, vol. 89 supplement: *Ancient Medical and Healing Systems: Their Legacy to Western Medicine*. Manchester: Manchester University Press, 181–202.

--- (2014). *The Role of the Lector in Ancient Egyptian Society*. Oxford: Archaeopress.

--- (2015). 'Dental infections in ancient Nubia.' In R. Metcalfe, J. Cockitt & R. David (eds), *Palaeopathology in Egypt and Nubia: A Century in Review*. Oxford: Archaeopress Egyptology, 69–81.

--- (2020). 'Why was a minor dislocation included amongst the more serious cases listed in the Edwin Smith papyrus?' In C. Graves (ed.), *BEC 4: Proceedings of the 4th British Egyptology Congress 7–9 September 2018, University of Manchester*. London: Egypt Exploration Society, 70–85.

Freemont, A. & Chasserini, D. (2021). 'Takabuti's health: techniques and findings.' In R. David & E. Murphy (eds), *The Life and Times of Takabuti in Ancient Egypt: Investigating the Belfast Mummy*. Liverpool: Liverpool University Press, 75–82.

Fritsch, K. O., Hamoud, H., Allam, A. H., Grossmann, A., Nur El-Din, A. H., Abdel-Maksoud, G., Soliman, M. A., Badr, I., Sutherland, J. D., Sutherland, M. L., Akl, M., Finch, C. E., Thomas, G. S., Wann, L. S. & Thompson, R. C. (2015). 'The orthopedic diseases of ancient Egypt.' *Anatomical Record (Hoboken NJ)* 298(6): 1036–46.

Frood, E. (2007). *Biographical Texts from the Ramesside Age*, Writings from the Biblical Age 26. Atlanta: Society of Biblical Literature.

--- (2010). 'Social structure and daily life: pharaonic.' In A. B. Lloyd (ed.), *A Companion to Ancient Egypt*, vol. 1. Oxford: Wiley-Blackwell, 469–90.

Fuchs, J. (1964). 'Physical alterations which occur in the blind and are illustrated on ancient Egyptians works of art.' *Annals of the New York Academy of Sciences* 117: 618–23.

Gardiner, A. H. (1938). 'The House of Life.' *Journal of Egyptian Archaeology* 24: 157–79.

--- (1955). *The Ramesseum Papyri*. Oxford: Oxford University Press.

Gardiner, A. H., Peet, T. E. & Černý, J. (1952). *The Inscriptions of Sinai. Part I. Introduction and plates*, 2nd revised edition. London: Egypt Exploration Society.

Garland, R. (2010). *The Eye of the Beholder: Deformity and Disability in the Graeco-Roman World*. London: BC Paperbacks.

Garner, R. (1979). 'Experimental mummification.' In R. David (ed.), *The Manchester Mummy Project*. Manchester: Manchester Museum, 19–24.

Gaumer, M. A. (2017). 'What difference did Islam make? Disease and disability in early medieval North Africa.' In C. Laes (ed.), *Disability in Antiquity*. Oxford, New York: Routledge, 403–20.

Gayet, A. (1894). *Le Temple de Louxor*, 1er fasc.: 'Constructions d'Amenophis III.' In U. Bouriant, *Mémoires publiés par les membres de la Mission archéologique française au Caire*. Tome Quinziéme. Paris: Ernest Leroux, 1–30.

Geldermalsen, A. A. V. (1993). 'Assault, a burden for a rural hospital in Lesotho.' *Tropical and Geographical Medicine* 45: 30–32.

Geller, M. J. (2010). *Ancient Babylonian Medicine: Theory and Practice*. Chichester: Wiley-Blackwell.

Germer, R. (1979). 'Untersuchung über Arzneimittelpflanzen in Altern Ägypten.' PhD thesis. University of Hamburg.

--- (1998). 'The plant remains found by Petrie at Lahun and some remarks on the problems of identifying Egyptian plant names.' In S. Quirke (ed.), *Lahun Studies*. Reigate: SIA Publishing, 84–91.

--- (2008). *Handbuch der Altägyptischen Heilpflanzen*. Wiesbaden: Harrassowitz Verlag.

Gevaert, B. (2017). 'Perfect Roman bodies: the Stoic view.' In C. Laes (ed.), *Disability in Antiquity*. Oxford, New York: Routledge, 213–21.

Ghalioungui, P. (1962). 'Some body swellings illustrated in two tombs of the ancient Empire and their possible relation to *âaâ*.' *Zeitschrift für Ägyptische Sprache und Altertumskunde* 87: 108–14.

--- (1963). *Magic and Medical Science in Ancient Egypt*. London: Hodder & Stoughton.

--- (1971). 'Did a dental profession exist in ancient Egypt?' *Medical History* 15(1): 92–94.

--- (1980). 'Medicine in ancient Egypt.' In J. E. Harris & E. F. Wente (eds), *An X-ray Atlas of the Royal Mummies*. Chicago, IL, London: University of Chicago Press, 52–98.

--- (1983). *The Physicians of Pharaonic Egypt*. Cairo: Al-Ahram Center for Scientific Translations.

--- (1987). *The Ebers Papyrus*. Cairo: Academy of Scientific Research and Technology.

Ghalioungui, P., Khalil, S. & Ammar, A. R. (1963). 'On an Ancient Egyptian method of diagnosing pregnancy and diagnosing foetal sex.' *Medical History* 7(3): 241–46.

Giovannetti, G., Guerrini, A., Carnieri, E. & Salvadori, P. A. (2016). 'Magnetic resonance imaging for the study of mummies.' *Magnetic Resonance Imaging* 34(6): 785–94.

Giunio, K. A. (2013). 'Isis – The Sea Star and the Ceremony of *Navigium Isidis*.' *Diadora: Journal of the Archaeological Museum in Zadar – Glasilo Arheološkog muzeja u Zadru* 26/27: 421–40.

Golénischeff, V. S. (1927). *Papyrus Hiératiques*. Cairo: Catalogue Général des Antiquités Égyptiennes du Musée du Caire 83.

Goudsmit, J. & Brandon-Jones, D. (1999). 'Mummies of olive baboons and Barbary macaques in the Baboon Catacomb of the Sacred Animal Necropolis at North Saqqara.' *Journal of Egyptian Archaeology* 85: 45–53.

Grapow, H., von Deines, H. & Westendorf, W. (1954–1973). *Grundriss der Medizin der alten Ägypter*, 11 vols. Berlin: Akademie-Verlag.

Gray, P. H. K. (1966a). 'Embalmers' restorations.' *Journal of Egyptian Archaeology* 52: 138–40.

--- (1966b). 'Radiological aspects of the mummies of ancient Egypt in the Rijksmuseum van Oudheden, Leiden.' *Oudheidkundige Mededelingen uit het Rijksmuseum van Oudheden te Leiden* 47: 1–30.

--- (1967). 'Radiography of ancient Egyptian mummies.' *Medical Radiography and Photography* 43: 34–44.

--- (1969). 'A case of osteogenesis imperfecta associated with dentinogenesis imperfecta, dating from antiquity.' *Clinical Radiology* 20: 106–08.

--- (1973). 'The radiography of mummies of ancient Egyptians.' *Journal of Human Evolution* 2(1): 51–53.

Grdseloff, B. (1938). 'La lecture et le sens du mot dbAx.' *Annales du Service des Antiquités de l'Égypte* 38: 353–54.

Griffith, F. Ll. (1897). *The Petrie Papyri: Hieratic Papyri from Kahun and Gurob, principally of the Middle Kingdom*. London: Quaritch.

--- (1898). *Hieratic Papyri from Kahun and Gurob*, vol. 1. London: Quaritch.

Griffith, F. Ll. & Thompson, H. (1904). *The Demotic Magical Papyrus of London and Leiden*. London: Grevel & Co.

Grove, C., Peschel, O. & Nerlich, A. G. (2015). 'A systematic approach to the application of soft tissue histopathology in paleopathology.' *BioMed Research International* 2557: 1–9.

Guiddotti, M. C. (2008). 'The burial furniture of Tjes-Ra-Peret, wet-nurse of Taharqa's daughter.' In R. Tiradritti (ed.), *Pharaonic Renaisssance: Archaism & the Sense of History in Ancient Egypt*. Budapest: Library of the Museum of Fine Arts, 130–35.

Guiffra, V., Fornaciari, G. & Ciranni, R. (2006). 'A new case of ancient restoration on an Egyptian mummy.' *Journal of Egyptian Archaeology* 92: 274–78.

Gunn, B. (1916). 'Religion of the poor in ancient Egypt.' *Journal of Egyptian Archaeology* 3: 81–94.

Gunther, R. (1934). *The Greek Herbal of Dioscorides*. Oxford: Oxford University Press.

Győry, H. (2010). '*Ꜣdt rnpt* or the "Pestilence of the Year".' In J. Cockitt & R. David (eds), *Pharmacy and Medicine in Ancient Egypt*. Oxford: Archaeopress, 81–84.

Győry, H. & Blázovics, A. (2020). 'Blessings or curse. The consumption of wine in ancient Egypt.' In H. Győry (ed.), *Aegyptus et Pannonia VI. Health and Life in Ancient Egypt. Mummies in Focus. Proceedings of the Conference held 27th–29th August 2019, Budapest*. Budapest: Hungarian–Egyptian Friendship Society, 111–16.

Győry, H., Horváth, B. Z. & Blákovics, A. (2020). 'Esthetical solution or useful prosthesis.' *Aegyptus et Pannonia VI. Health and Life in Ancient Egypt. Mummies in Focus. Proceedings of the Conference held 27–29 August 2019, Budapest*. Budapest: Hungarian–Egyptian Friendship Society, 75–109.

Habicht, M. E., Eppenberger, P. E. & Rühli, F. (2021). 'A critical assessment of proposed outbreaks of plague and other epidemic disease in ancient Egypt.' *International Journal of Infectious Diseases* 103: 217–19.

Halioua, B. & Ziskind, B. (2005). *Medicine in the Days of the Pharaohs.* Cambridge, MA: Harvard University Press.

Hamlyn, P. F. & Schmidt, R. J. (1994). 'Potential therapeutic application of fungal filaments in wound management.' *Mycologist* 8(4): 147–52.

Harer, W. B. (1985). 'Pharmacological and biological properties of the Egyptian Lotus.' *Journal of the American Research Center in Egypt* 22: 49–54.

Harris, J. E. & Weeks, K. R. (1973). *X-raying the Pharaohs.* New York: Charles Scribner's Sons.

Harris, J. E. & Wente, E. F. (eds) (1980). *An X-Ray Atlas of the Royal Mummies.* Chicago, IL, London: University of Chicago Press.

Harris, J. R. (1987). 'Medicine.' In J. R. Harris (ed.), *The Legacy of Egypt.* Oxford: Clarendon Press, 112–37.

Harrison, R. G., Connolly, R. C., Ahmed, S., Abdalla A. B. & el-Ghawaby, M. (1979). 'A mummified foetus from the Tomb of Tutankamun.' *Antiquity* 53: 19–21.

Hart, G. D. (1977). 'Autopsy of an Egyptian mummy (Nakht – ROM 1).' *Canadian Medical Association Journal* 117: 461–76.

Hawass, Z., Gad, Y. Z., Ismail, S., Khairat, R., Fathalla, D., Hasan, N., Ahmed, A., Elleithy, H., Ball, M., Gaballah, F., Wasef, S., Fateen, M., Amer, H., Gostner, P., Selim, A., Zink, A. & Pusch, C. M. (2010). 'Ancestry and pathology in King Tutankhamun's family.' *Journal of the American Medical Association* 303(7): 638–47.

Hawass, Z. & Saleem, S. N. (2011). 'Mummified daughters of King Tutankhamun.' *American Journal of Roentgenology* 197(5): 829–36.

Heilport, P. & Worp, K. A. (2007). 'A wet-nurse contract with unusual provenance.' *Chronique d'Égypte* 82: 218–26.

Herbin, Fr.-R. (1988). 'Les premières pages du papyrus Salt 825.' *Bulletin de l'Institut Français d'Archéologie Orientale* 88: 95–112.

Herodotus (translated A. de Sélincourt, 2003). *The Histories.* London: Penguin Books.

Héthelyi, É. B. & Györy, H. (2020). 'Anise and ancient Egyptian pharmacopoeia.' In H. Györy (ed.), *Aegyptus et Pannonia VI. Health and Life in Ancient Egypt. Mummies in Focus. Proceedings of the Conference held 27th–29th August 2019, Budapest.* Budapest: Hungarian–Egyptian Friendship Society, 183–237.

Hickson, J. F. (1971). 'Medicine in ancient Egypt and its relevance today.' *Journal of the Royal College of General Practitioners* 21: 511–16.

Hierakonpolis Expedition (2012). *Hierakonpolis Online* (accessed February 3, 2022) <http://www.hierakonpolis-online.org/>.

Hillson, S. (1979). 'Diet and dental disease.' *World Archaeology* 11: 147–62.

Hoffman, M. A. (1993). *Egypt before the Pharaohs.* New York: Barnes & Noble.

Hoffman-Axthelm, W. (1979). 'Is the practice of dentistry in ancient Egypt an archaeological fact?' *Bulletin of the History of Dentistry* 27(2): 71–78.

Höflmayer, F. (2016). 'Radiocarbon dating and Egyptian chronology – From the "Curve of Knowns" to Bayesian Modeling.' In *The Oxford Handbook of Topics in Archaeology*. Oxford: Oxford University Press, https://doi.org/10.1093/oxfordhb/9780199935413.013.64.

Homer (translated R. Fitzgerald, 1990). *The Odyssey*. New York: Vintage Books.

Hooton, E. A. (1917). 'Oral surgery in Egypt during the Old Empire.' *Harvard African Studies* 1: 29–32.

Hornung, E. (1992). *Idea into Image: Essays on Ancient Egyptian Thought*. New York: Timken, 59–60.

--- (1996). *Conceptions of God in Ancient Egypt: The One and the Many*. Ithaca, NY: Cornell University Press.

Houlihan, P. F. (1996). *The Animal World of the Pharaohs*. London: Thames & Hudson.

Huchet, J. B., Callou, C., Lichtenburg, R. & Dunand, F. (2013). 'The dog mummy, the ticks and the louse fly: archaeological report of severe ectoparasitosis in ancient Egypt.' *International Journal of Paleopathology* 3: 165–75.

Hussien, F., El Banna, R., Kandeel, W. & Sarry El Din, A. (2010). 'Similarity of fracture treatment of workers and high officials of the pyramid builders.' In J. Cockett & R. David (eds), *Pharmacy and Medicine in Ancient Egypt. Proceedings of the Conferences held in Cairo (2007) and Manchester (2008)*. Oxford: Archaeopress, 85–89.

Ikram, S. (ed.) (2015). *Divine Creatures: Animal Mummies in Ancient Egypt*. Cairo: American University in Cairo Press.

Ikram, S., Nicolson, P., Bertini, L. & Hurley, D. (2014). 'Killing man's best friend?' *Archaeological Review from Cambridge* 28(2): 48–66.

Isherwood, I., Jarvis, H. & Fawcitt, R. A. (1979). 'Radiology of the Manchester Mummies.' In David, A. R. (ed.), *The Manchester Museum Mummy Project: multidisciplinary research on ancient Egyptian mummified remains*. Manchester: Manchester Museum, 25–64.

Isidro, A., Malgosa, A. & Prats-Muñoz, G. (2014). 'Anthracosis in a Coptic mummy.' *Archivos de Bronconeumologia* 50(8): 368–69.

Iskander, Z., Harris, J. E. & Farid, S. (1979). 'Further evidence of dental prosthesis in ancient Egypt.' *Annales du Service des Antiquités de l'Égypte* 63: 93–122.

Isocrates: *Busiris* (translated La Rue Von Hoch, 1945), vol. 3. Boston, MA: Harvard University Press.

Ivanov, S. V. (2018). 'The Tomb of Tjay (TT 23). Progress Report.' *Egypt and Neighbouring Countries: Online Journal* 2: file:///C:/Users/drdem/Downloads/the-tomb-of-tjay-tt-23-progress-report.pdf.

Iversen, E. (1939). 'Papyrus Carlsberg no. VIII, with some remarks on the Egyptian origin of some popular birth prognoses.' In Det Kongelige Danske Videnskabernes Selskab (ed.), *Historisk-filologiske Meddelelser* 26/5. Copenhagen: Ejnar Munksgaard.

Jackson, R. (1990). 'Roman doctors and their instruments: recent research into ancient practice.' *Journal of Roman Archaeology* 3: 5–27.

Jacobs, S. W. & Culbertson, E. J. (2018). 'Effects of topical mandelic acid treatment on facial skin viscoelasticity.' *Facial Plastic Surgery* 34(6): 651–56.

James, T. G. H. (1953). *The Mastaba of Khentika Called Ikhekhi*. London: Oxford University Press.

Janssen, J. J. (1980). 'Absence from Work by the Necropolis Workmen of Thebes.' *Studien zur Altägyptischen Kultur* 8: 127–52.

Janssen, R. M. & Janssen, J. J. (2007). *Growing Up and Getting Old in Ancient Egypt*. London: Golden House Publications.

Jantzen, G. (1968). 'Der blinde Harfner auf dem Grabrelief.' *Materia Medica Nordmark* 20: 689–94.

Jeffreys, D. & Tait, J. (2000). 'Social exclusion in dynastic Egypt.' In J. Hubert (ed.), *Madness, Disability and Social Exclusion: The Archaeology and Anthropology of 'Difference.'* London: Routledge, 87–95.

Joachim, H. (translator) (1890). *Papyros Ebers. Das älteste buch über heilkunde*. Berlin: G. Reimer.

Johnston, I. (2018). 'Galen and his system of medicine.' In P. T. Keyser & J. Scarborough (eds), *Science and Medicine in the Classical World*. Oxford: Oxford University Press, 765–88.

Johnson, W. R. (1992). 'An Asiatic battle scene of Tutankhamun from Thebes: A late Amarna antecedent of the Ramesside battle-narrative tradition.' PhD thesis, University of Chicago.

Jonckheere, F. (1945). 'Coup d'Oeil sur la médecine Égyptienne: l'Intérêt des documents non medicaux.' *Chronique d'Égypte* 20: 24–32, note 6.

--- (1950). 'La place du prêtre de Sekhmet dans le corps médical de l'ancienne Egypte.' In *Actes du Vie Congrès d'Histoire des Sciences*. Amsterdam, 324–33.

--- (1954). *Prescriptions Médicales sur Ostraca Hiératiques*. Brussels: Fondation Égyptologique Reine Elisabeth.

--- (1955). 'Le "préparateur de remèdes" dans l'organisatioon de la pharmacie Égyptienne.' In O. Firchow (ed.), *Äegyptologische Studien*. Deutsche Akademie de Wissenschaften zu Berlin 29, 160–61.

--- (1958). *Les Médecins de l'Égypte Pharaonique, essai des Prosopographie*. Brussels: Edition de la Fondation Égyptologique Reine Elizabeth.

Jones, D. (2000). *An Index of Ancient Egyptian Titles, Epithets and Phrases of the Old Kingdom*, I. Oxford: Archaeopress.

Jones, J. (2007). 'New perspectives on the development of mummification practices during the Pre- and Early Dynastic Periods.' In J.-C. Goyon & C. Cardin (eds), *Proceedings of the Ninth International Congress of Egyptologists. Grenoble 6–12 September 2004*. Leuven: Orientalia Lovaniensia Analecta 150: 979–99.

Jørgensen, M. (1998). *Catalogue: Egypt II (1550–1080 B.C.) Ny Carlsberg Glyptotek*. Copenhagen: Ny Carlsberg Glyptotek, 118–19, no. 39 (stela ÆIN 134).

Joshel, S. R. (1986). 'Nurturing the master's child: slavery and the Roman child-nurse.' *Signs* 12(1): 3–22.

Jouanna, J. (2012). *Greek Medicine from Hippocrates to Galen*. Leiden, Boston: Brill, 3–20.

Judd, M. (2008). 'The parry problem.' *Journal of Archaeological Science* 35(6): 1658–66.

Judd, T. (2009). *Rock Art of the Eastern Desert: Content, Comparisons, Dating and Significance*. Oxford: Archaeopress.

Junker, H. (1927). 'Die Stele des Hofarztes Irj.' *Zeitschrift für Ägyptische Sprache und Altertumskunde* 63: 53–70.

--- (1929). *Giza I: Die mastabas der IV. Dynastie Auf Dem Westfriedhof.* Wien: Hölder-Pichler-Tempsky A.-G.

Kamal, H. (1967). *Dictionary of Pharaonic Medicine.* Cairo: The National Publication House.

Kanawati, N., Woods, A., Shafik, S. & Alexakis, E. (2010). *Mereruka and his Family. III: 1 The Tomb of Mereruka.* Oxford: Aris and Phillips Ltd.

Kaplony, P. (1963). *Die Inschriften der ägyptischen Frühzeit*, 1. Wiesbaden: O. Harrassowitz.

Katz, M. H. (2005). 'Cleanliness and ablution.' In J. D. McAuliffe (ed.), *Encyclopaedia of the Qu'ran.* Leiden: Brill, 341–44.

Kelder, J. M., Cole, S. E. & Cline, E. H. (2018). 'Memphis, Minos, and Mycenae: Bronze Age contact between Egypt and the Aegean.' In J. Spier, T. Potts and S. E. Cole (eds), *Beyond the Nile: Egypt and the Classical World.* Los Angeles: The Paul Getty Museum, 9–17.

Kellenberger, E. (2013). 'Children and adults with intellectual disability in antiquity and modernity: towards a Biblical and sociological model.' *CrossCurrents: Association for Religion and Intellectual Life* (December): 449–72.

--- (2017). 'Mesopotamia and Israel.' In C. Laes (ed.), *Disability in Antiquity.* Abingdon, Oxon. and New York: Routledge, 47–60.

Kemp, B. J. & Merrillees, R. (1980). *Minoan Pottery in Second Millennium Egypt.* Mainz Am Rhein: Verlag Philipp von Zabern.

Kenawy, M. A. & Abdel-Hamid, Y. M. (2015). 'Insects in ancient (Pharaonic) Egypt: a review of fauna, their mythological and religious significance and associated diseases.' *Egyptian Academic Journal of Biological Sciences. A, Entomology* 8(1): 15–32.

Khairat, R., Ball, M., Chang, C. C., Bianucci, R., Nerlich, A. G., Trautmann, M., Ismail, S., Shanab, G. M., Karim, A. M., Gad, Y. Z. & Pusch, C. M. (2013). 'First insights into the metagenome of Egyptian mummies using next-generation sequencing.' *Journal of Applied Genetics* 54: 309–25.

Kitchen, K. A. (1982). *Pharaoh Triumphant: The Life and Times of Ramesses II.* Warminster: Aris & Phillips Ltd.

--- (1983). *Ramesside Inscriptions*, VI. Oxford: Blackwell.

Klasens, A. (1952). *A Magical Statue Base (Socle Béhague) in the Museum of Antiquities at Leiden.* Leiden: Brill.

Klemm, R. & Klemm, D. (2013). *Gold and Gold Mining in Ancient Egypt and Nubia.* Berlin, Heidelberg: Springer.

Kloos, H. & David, R. (2002). 'The paleoepidemiology of schistosomiasis in ancient Egypt.' *Human Ecology Review* 9(1): 14–25.

Koenig, Y. (2001). 'À propos de la conspiration du harem.' *Bulletin de l'Institut Français d'Archéologie Orientale* 101: 293–314.

Konigsberg, L. & Frankenberg, S. (2013). 'Demography.' In E. DiGangi & M. Moore (eds), *Research Methods in Human Skeletal Biology.* New York: Academy Press, 293–322.

Koschel, K. (1996). 'Opium alkaloids in a Cypriote Base Ring I vessel (bilbil) of the Middle Bronze Age from Egypt.' *Ägypten und Levante* 6: 159–66.

Kozieradzka-Ogunmakin, I. (2015). 'A case of metastatic carcinoma in an Old Kingdom-period skeleton from Saqqara.' In S. Ikram, J. Kaiser & R. Walker (eds), *Egyptian Bioarchaeology: Humans, Animals and the Environment.* Leiden: Sidestone Press, 77–85.

Kozloff, A. P. (2006). 'Bubonic plague during the reign of Amenhotep III?' *KMT* 17(3): 36–46.

Kozma, C. (2006). 'Dwarfs in ancient Egypt.' *American Journal of Medical Genetics* 140A: 303–11.

Kruchten, J.-M. (2001). 'Oracles.' In D. B. Redford (ed.), *The Oxford Encyclopedia of Ancient Egypt*, vol. 2. Oxford: Oxford University Press, 609–12.

Kuhrt, A. (1995). *The Ancient Near East c.3000–330 BC*, vol I. London, New York: Routledge.

Laes, C. (ed.) (2017). *Disability in Antiquity.* London, New York: Routledge.

Lajtar, A. (2008). 'The cult of Amenhotep Son of Hapu and Imhotep in Deir el-Bahari in the Hellenistic and Roman Periods.' In A. Delattre & P. Heilporn (eds), *<Et maintenant ce ne cont plus que des villages ...>. Thèbes et sa région aux époques Hellénistique, Romaine et Byzantine.* Actes Du Colloque Tenu À Bruxelles les 2 et 3 Décembre 2005. Brussels: Association Égyptologique Reine Élisabeth, 113–23.

Lalremruata, A., Ball, M., Bianucci, R., Welte, B., Nerlich, A. G., Kun, J. F. & Pusch, C. M. (2013). 'Molecular identification of falciparum malaria and human tuberculosis co-infections in mummies from the Fayum depression (lower Egypt).' *PLoS One* 8: https://doi.org/10.1371/journal.pone.0060307.

Lambert-Zazulak, P. I. (2000). 'The international ancient Egyptian mummy tissue bank at the Manchester Museum.' *Antiquity* 74: 44–48.

Lang, P. (2013). *Medicine and Society in Ptolemaic Egypt.* Leiden: Brill.

Leake, C. (1952). *The Old Egyptian Medical Papyri.* Kansas: University of Kansas Press.

Leblanc, C. (2004). 'L'ecole du temple (at-sebait) et le per-ankh (maison de vie) a propos de recentes decouvertes effectuees dans le contexte du Ramesseum.' *Memnonia* 15: 93–101.

Leca, A. P. (1988). *La Médecine Égyptienne au Temps des Pharaons.* Paris: Roger Dacosta.

Leek, F. F. (1966). 'Observations of the dental pathology seen in ancient Egyptian skulls.' *Journal of Egyptian Archaeology* 52: 59–64.

--- (1967a). 'The practice of dentistry in ancient Egypt.' *Journal of Egyptian Archaeology* 53: 51–58.

--- (1967b). 'Reputed early Egyptian dental operation, an appraisal.' In D. R. Brothwell & A. T. Sandison (eds), *Diseases in Antiquity.* Springfield, IL: Charles C. Thomas, 702–05.

--- (1972). 'Did a dental profession exist in ancient Egypt during the 3rd millennium B.C.?' *Medical History* 16(4): 404–06.

--- (1986). 'Cheops' courtiers: their skeletal remains.' In R. David (ed.), *Science in Egyptology.* Manchester: Manchester University Press, 183–99.

Lefebvre, M. G. (1952). 'Les prêtres de Sekhmet.' *Archiv Orientální* 20: 57–64; pls. I–II.

--- (1956). *Essai sur la Médecine Égyptienne de l'Époque Pharaonique*. Paris: Presses Universitaires de France.

Leitz, C. (1999). *Magical and Medical Papyri of the New Kingdom*, Hieratic Papyri in the British Museum 7. London: British Museum.

Lesko, B. S. (2001). 'Private cults.' In D. B. Redford (ed.), *The Oxford Encyclopedia of Ancient Egypt*, vol. 1. Oxford: Oxford University Press, 336–39.

--- (2002). *Women and Religion in Ancient Egypt*. New York: Brown University Press.

Lewis-Williams, J. D. (2002). 'Three-dimensional puzzles: Southern Africa and upper Palaeolithic rock art.' *Ethnos* 67(2): 245–64.

Liao, J. B. (2006). 'Viruses and human cancer.' *Yale Journal of Biology and Medicine* 79(3–4): 115–22.

Lichtheim, M. (1975, 1976, 1980). *Ancient Egyptian Literature*, vols 1–3. Berkeley, Los Angeles: University of California Press.

Lisowski, F. P. (1967). 'Prehistoric and early historic trepanation.' In D. Brothwell & E. T. Sandison (eds), *Diseases in Antiquity: A Survey of the Diseases, Injuries, and Surgery of Early Populations*. Springfield, IL: Charles C. Thomas, 651–72.

Lloyd, A. B. (1982). 'The inscription of UdjaHorresnet: a collaborator's testament.' *Journal of Egyptian Archaeology* 68: 166–80.

Loktionov, A. A. (2017). 'May my nose and ears be cut off: practical and "supra-practical" aspects of mutilation in the Egyptian New Kingdom.' *Journal of the Economic and Social History of the Orient* 60: 263–91.

Lopez, F. (2015). *Democede di Crotone e Udjahorresnet di Sais. Medici primari alla corte achemenide di Dario il Grande*. Pisa: Pisa University Press.

Loprieno-Gnirs, A. (ed.) (2020). *Transhuman: Von der Prothetik zum Cyborg*. Germany: Museum Ulm, 23–28.

Lorand, D. (2009). *Le Papyrus Dramatique du Ramesseum*. Leuven: Peeters.

Lord, C. (2016). 'One and the same? An investigation into the connection between veterinary and medical practice in ancient Egypt.' In C. Price, R. Forshaw, A. Chamberlain & P. Nicholson (eds), *Mummies, Magic and Medicine in Ancient Egypt: Multidisciplinary Essays for Rosalie David*. Manchester: Manchester University Press, 142–56.

Lorton, D. (1977). 'The treatment of criminals in ancient Egypt: through the New Kingdom.' *Journal of the Economic and Social History of the Orient* 20(1): 2–64.

Lowenstein, E. J. (2009). 'Osteogenesis imperfecta in a 3,000-year-old mummy.' *Child's Nervous System* 25(5): 515–16.

Loynes, R. D. (2015). *Prepared for Eternity: A Study of Human Embalming Techniques in Ancient Egypt Using Computerised Tomography Scans of Mummies*. Oxford: Archaeopress.

Loynes, R. D. & Bianucci, R. (2021). 'Medical imaging in mummy studies.' In D. H. Shin & R. Bianucci (eds), *The Handbook of Mummy Studies: New Frontiers in Scientific and Cultural Perspectives*. Singapore: Springer, 259.

Lucas, A. & Harris, J. R. (1962). *Ancient Egyptian Materials and Industries*. London: Edward Arnold (Publishers) Limited.

Maccheroni, M. & Fillios, M. (2019). 'Replication of ancient Egyptian oral surgical procedures using stone and bronze hand drills.' *Journal of the History of Dentistry* 67(1): 31–39.

McCreesh, N. & Gize, A. (2021). 'Takabuti's hair.' In R. David & E. Murphy (eds), *The Life and Times of Takabuti in Ancient Egypt: Investigating the Belfast Mummy*. Liverpool: Liverpool University Press, 58–64.

McDermott, B. (2004). *Warfare in Ancient Egypt*. Stroud: Sutton Publishing.

McDowell, A. G. (1990). *Jurisdiction in the Workmen's Community of Deir el-Medineh*. Leiden: Nederlands Instituut voor Het Nabije.

--- (1998). 'Legal aspects of care of the elderly in Egypt to the end of the New Kingdom.' In M. Stol & S. P. Vleeming (eds), *The Care of the Elderly in the Ancient Near East*. Leiden, Boston, Cologne: Brill, 199–221.

--- (1999). *Village Life in Ancient Egypt: Laundry Lists and Love Songs*. Oxford, New York: Oxford University Press.

McKnight, L. & Atherton-Woolham, S. (eds) (2015). *Gifts for the Gods: Ancient Egyptian Animal Mummies and the British*. Liverpool: Liverpool University Press.

McKnight, L. M., Atherton, S. D. & David, R. (2011). 'Introducing the ancient Egyptian animal bio bank at the KNH Centre for biomedical Egyptology, University of Manchester.' *Antiquity Project Gallery* 85(329): http://www.antiquity.ac.uk/projgall/mcknight329.

Maixner, F., Overath, T., Linke, D., Janko, M., Guerriero, G., van den Berg, B. H., Stade, B., Leidinger, P., Backes, C., Jaremek, M., Kneissl, B., Meder, B., Franke, A., Egarter-Vigl, E., Meese, E., Schwarz, A., Tholey, A., Zink, A. & Keller, A. (2013). 'Paleoproteomic study of the Iceman's brain tissue.' *Cellular and Molecular Life Sciences* 70(19): 3709–22.

Majno, G. (1975). *The Healing Hand: Man and Wound in the Ancient World*. Cambridge, MA: Harvard University Press.

Manetho (translated W. G. Waddell, 1940). *Aegyptiaca*, The Loeb Classical Library. Cambridge, MA: Harvard University Press.

Manniche, L. (1978). 'Symbolic blindness.' *Chronique d'Égypte* 53(105): 13–21.

--- (1989). *An Ancient Egyptian Herbal*. Austin: University of Texas Press; London: British Museum Publications.

Marchant, J. (2013). *The Shadow King*. Boston, MA: Da Capo Press.

Marganne, M.-H. (1993). 'Links between Egyptian and Greek medicine.' *Forum Trends in Experimental and Cultural Medicine* 3(5): 35–43.

Mariette, A. (1889). *Les Mastabas de l'Ancien Empire. Mastaba D62, le tombeau de Ptah-Hotep*. Paris: Vieweg.

Marshall, A. (2022). *Childhood in Ancient Egypt*. Cairo: The American University in Cairo Press.

Martin, D. C. (2013). 'Like you need a hole in the head: tool innovation a possible cause of trepanation. A case from Kerma, Nubia.' *International Journal of Osteoarchaeology* 23: 545–56.

Martin, G. T. (1981). *The Sacred Animal Necropolis at North Saqqara*. London: Egypt Exploration Society.

Martindale, W. (1977). *The Extra Pharmacopoeia*, 27th edition. London: The Pharmaceutical Press.

Masali, M. & Chiarelli, B. (1972). 'Demographic data on the remains of ancient Egyptians.' *Journal of Human Evolution* 1: 161–69.

Maspero, G. (1875). *Mémoires sur quelques Papyrus du Louvre*. Paris: Franck.

Matheson, C. D., David, R., Spigelman, M. & Donoghue, H. D. (2014). 'Molecular confirmation of schistosoma and family relationship in two ancient Egyptian mummies.' In H. Gill-Frerking, W. Rosendahl, A. R. Zink & A. Alterauge (eds), *Yearbook of Mummy Studies*, vol. 2. Munich: Verlag Dr Friederich Pfeil, 39–47.

Matthew, P. K., Kapua, F., Soaki, P. J. & Watters, K. A. K. (1996). 'Trauma admissions in the southern highlands of Papua New Guinea.' *ANZ Journal of Surgery* 66: 659–63.

Megahed, M., & Vymazalová, H. (2011). 'Ancient Egyptian royal circumcision from the pyramid complex of Djedkare.' *Anthropologie* (Czech Republic) 49(2): 157–66.

Merrillees, R. (1962). 'Opium trade in the Bronze Age Levant.' *Antiquity* 36: 287–92.

--- (1979). 'Opium again in antiquity.' *Levant* 11: 167–71.

Meskell, L. (1999). *Archaeologies of Social Life*. Oxford: Blackwell Publishers.

Metcalfe, R. M. (2010). 'Molecular methods for the study of ancient pharmacy.' In J. Cockitt & R. David (eds), *Pharmacy and Medicine in Ancient Egypt: Proceedings of the conferences held in Cairo (2007) and Manchester (2008)*. Oxford: Archaeopress, 110–12.

Millar, M. I. & Lane, S. D. (1988). 'Ethno-ophthalmology in the Egyptian delta: an historical systems approach to ethnomedicine in the Middle East.' *Social Science and Medicine* 26: 651–57.

Miller, J. (2008). *An appraisal of the skulls and dentition of ancient Egyptians, highlighting the pathology and speculating on the influence of diet and environment*. Oxford: Archaeopress.

Miller, R. L. (1989). '*Dqr*, spinning and treatment of guinea worm in P. Ebers 875.' *Journal of Egyptian Archaeology* 75: 249–54.

--- (1991). 'Palaeoepidemiology, literacy, and medical tradition among necropolis workmen in New Kingdom Egypt.' *Medical History* 35: 1–24.

Miller, R. L., Armelagos, G. J., Ikram, S., De Jonge, N., Krijer, F. W. & Deelder, A. M. (1993). 'Predynastic schistosomiasis.' In W. V. Davies & R. Walker (eds), *Biological Anthropology and the Study of Ancient Egypt*. London: British Museum Press, 55–60.

Miller, R. L., Ikram, S., Armelagoss, G. J., Walker, R., Harer, W. B., Shiff, C. J., Baggett, D., Carrigan, M. & Maret, S. M. (1994). 'Diagnosis of plasmodium falciparum infections in mummies using the rapid manual ParaSightTM-F test.' *Transactions of the Royal Society of Tropical Medicine and Hygiene* 88(1): 31–32.

Millet, N. B., Hart, G. D., Reyman, T. A., Zimmerman, M. R. & Lewin, P. K. (1980). 'ROM 1: mummification for the common people.' In A. Cockburn & E. Cockburn (eds), *Mummies, Disease and Ancient Cultures*. Cambridge: Cambridge University Press, 71–84.

Milne, J. G. (1914). 'The sanatorium of Dêr el-Bahri.' *Journal of Egyptian Archaeology* 1: 96–98.

Miniaci, G. (2020). *The Middle Kingdom Ramesseum Papyri Tomb and its Archaeological Context*, Kitab – Egyptology in Focus 1. London: Nicanor Books.

Mitchell, J. K. (1900). 'Study of a mummy affected with anterior poliomyelitis.' *Philadelphia Medical Journal* 6: 414–15.

Moissidou, D., Day, J., Shin, D. D. & Bianucci, R. (2015). 'Invasive versus non-invasive methods applied to mummy research: will this controversy ever be solved?' *BioMed Res Int* doi: 10.1155/2015/192829.

Molto, E. & Sheldrick, P. (2018). 'Paleo-oncology in the Dakhleh Oasis, Egypt: case studies and a paleoepidemiological perspective.' *International Journal of Paleopathology* 21: 96–110.

Molto, J. E. (1989). 'Spina bifida occulta in skeletal samples from the Dakhleh Oasis.' *Paleopathology Newsletter* (abstract) 66 (supplement): 8.

Monot, M., Honoré, N., Garnier, T., Araoz, R., Coppée, J. Y., Lacroix, C. *et al.* (2005). 'On the origin of leprosy.' *Science* 308(5724): 1040–42.

Montserrat, M. G. (2021). 'An approach to translating *shrt* and *ḏ3rt*. Compared methods.' In R. D. Sola, M. F. Georges & M. Guasch-Jané (eds), *Pharmacy and Medicine in Ancient Egypt. Proceedings of the conference held in Barcelona (2018)*. Oxford: Archaeopress, 30–37.

Moran, W. L. (1992). *The Amarna Letters*. Baltimore, MD, London: The John Hopkins University Press.

Morenz, L. D. (2003). 'Schamanismus in der Frühzeit Agypten?' *Archiv für Religionsgeschichte* (Arg 5). Munchen, Leipzig: Wissenschaftlicher Aufsetz: 212–26.

Morrow, M., Morrow, M., Judd, T. & Phillipson, G. (2010). *Desert Rats: Rock Art Topographical Survey in Egypt's Eastern Desert*. Oxford: Archaeopress.

Morse, D., Brothwell, D. R. & Ucko, P. J. (1964). 'Tuberculosis in ancient Egypt.' *American Review of Respiratory Disease* 90: 524–41.

Moussa, A. M. & Altenmüller, H. (1977). 'Das Grab des Nianchchnum und Chnumhotep.' *Archäologische Veröffentlichungen, Deutschen Archäologisches Institut, Abteilung Kairo* 21: 25–29.

Murray, M. A. (1910). *The Tomb of the Two Brothers*. Manchester: Sherratt & Hughes; London: Dulau & Co.

Naville, E. (1892). *The Festival-Hall of Osorkon II in the Great Temple of Bubastis*, The Egypt Exploration Fund, 10th Memoir. London: Kegan Paul, Trench, Trübner & Co., Ltd.

--- (1896). *The Temple of Deir el-Bahri*, Part II. London: The Egypt Exploration Fund.

Nerlich, A. G. & Bianucci, R. (2021). 'Palaeo-oncology and mummies.' In D. H. Shin & R. Bianucci (eds), *The Handbook of Mummy Studies: New Frontiers in Scientific and Cultural Perspectives*. Singapore: Springer, 131–46.

Nerlich, A. G., Zink, A., Haghedorn, H. G., Szeimies, U. & Weyss, C. (2000a). 'Anthropological & palaeopathological analysis of the human remains from three "Tombs of the Nobles" of the necropolis of Thebes-West, Upper Egypt.' *Anthropologischer Anzeiger* 58(4): 321–43.

Nerlich, A. G., Zink, A., Szeimies, U. & Haghedorn, H. G. (2000b). 'Ancient Egyptian prosthesis of the big toe.' *Lancet* 356: 2176–79.

Nerlich, A. G., Zink, A., Szeimies, U., Hagedorn, H. G. & Rösing, F. W. (2003). 'Perforating skull trauma in ancient Egypt and evidence for early neurosurgical therapy.' In R. Arnott, S. Finger & C. U. M. Smith (eds), *Trepanation, History, Discovery, Theory*. Lisse: Swets & Zeitlinger BV, 191–201.

Nerlich, A. G., Rohrbach, H., Bachmeier, B. & Zinc, A. (2006). 'Malignant tumors in two ancient populations: an approach to historical tumor epidemiology.' *Oncology Reports* 16(1): 197–202.

Nerlich, A. G., Schraut, B., Dittrich, S., Jelinek, T. & Zink, A. R. (2008). '*Plasmodium falciparum* in ancient Egypt.' *Emerging Infectious Diseases* 14(8): 1317–19.

Nerlich, A. G., Panzer, S., Hower-Tilmann, E. & Lösch, S. (2010a) 'Palaeopathological–radiological evidence for cerebral-palsy in an ancient Egyptian female mummy from a 13th Dynasty tomb.' In J. Cockitt & R. David, *Pharmacy & Medicine in Ancient Egypt: Proceedings of the conferences held in Cairo (2007) & Manchester (2008)*. Oxford: Archaeopress, 113–16.

Nerlich, A. G., Panzer, S. and Lösch, S. (2010b). 'Surgery in ancient Egypt – palaeopathological evidence for successful medical treatment by surgery.' In J. Cockitt and R. David (eds), *Pharmacy and Medicine in Ancient Egypt: Proceedings of the Conferences Held in Cairo (2007) and Manchester (2008)*. Oxford: Archaeopress, 117–21.

Neukamm, J., Pfrengle, S., Molak, M., Seitz, A., Francken, M., Eppenberger, P., Avanzi, C., Reiter, E., Urban, C., Welte, B., Stockhammer, P. W., Teßmann, B., Herbig, A., Harvati, K., Nieselt, K., Krause, J. & Schuenemann, V. J. (2020). '2000-year-old pathogen genomes reconstructed from metagenomic analysis of Egyptian mummified individuals.' *BMC Biology* 18: 108. https://doi.org/10.1186/s12915-020-00839-8.

Nuki, G. & Simkin, P. A. (2006). 'A concise history of gout and hyperuricemia and their treatment.' *Arthritis Research and Therapy* 8 (Suppl. 1): https://doi.org/10.1186/ar1906.

Nunn, J. (1996). *Ancient Egyptian Medicine*. London: British Museum Press.

O'Connor, D. (2002). 'Function and program: understanding ceremonial slate palettes.' *Journal of the American Research Center in Egypt* 39: 5–25.

Ollabarria, L. (2022). 'XX-Cavations: women in ancient Egypt and modern Egyptology.' *Interdisciplinary Egyptology* S 1(1): 13.

Onstine, S., Herrerin, J., Sánchez, M. & Dinares, R. (2018). 'Two cases of possible childbirth related death from Theban Tomb 16 in Luxor, Egypt.' In *Athanatos: Program & Abstracts, Extraordinary World Congress on Mummy Studies 2018*. Tenerife: Museos de Tenerife La Naturaleza y El Hombre: 62.

Oras, E., Anderson, J., Tõrv, M., Signe, V., Riina, R., Sünne, R., Maarja, M., Martin, M., Saag, L., Saage, R., Teearu-Ojakäär, A., Pilleriin, P., Tambets, K., Metspalu, M., Lees, D. C., Maxwell, V. L., Barclay, M. V. L., Hall, M. J. R., Ikram, S. & Piombino-Mascali, D. (2020). 'Multidisciplinary investigation of two Egyptian child mummies curated at the University of Tartu Art Museum, Estonia (Late/Graeco-Roman Periods).' *PLoS One*: https://doi.org/10.1371/journal.pone.0227446.

Orriols-Llonch, M. (2016). 'Women's role in sexual intercourse in ancient Egypt.' In S. L. Budin & J. MacIntosh Turfa (eds), *Women in Antiquity*. London, New York: Routledge, 194–203.

Pain, S. (2007). 'The Pharaohs' pharmacists.' *New Scientist* 196(2634): 40–43.

Panagiotakopulu, E. (2004). 'Pharaonic Egypt and the origins of plague.' *Journal of Biogeography* 31: 269–75.

Panagiotakopulu, E. & Buckland, P. C. (1999). '*Cimex lectularius* L., the common bed bug from Pharaonic Egypt.' *Antiquity* 73: 908–11.

Pantazis, I., Tourna, E., Maravelia, A., Kalampoukas, K., Michailidis, G., Kalogerakou, K., Kyriazi, S., Couvaris, C., Geroulanos, S. & Bontozoglou, N. A. (2020). 'A Ptolemaic mummy reveals evidence of invasive dentistry in ancient Egypt.' *Anatomical Record (Hoboken NJ)* 303(12): 3129–35.

Panzer, S., Treitl, M., Zesch, S., Rosendahl, W., Helmbold-Doyé, J., Thompson, R. C. & Zink, A. R. (2022). 'Radiological evidence of purulent infections in ancient Egyptian child mummies.' *International Journal of Paleopathology* 36: 30–35.

Papagrigorakis, M. J., Yapijakis, C., Synodinos, P. N. & Baziotopoulou-Valavani, E. (2006). 'DNA examination of ancient dental pulp incriminates typhoid fever as a probable cause of the Plague of Athens.' *International Journal of Infectious Diseases* 10(3): 206–14.

Parkinson, R. B. (1991). *Voices from Ancient Egypt.* Norman, OK: University of Oklahoma Press.

--- (1997). *The Tale of Sinuhe and Other Ancient Egyptian Poems 1940–1640 BC.* Oxford: Oxford University Press, 27–43.

--- (2001). 'Papyrus Westcar.' In D. B. Redford (ed.), *The Oxford Encyclopedia of Ancient Egypt*, vol. 3. Oxford: Oxford University Press, 24–25.

--- (2002). *Poetry and Culture in Middle Kingdom Egypt.* London, New York: Continuum.

--- (2009). *Reading Ancient Egyptian Poetry.* Chichester: Wiley-Blackwell.

--- (2019). 'Libraries in ancient Egypt, c.2600-1600 BCE'. In K. Ryholt & G. Barjamovic (eds), *Libraries before Alexandria.* Oxford: Oxford University Press, 115–67.

Parsche, F., Balabanova, S. & Pirsig, W. (1993). 'Drugs in ancient populations.' *Lancet* 341: 503.

Partridge, R. B. (2002). *Fighting Pharaohs: Weapons and Warfare in Ancient Egypt.* Manchester: Peartree Publishing.

Petrie, W. M. F. (1890). *Kahun, Gurob and Hawara.* London: Kegan Paul, Trench, Trubner & Co.

--- (1891 [1974]). *Illahun, Kahun and Gurob.* London, republ. Warminster: Aris & Phillips Ltd.

--- (1920 [rev. ed. 1974]). *Prehistoric Egypt.* London: British School of Archaeology in Egypt & Egyptian Research Account; Warminster: Aris & Phillips.

--- (1953). *Ceremonial Slate Palettes.* London: British School of Archaeology in Egypt & B. Quaritch.

Picardo, N. S. (2010). '(Ad)dressing Washptah: illness or injury in the Vizer's death, as related in his tomb biography.' In Z. Hawass & J. Houser (eds), *Millions of Jubilees: Studies in Honor of David P. Silverman* 2. Cairo: Conseil Suprême des Antiquités, 93–104.

Pinch, G. (1983). 'Childbirth and female figurines at Deir el-Medina & el-Amarna.' *Orientalia. Commentarii periodici Pontificii instituti biblici, Nova Series (Rome)* 52: 405–14.

--- (2006). *Magic in Ancient Egypt*, 2nd rev. ed. London: British Museum Press.

Pliny the Elder (translated H. Rackham, W. H. S. Jones & D. E. Eichholz, 1991). *Natural History*, Loeb Classical Library. Cambridge, MA: Harvard University Press.

Poinar, H., Kuch, M., McDonald, G., Martin, P. & Pääbo, S. (2003). 'Nuclear gene sequences from a late Pleistocene sloth coprolite.' *Current Biology* 13(13): 1150–52.

Policard, A. & Collet, A. (1952). 'Deposition of siliceous dust in the lungs of the inhabitants of the Sahara Desert.' *International Archives of Occupational and Environmental Health* 5: 527.

Pommerening, T. (2010). 'Healing measures: *dja* and *oipe* in ancient Egyptian pharmacy and medicine.' In J. Cockitt & R. David (eds), *Pharmacy and Medicine in Ancient Egypt. Proceedings of the conferences held in Cairo (2007) and Manchester (2008)*. Oxford: Archaeopress, 132–37.

--- (2017a). 'Medical re-enactments: ancient Egyptian prescriptions from an emic view.' In G. Rosali & M. C. Guidotti (eds), *Proceedings of the XIth Congress of Egyptologists, Florence, Italy 23–30, 2015*. Oxford: Archaeopress, 519–26.

--- (2017b). 'Classification in ancient Egyptian medical formulae and its role in rediscovering comprehensive and specific concepts of drugs and effects.' In T. Pommerening & W. Bisang (eds), *Classification from Antiquity to Modern Times. Sources, Methods, and Theories from an Interdisciplinary Perspective*. Berlin, Boston: De Gruyter, 167–98.

--- (2020). 'Egyptian medicine.' In D. C. Snell (ed.), *A Companion to the Ancient Near East*. Chichester: Wiley-Blackwell.

Porter, B. & Moss, R. (1994). *Topographical Bibliography of Ancient Egyptian Hieroglyphic Texts, Reliefs and Paintings*, 2nd ed., Tome 1. Oxford: Griffith Institute, Ashmolean Museum.

Posener-Kriéger, P. (1976). 'Les archives du temple funéraires de Neferirkare-Kakai (Les papyrus d'Abousir): traduction et commentaire.' *Bibliothèque d'Étude*, Cairo 65.

Price, C. (2016). 'On the function of "healing" statues.' In C. Price, R. Forshaw, A. Chamberlain, & P. Nicholson (eds), *Mummies, Magic and Medicine in Ancient Egypt: Multidisciplinary Essays for Rosalie David*. Manchester: Manchester University Press, 269–83.

Pritchard, J. B. (1955). *Ancient Near Eastern Texts Relating to the Old Testament*, 2nd edition. Princeton, NJ: Princeton University Press.

Pusch, C. M., Broghammer, M., Nicholson, G. J., Nerlich, A. G., Zink, A., Kennerknecht, L., Bachmann, N. & Blin, N. (2004). 'PCR-induced sequence alterations hamper the typing of prehistoric bone samples for diagnostic achondroplasia mutations.' *Molecular Biology and Evolution* 21: 2005–11.

Quack, J. F. (2006). 'Zur lesung und deutung des Dramatischen Ramesseum papyrus', *Zeitschrift für Ägyptische Sprache und Altertumskunde* 133: 72–89.

Quibell, J. E., Pirie, A. A., Spiegelberg, W., Paget, R. F. E. & Griffith, F. Ll. (1898). *The Ramesseum; and The Tomb of Ptah-hetep; copied by R. F. E. Paget and A. A. Pirie: With commets by F. Ll. Griffith*. London: B. Quaritch.

--- (1913). *Excavations at Saqqara, 1911–12: the tomb of Hesy*, Service des Antiquités de l'Égypte. Cairo: l'Institut Francais d'Archéologie Orientale.

Quirke, S. (1992). *Ancient Egyptian Religion*. London: British Museum Press.

--- (ed.) (1998). *Lahun Studies*. New Malden: SIA Publishing.

--- (2002). *Manuscript for Health of Mother & Child. The Kahun Medical Papyrus or Gynaecological Papyrus*. London: Petrie Museum of Egyptian Archaeology, UC 32057.

--- (2005). *Lahun: A Town in Egypt 1800 BC and the History of its Landscape*. London: Golden House Publications.

--- (2016). *Birth Tusks: The Armoury of Health in Context – Egypt 1800 BC*. London: Golden House Publications.

Rabino Massa, E. (1979). 'Two cases of spina bifida in Egyptian mummies.' Paper presented at the 2nd European Meeting of the Paleopathology Association, Turin. *Paleopathology Newsletter* (abstract) 25 (supplement) (178): 13.

Rabino Massa, E., Cerutti, N. & Savoia D. (2000). 'Malaria in ancient Egypt: paleoimmunological investigations in predynastic mummified remains.' *Chungara Revista de Antropología Chilena* 32: 7–9.

Rateitshak-Pluss, E. M. & Guggenheim, B. (1982). 'Effects of a carbohydrate free diet and sugar substitutes on dental plaque accumulation.' *Journal of Clinical Periodontology* 9: 239–51.

Ravagan, A. M. & Grossi, E. (2009). 'The oldest pregnancy test of human history invented by ancient Egyptians has a precise scientific basis.' In *'Erotic, Erotism and Sexuality in Ancient Egypt'*, Proceedings of the Second International Congress for Young Egyptologists – Lisbon – 23–26 October 2006. Lisbon: Lisbon University Press, 54–65.

Raven, M. J. & Taconis, W. K. (2005). *Egyptian Mummies: Radiological Atlas of the Collections in the National Museum of Antiquities at Leiden*. Turnhout: Brepols.

Ravishankar, P., Multari, D., Power, R., & Haynes, P. (2020). 'Bioarchaeological proteomic analysis of skin samples from an ancient Egyptian child mummy.' *Proceedings of the 68th American Society for Mass Spectrometry Conference on Mass Spectrometry and Allied Topics, 1 Jun 2020–12 Jun 2020*. Santa Fe, NM: American Society for Mass Spectrometry.

Rawlinson, G. (1956). *The History of Herodotus*. New York: Tudor Publishing Company.

Reeves, N. (1999). 'New light on ancient Egyptian prosthetic medicine.' In W. V. Davies (ed.), *Studies in honour of Egyptian antiquities: a tribute to Thomas Garnet Henry James*. London: British Museum, Occasional Paper 123: 73–77. Pl. XVII.

--- (2001). *Akhenaten: Egypt's False Prophet*. London: Thames & Hudson.

Reyman, T. A., Zimmerman, M. R. & Lewin, P. K. (1977). 'Autopsy of an Egyptian mummy. 5. Histopathologic investigation.' *Canadian Medical Association Journal* 117(5): 7.

Reymond, E. A. E. (ed.) (1976). *From the Contents of the Libraries of the Suchos Temples in the Fayyum. Part 1. A Medical Book from Crocodilopolis. P. Vindob. D. 6257*. Vienna: Brüder Hollinek.

Richards, M. P. & Britton, K. (2020). *Archaeological Science: An Introduction*. Cambridge: Cambridge University Press.

Ring, M. E. (1985). *Dentistry: An Illustrated History*. New York: Harry N. Abrahams.

Ritner, R. K. (1993). *The Mechanics of Ancient Egyptian Magical Practice*, Studies in Ancient Oriental Civilisation, vol. 54. Chicago, IL: The University of Chicago.

--- (2000). 'Innovations and adaptations in ancient Egyptian medicine.' *Journal of Near Eastern Studies* 59(2): 107–17.

--- (2001a). 'Magic.' In D. B. Redford (ed.), *The Oxford Encyclopedia of Ancient Egypt*, vol. 2. Oxford: Oxford University Press, 321–36.

--- (2001b). 'Medicine.' In D. B. Redford (ed.), *The Oxford Encyclopedia of Ancient Egypt*, vol. 2. Oxford: Oxford University Press: 353–56.

Roberts, C. A. & Manchester, K. (2005). *Archaeology of Disease*. Stroud: Sutton Publishing.

Robins, G. (1993). *Women in Ancient Egypt*. London: British Museum Press.

Robinson, J.-M. (2017). *'"Blood is thicker than water." Non-Royal Consanguineous Marriage in Ancient Egypt: An Exploration of Economic and Biological Outcomes.* Oxford: Archaeopress.

Roehrig, C. H. (2005). 'Senenmut, royal tutor to princess Neferure.' In C. H. Roehrig, R. Dreyfus & C. A. Keller (eds), *Hatshepsut from Queen to Pharaoh*. New Haven, CT, London: Yale University Press, 112–13.

Rollo, F., Ubaldi, M., Ermini, L. & Marota, I. (2002). 'Ötzi's last meals: DNA analysis of the intestinal content of the Neolithic glacier mummy from the Alps.' *Proceedings of the National Academy of Sciences of the United States of America* 99(20): 12594–99.

Rose, M. L. (2017). 'Ability and disability in classical Athenian oratory.' In C. Laes (ed.), *Disability in Antiquity*. Oxford, New York: Routledge, 139–53.

Roth, A. M. (1991). *Egyptian Phyles in the Old Kingdom: The Evolution of a System of Social Organization*, Studies in Ancient Oriental Civilization, no. 48. Chicago, IL: The Oriental Institute of the University of Chicago.

Rowling, J. T. (1989). 'The rise and decline of surgery in dynastic Egypt.' *Antiquity* 63: 312–19.

Ruffer, M. A. (1910a). *Studies in the Paleopathology of Egypt*, ed. R. L. Moodie. Chicago, IL: Chicago University Press.

--- (1910b). 'Notes on the presence of Bilharzia haematobium in Egyptian mummies of the XXth Dynasty.' *British Medical Journal* 1: 16.

--- (1910c). 'Remarks on the histology and pathological anatomy of two Egyptian mummies.' *Cairo Scientific Journal* 4: 1–5.

--- (1911). 'On arterial lesions found in Egyptian mummies (1580 BC–535 AD).' *Journal of Pathology and Bacteriology* 16: 453–62.

--- (1920). 'A study of abnormalities and pathology of ancient Egyptian teeth.' *American Journal of Physical Anthropology* 3: 335–82.

Rutherford, P. (2008a). 'The use of immunocytochemistry to diagnose disease in mummies.' In R. David (ed.), *Egyptian Mummies and Modern Science*. Cambridge: Cambridge University Press, 99–115.

--- (2008b). 'DNA identification in mummies and associated material.' In R. David (ed.), *Egyptian Mummies and Modern Science*. Cambridge: Cambridge University Press, 116–32.

Ryholt, K. (2019). 'Libraries from the Late Period and Graeco-Roman Egypt, *c.* 800 BCE–250 CE.' In K. Ryholt & G. Barjamovic (eds), *Libraries before Alexandria: Ancient Near Eastern Traditions*. Oxford: Oxford University Press, 390–458.

Ryholt, K. & Barjamovic, G. (2019). 'Libraries before Alexandria.' In K. Ryholt & G. Barjamovic (eds), *Libraries before Alexandria: Ancient Near Eastern Traditions*. Oxford: Oxford University Press, 1–66.

Sadek, A. I. (1988). *Popular Religion in Egypt during the New Kingdom*. Hildesheim: Gerstenberg Verlag.

Saleem, S. N. (2022). 'A radiological assessment of the "pregnant mummy": a comment to Ejsmond *et al.*, 2021.' *Journal of Archaeological Science* 137(6): https://doi.org/10.1016/j.jas.2021.105508.

Sales, J. & Das, C. (2018). 'Healing practices in ancient Egypt: the incubation of dreams at the Sanatorium of the Temple of Hathor in Dendara.' In C. E. Soares, C. Ruffio, F. Isaac & J. M. Malheiro (eds), *From the Fight against Sickness to the Invention of Immortality*. Porto: Universidade do Porto, Faculdade de Letras, 13–24.

Sales, J. C. (2018). 'Strike, smite and terrify: reflections on physical, ritual and psychological violence in Ancient Egypt.' In M. C. Pimentel & N. S. Rodrigues (eds), *Violence in the Ancient and Medieval Worlds*. Leuven, Paris, Bristol: Peeters, 295–313, 529–82.

Sanchez, G. M. (2000). 'A neurosurgeon's view of the battle of reliefs of King Sety I: aspects of neurological importance.' *Journal of the American Research Center in Egypt* 37: 143–65.

--- (2003). 'Injuries in the battle of Kadesh.' *KMT* 14(1): 58–65.

Sanchez, G. M. & Meltzer, E. S. (2012). *The Edwin Smith Papyrus: Updated Translation of the Trauma Treatise and Modern Medical Commentaries*. Atlanta, GA: Lockwood Press.

Sandison, A. T. (1967). 'Diseases of the eyes.' In D. Brothwell & A. T. Sandison (eds), *Diseases in Antiquity*. Springfield, IL: C. C. Thomas, 457–83.

Sandmann, M. (1938). *Texts from the Time of Akhenaten*. Brussels: Bibliotheca Aegyptiaca VIII.

Sauneron, S. (2000). *The Priests of Ancient Egypt* (translated D. Lorton). Ithaca and London: Cornell University Press.

--- (1962). 'Le germe dans les os.' *Bulletin de l'Institut Français d'Archéologie Orientale* 60: 19–27.

--- (1989). *Un traité égyptien d'ophiologie: Papyrus du Brooklyn Museum nos 47.218.48 et 85*. Cairo: Institut Français d'Archéologie Orientale.

Säve-Söderbergh, T. (1957). *Private Tombs at Thebes Volume 1: Four Eighteenth Dynasty Tombs*. Oxford: Griffith Institute.

Scanlan, B. (2004). 'Animals: the hunted and domestic.' In L. Donovan & K. McCorquodale (eds), *Egyptian Art: Principles and Themes in Wall Scenes*. Sydney: Macquarie University Press, 83–100.

Scarborough, J. (1976). 'Celsus on human vivisection at Ptolemaic Alexandria.' *Clio Medica* 11: 25–38.

--- (2018). 'Pharmacology in the Early Roman Empire: Dioscorides and his multicultural gleanings.' In P. T. Keyser & J. Scarborough (eds), *Science and Medicine in the Classical World*. Oxford: Oxford University Press, 519–42.

Scavenius, M. & Sloth, C. (1996). 'Fractures of the scapula.' *Acta Orthopaedica Belgica* 62: 129–32.

Schäfer, H. (1899). 'Die Wiedereinrichtung einer Ärzteschule in Sais unter König Darius I.' *Zeitschrift für Ägyptische Sprache und Altertumskunde* 37: 72–74.

Scheidel, W. D. (2001). *Death on the Nile: Disease and the Demography of Roman Egypt*. Leiden: Brill.

Schultz, A. H. (1967). 'Notes on diseases and healed fractures of wild apes.' In D. Brothwell & A. T. Sandison (eds), *Diseases in Antiquity: A Survey of the Diseases, Injuries and Surgery of Early Populations*. Springfield, IL: Charles C. Thomas, 47–55.

Scurlock, J.-A. (2018). 'Mesopotamian beginnings for Greek science?' In P. T. Keyser & J. Scarborough (eds), *Science and Medicine in the Classical World*. Oxford: Oxford University Press, 35–46.

Seath-Burrows, J. H. (2010). 'A Non-Destructive Analytical Study of Predynastic Period Unguents from Ancient Egypt.' Unpublished PhD thesis, The University of Manchester.

Senti, S., Habicht, M. E., Rayo, E., Eppenberger, P. E., Rühli, F. J. & Galassi, F. M. (2018). 'Egyptian canopic jars at the crossroad of medicine and archaeology: overview of 100 years of research and future scientific expectations.' *Pathobiology* 85: 267–75.

Sethe, K. (1903/1933). *Urkunden des Alten Reichs. Erster Band*. Urkunden des Ägyptischen Altertums Abteilung 1, Hft. 1–4. Leipzig: J. C. Hinrichs'sche Buchhandlung

Seyfried, K. J. (1981). *Beiträge zu den Expeditionen des Mittleren Reiches in die Ost-Wüste*. Hildesheim: Gerstenberg Verlag.

Shapiro, B., Rambaut, A. & Gilbert, M. T. P. (2006). 'No proof that typhoid caused the Plague of Athens (a reply to Papagrigorakis *et al.*) (2006).' *International Journal of Infectious Diseases* 10(4): 334–35.

Shaw, A. F. B. (1938). 'The histological examination of mummified material.' *Journal of Pathology and Bacteriology* 47: 115.

Shaw, I. (ed.) (2000). *The Oxford History of Ancient Egypt*. Oxford: Oxford University Press.

Sherman, E. J. (1967). 'Djedhor the saviour statue base 01 10589.' *Journal of Egyptian Archaeology* 81: 82–102.

Shirley, J. J. (2007). 'The life and career of Nebamun, the physician of the king in Thebes.' In J. Richards & Z. Hawass (eds), *The Archaeology and Art of Ancient Egypt: Essays in Honor of David B. O'Connor*, vol. 2. Annales du Service des Antiquités de l'Égypte, Cahier no. 36. Cairo: Supreme Council of Antiquities, 381–401.

Siculus, Diodorus (translated C. H. Oldfather, 1933). *Bibliotheca Historica* Bk 1, Loeb Classical Library. Cambridge, MA: Harvard University Press.

Sigerist, H. E. (1958). 'The Latin medical literature of the Early Middle Ages.' *Journal of the History of Medicine and Allied Sciences* 13(2): 127–46.

Simpson, W. K. (1976). *The Mastabas of Qar and Idu*. Boston, MA: Museum of Fine Arts.

--- (2003). *The Literature of Ancient Egypt*. New Haven, CT, London: Yale University Press.

Singer, G. G. (2016). 'Shaushka, the traveling Goddess.' *Trabajos de Egiptología* 7: 43–58.

Smith, G. E. (1908). 'The most ancient of splints.' *British Medical Journal* 1: 732–34.

--- (1912). *The Royal Mummies: Catalogue Général des Antiquités Égyptiennes du Musée du Caire, Nos. 61051–61100*. Cairo: Service des Antiquités de l'Égypte.

Smith, G. E. & Dawson, W. R. (1924, this edition 1991). *Egyptian Mummies*, 3rd edition. London, New York: Kegan Paul International.

Smith, G. E. & Wood Jones, F. (1910). 'Report on the human remains.' In G. A. Reisner (ed.), *The Archaeological Survey of Nubia: Report for 1907–1908*. Cairo: National Printing Department, vol. 2, 7–367.

Smith, M. (2009). *Traversing Eternity: Texts from the Afterlife from Ptolemaic and Roman Egypt*. Oxford: Oxford University Press.

Smith, M. O. (1997). 'Osteological indications of warfare in the Archaic period of the western Tennessee valley.' In D. L. Martin & D. W. Frayer (ed.), *Troubled Times: Violence and Warfare in the Past*. Amsterdam: Gordon & Breach, 241–66.

Sosztarits, O. (2013). 'Water in the Isis Sanctuary of Savaria.' *GEOszkóp* 16:13/11 (in Hungarian).

Sousa, R. (2019). *Gilded Flesh*. Oxford: Oxbow Books.

Sperati, G. (2009). 'Amputation of the nose throughout history.' *Acta Otorhinolaryngologica Italica* 29: 44–50.

Stannard, J. (1999). 'Diseases in Western Antiquity.' In K. F. Kiple (ed.), *The Cambridge World History of Human Disease*. Cambridge: Cambridge University Press.

Steuer, R. O. & de C. M. Saunders, J. B. (1959). *Ancient Egyptian and Cnidian Medicine: The Relationship of their Aetiological Concepts of Disease*. Berkeley, CA: University of California Press.

Stevens, A. & Dabbs, G. (2018). 'The North Tombs cemetery excavations and skeletal analysis.' *Journal of Egyptian Archaeology* 104(2): 121–44.

Stevens, J. M. (1975). 'Gynaecology from ancient Egypt: the papyrus Kahun: a translation of the oldest treatise on gynaecology that has survived from the ancient world.' *Medical Journal of Australia* 2: 949–52.

Stok, F. (2018). 'Medical Sects: Herophilus, Erasistratus, Empiricists.' In P. T. Keyser & J. Scarborough (eds), *Science and Medicine in the Classical World*. Oxford: Oxford University Press, 359–80.

Strabo (translated H. L. Jones, 1932). *Geography*, Loeb Classical Library. Cambridge, MA: Harvard University Press.

Strouhal, E. (1996). 'Traces of a smallpox epidemic in the family of Ramesses V of the Egyptian 20th Dynasty.' *Anthropologie* 34(3): 315–19.

--- (1997). *Life of the Ancient Egyptians*. Liverpool: Liverpool University Press.

Strouhal, E., Vachala, B. & Vymazalová, H. (2014). *The Medicine of the Ancient Egyptians, 1, Surgery, Gynecology, Obstetrics, and Pediatrics*. Cairo: The American University in Cairo Press.

--- (2021). *The Medicine of the Ancient Egyptians, 2, Internal Medicine*. Cairo: The American University in Cairo Press.

Strudwick, N. C. (2005). *Texts from the Pyramid Age*, ed. R. J. Leprohon. Writings from the Ancient World. Atlanta: Society of Biblical Literature.

Stuhr, M. (2002). *Medical Writings of the Ancient Egyptians* (accessed May 24, 2021) <https://www.medizinische-papyri.de/PapyrusBerlin3038/>.

Suddick, R. P. & Harris, N. O. (1990). 'Historical perspectives of oral biology: a series.' *Critical Reviews in Oral Biology and Medicine* 1: 135–51.

Sudhoff, K. (1917). 'Der Stelzfuss aus Capua.' *Mitteilungen zur Naturwissenschaften* 16: 291–93.

Sullivan, R. (1997). 'Divine and rational: the reproductive health of women in ancient Egypt.' *Obstetrical and Gynecological Survey* 52(10): 635–42.

--- (1998). 'Proto-surgery in ancient Egypt.' *Acta Medica* (Hradec Králové) 41: 109–20.

Szpakowska, K. (2003). *Behind Closed Eyes: Dreams and Nightmares in Ancient Egypt*. Swansea: Classical Press of Wales.

Tapp, E. (1979). 'Disease in the Manchester Mummies.' In A. R. David (ed.), *The Manchester Museum Mummy Project: Multidisciplinary Research on Ancient Egyptian Mummified Remains*. Manchester: Manchester Museum, 95–102.

Tapp, E. & Wildsmith, K. (1992). 'The autopsy and endoscopy of the Leeds Mummy.' In A. R. David & E. Tapp (eds), *The Mummy's Tale: The Scientific and Medical Investigation of Natsef-Amun, Priest in the Temple of Karnak*. London: Michael O'Mara Books, 132–53.

Teeter, E. (2011). *Religion and Ritual in Ancient Egypt*. Cambridge: Cambridge University Press.

Theophrastus (translated A. F. Hort, 1916). *Enquiry into Plants*, Loeb Classical Library. Cambridge, MA: Harvard University Press.

The Tebtunis Papyri (2001). *Center for the Tebtunis Papyri*. Berkeley: University of California (accessed March 18, 2022) <https://www.tebtunis.berkeley.edu>.

Thomas, S. (2013). 'The *Pastophorion*: "Priests' Houses" in legal texts from Ptolemaic Pathyris and elsewhere in Egypt.' *Journal of Egyptian Archaeology* 99: 155–70.

--- (2014). 'The *Pastophorion* revisited: owners and users of "Priests' Houses" in Ptolemaic Pathyris and elsewhere in Egypt.' *Journal of Egyptian Archaeology* 100: 111–32.

Thomas, S., Fisher, B., Fram, P. & Waring, M. (1998). 'Odour absorbing dressings: a comparative laboratory study.' *World Wide Wounds* (accessed August 7, 2022) <http://www.worldwidewounds.com/1998/march/Odour-Absorbing-Dressings/odour-absorbing-dressings.html>.

Tobin, V. A. (2003). 'The admonitions of an Egyptian sage.' In W. K. Simpson (ed.), *The Literature of Ancient Egypt*. New Haven, CT, London: Yale University Press, 188–210.

Töpfer, S. (2014). 'The physical activity of parturition in ancient Egypt: textual and epigraphical sources.' *Dynamis* 34(2): 317–35.

--- (2017). 'Burial and mortuary practices in Late Period and Graeco-Roman Egypt.' In K. A. Kóthay (ed.), *Proceedings of the International Conference held at Museum of Fine Arts, Budapest, 17–19 July 2014*. Budapest: Museum of Fine Arts, 23–34.

Torras, N. B. (2021). 'The Pure Priest of Sekhmet, between health and disease.' In R. D. Solà, M. F. Georges & M. R. Guasch-Jané (eds), *Pharmacy and Medicine in Ancient Egypt*. Oxford: Archaeopress Egyptology 54, 116–24.

Trevisanato, S. I. (2006). 'Treatments for burns in the London Medical Papyrus show the first seven biblical plagues of Egypt are coherent with Santorini's volcanic fallout.' *Medical Hypotheses* 66(1): 193–96.

Turnbull, C. & Hodgson, D. M. (2005). 'Genetic predisposition to cancer.' *Clinical Medicine (London)* 5(5): 491–98.

van de Walle, B. & de Meulenaere, H. (1973). 'Compléments à la prosopographie médicale.' *Revue d'Égyptologie* 25: 58–83.

Veldmeijer, A. & Ikram, S. (2020). 'Tutankhamun's sticks and staves. The importance of deceptively simple objects.' *Scribe* 5: 8–13.

Verbrugghe, G. P. & Wickersham, J. M. (2001). *Berossos and Manetho, Introduced and Translated: Native Traditions in Ancient Mesopotamia and Egypt*. Ann Arbor: University of Michigan Press.

Vercoutter, J. (ed.) (1980). *Livre du Centenaire 1880–1980 Memoires de l'Insitut français d'archéologie orientale du Caire*, 104. Cairo: Institut Français d'Archéologie Orientale.

Vlachojannis, J., Magora, F. & Chrubasi, S. (2011). 'Willow species and aspirin: different mechanism of actions.' *Phytotherapy Research* 25: 1102–04.

von Känel, F. (1984). *Les prêtres-ouâb de Sekhmet et les conjurateurs de Serket*, Bibliothèque de l'École des Hautes Études 87. Paris: Presses Universitaires de France.

von Lieven, A. (2007). *Grundriss des Laufes der Sterne. Das sogenannte Nutbuch*, CNI Publications 31. Copenhagen: Museum Tusculanum Press.

von Staden, H. (1989). *Herophilus: The Art of Medicine in Early Alexandria*. Cambridge: Cambridge University Press.

Wade, A. D. & Nelson, A. J. (2013). 'Radiological evaluation of the evisceration tradition in ancient Egyptian mummies.' *HOMO – Journal of Comparative Human Biology* 64: 1–28.

Wade, A. D., Hurnanen, J., Lawson, B., Tampieri, D. & Nelson, A. J. (2012). 'Early dental intervention in the Redpath Ptolemaic Theban Male.' *International Journal of Paleopathology* 2(4): 217–22.

Walker, J. (1990). 'The place of magic in the practice of medicine in ancient Egypt.' *Bulletin of the Australian Centre for Egyptology* 1: 85–95.

Walker, P. L. (1997). 'Wife beating, boxing, and broken noses: skeletal evidence for the cultural patterning of violence.' In D. L. Martin & D. W. Frayer (eds), *Troubled Times: Violence and Warfare in the Past*. Amsterdam: Gordon and Breach, 145–80.

Walker, R. E. (1964). 'The Veterinary Papyrus of Kahun: a revised translation and interpretation of the ancient Egyptian treatise known as the Veterinary Papyrus of Kahun.' *Veterinary Record* 75: 198–200.

Wall, L. L. (1988). *Hausa Medicine: Illness and Wellbeing in a West African Culture*. Durham, NC, London: Duke University Press.

Wasmuth, M. & Creasman, P. P. (eds) (2020). 'Udjahorresnet and his world.' *Journal of Ancient Egyptian Interconnections* 26.

Watterson, B. (1991). *Women in Ancient Egypt*. Stroud: Sutton Publishing.

Weeks, K. R. (1980). 'Ancient Egyptian dentistry.' In J. E. Harris & J. E. Wente (eds), *An X-Ray Atlas of the Royal Mummies*. Chicago, IL, London: University of Chicago Press, 99–121.

--- (1995). 'Medicine, surgery and public health in ancient Egypt.' In J. M. Sasson (ed.), *Civilizations of the Ancient Near East* 3. Peabody, MA: Hendrickson Publishers, 1787–98.

Wente, E. F. (1980). 'Age of death of pharaohs of the New Kingdom, determined from historical sources.' In J. E. Harris & E. F. Wente (eds), *An X-Ray Atlas of the Royal Mummies*. Chicago, IL, London: Chicago University Press, 234–85.

--- (1990). *Letters from Ancient Egypt*. Atlanta: Scholars Press.

West, S. (1998). 'Whose baby? A note on P. Oxy. 744.' *Zeitschrift für Papyrologie und Epigraphik* 120: 167–72.

Westendorf, W. (1980). 'Isiknoten.' In W. Helck, E. Otto, & W. Westendorf (eds.) (1972–92), *Lexikon der Agyptologie*, 7 vols. Wiesbaden: Otto Harrassowitz 3: 204.

--- (1992). *Erwachen der Heilkunst. Die Medizin im Alten Ägypten*. Zurich: Artemis & Winkler.

Wildung, D. (1977). *Egyptian Saints: Deification in Pharaonic Egypt*. New York: New York University Press.

Williams, H. V. (1929). 'Human paleopathology.' *Archives of Pathology* 7: 839–902.

Williams, R. J. (1972). 'Scribal training in ancient Egypt.' *Journal of the American Oriental Society* 92(2): 214–21.

Wilson, A. B. (1992). 'History of amputation surgery and prosthetics.' In H. K. Bowker & J. W. Michael (eds), *Atlas of Limb Prosthetics: surgical, prosthetic & rehabilitation principles*. St. Louis: Mosby Year Book.

Winkler, H. A. (1938). *Rock Drawings of Southern Upper Egypt 1938–9: Sir Robert Mond Desert Expedition*. London: Egypt Exploration Society.

Wood Jones, F. (1908). 'Some lessons from ancient fractures.' *British Medical Journal* (2486): 455–58.

Worth Estes, J. (1993). *The Medical Skills of Ancient Egypt*. Rev. ed. Canton, MA: Science History Publications.

Wreszinski, W. (1909). *Der Grosse Medizinische Papyrus des Berliner Museums*. Leipzig: J. C. Hinrichs.

--- (1912). *Der Londoner medizinische Papyrus (Brit. Museum Nr. 10059) und der Papyrus Hearst: in Transkription, Übersetzung und Kommentar mit Facsimile des Londoner Papyrus*. Leipzig: J. C. Hinrichs'sche Buchhandlung.

Wróbel, J. T. (1977). 'Nuphar Alkaloids.' In R. H. F. Manske (ed.), *The Alkaloids* 16. New York: Academic Press, 181–214.

Zaki, M. E., Sarry El-Din, A. M. & Asaad, H. (2000). 'Histomorphometric analysis of skeletal remains from ancient Egyptians from Giza Old Kingdom.' *Medical Journal of Cairo University* 25: 14–34.

Zaki, M. E., Hussien, F. H. & Abd El-Shafy El Banna, R. (2009). 'Osteoporosis among ancient Egyptians.' *International Journal of Osteoarchaeology* 19: 78–89.

Zaki, M. E., Sarry El-Din, A. M., Al-Tohamy Soliman, M., Mahmoud, N. H. & Basha, W. A. (2010). 'Limb amputation in ancient Egypt from Old Kingdom.' *Journal of Applied Sciences Research* 6: 913–17.

Zaki, M. E., Abd El-Fattah, F. A. & Mohie, M. A. (2017). 'Examination of ancient Egyptian mummy with foot deformity from the New Kingdom Period.' *Journal of Orthopaedics Trauma Surgery and Related Research* 12(2): 29–31.

Zakrzewski, S. (2015). 'Life expectancy.' In E. Frood & W. Wendrich (eds), *UCLA Encyclopedia of Egyptology*, Los Angeles (accessed June 30, 2023) <https://escholarship.org/uc/nelc_uee>.

Zibelius-Chen, K. (1994). 'Die Kubanstele Ramses' II. und die nubischen Goldregionen.' In C. Berger, G. Clerc & N. Grimal (eds), *Hommages à Jean Leclant*, vol. 2. Cairo: L'Institut Français d'Archéologie Orientale du Caire, 411–17.

Zimmerman, M. R. (1977). 'An experimental study of mummification pertinent to the antiquity of cancer.' *Cancer* 40(3): 1358–62.

Zink, A. R., Rohrbach, H., Szeimies, U., Hagedorn, H. G., Haas, C. J., Weyss, C., Bachmeier, B. & Nerlich, A. G. (1999). 'Malignant tumors in an ancient Egyptian population.' *Anticancer Research* 19: 4273–77.

Zink, A. R, Reischl, U., Wolf, H. & Nerlich, A. G. (2000). 'Molecular evidence of bacteremia by gastrointestinal pathogenic bacteria in an infant mummy from ancient Egypt.' *Archives of Pathology and Laboratory Medicine* 124: 1614–18.

Zink, A. R., Haas, C. J., Reischl, U., Szeimies, U. & Nerlich, A. G. (2001). 'Molecular analysis of skeletal tuberculosis in an ancient Egyptian population.' *Journal of Medical Microbiology* 50: 355–66.

Zink, A. R., Spigelman, M., Schraut, B., Greenblatt, C. L., Nerlich, A. G. & Donoghue, H. D. (2006). 'Leishmaniasis in ancient Egypt and Upper Nubia.' *Emerging Infectious Diseases* 12(10): 1616–17.

Ziskind, B. (2009). 'Urinary schistosomiasis in ancient Egypt.' *Néphrologie et Thérapeutique* 5(7): 658–61.

Zorab, P. A. (1961). 'The historical and prehistorical background of ankylosing spondylitis.' *Proceedings of the Royal Society of Medicine* 54: 415–20.

Index

Italic numerals indicate an illustration caption

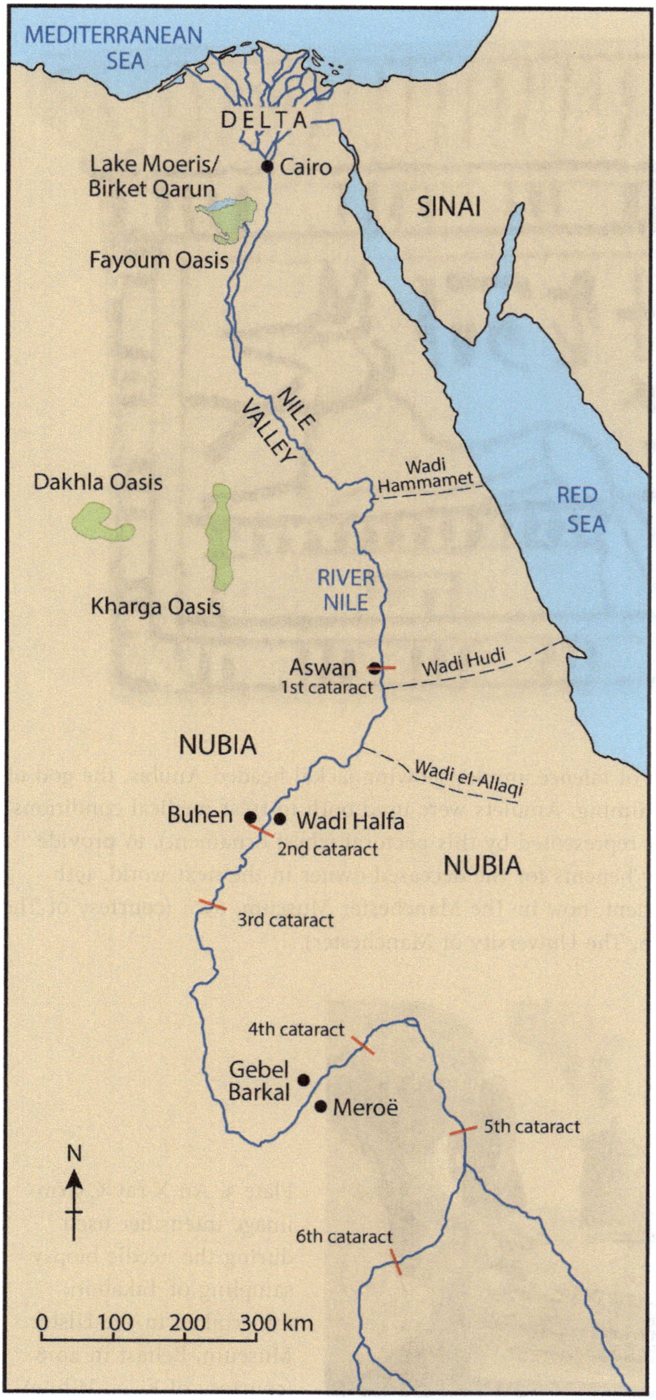

Plate 1. Map of Egypt showing main geographical features. Redrawn by L. Mulqueeny based on Partridge (2002: 391) and Baines and Málek (1980: 13, 41).

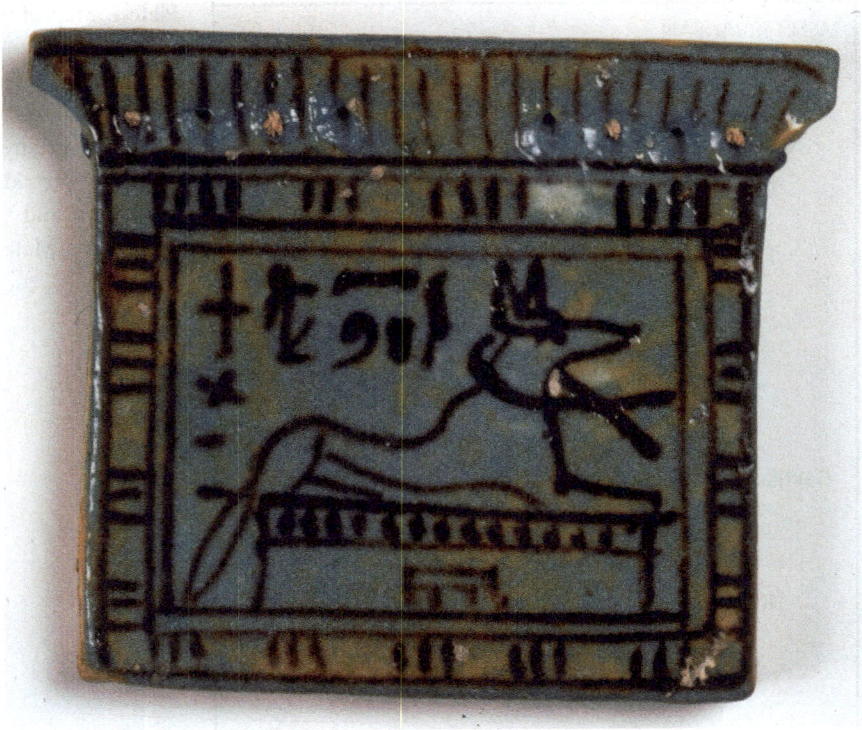

Plate 2. Reverse side of faience amulet showing jackal-headed Anubis, the god of cemeteries and embalming. Amulets were used both to treat medical conditions in the living and, as represented by this pectoral (chest ornament), to provide protection and other benefits for the deceased owner in the next world. 19th Dynasty. From Sedment, now in The Manchester Museum, 6961 (courtesy of The Manchester Museum, The University of Manchester).

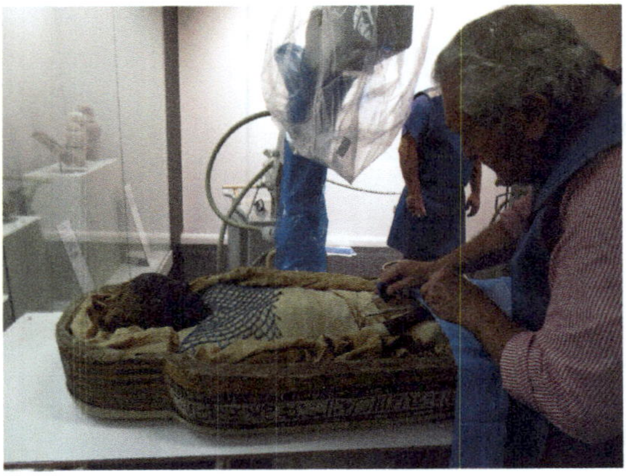

Plate 3. An X-ray C-arm image intensifier used during the needle biopsy sampling of Takabuti, undertaken in the Ulster Museum, Belfast in 2018 (courtesy of K. N. White).

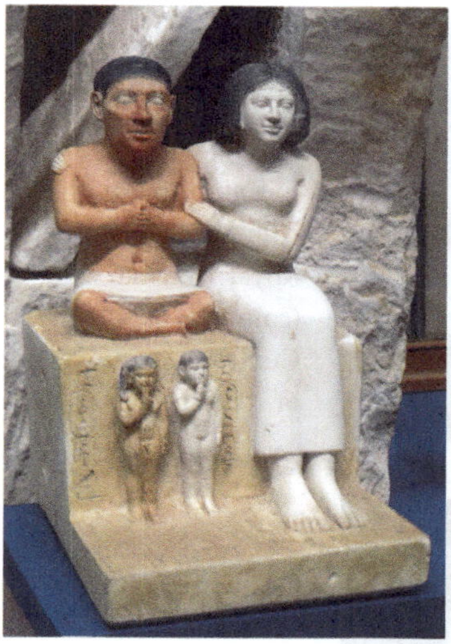

Plate 4. 6th Dynasty statue of Seneb showing him with his wife, Senetites, and their son and daughter. The statue depicts him as a classic example of an achondroplastic dwarf, in which the head and trunk are normal but the limbs are short. Limestone. Found at Giza, now in the Egyptian Museum, Cairo, JE 51281 (courtesy of A. Dodson).

Plate 5. Edwin Smith Papyrus, recto Column 6 (right) and 7 (left). The text describes anatomical observations and the examination, diagnosis, treatment and prognosis of forty-eight types of medical condition. Discovered in Luxor and dated to *c.* 1650–1550 BC. New York Academy of Medicine (Wikimedia Commons. Public Domain).

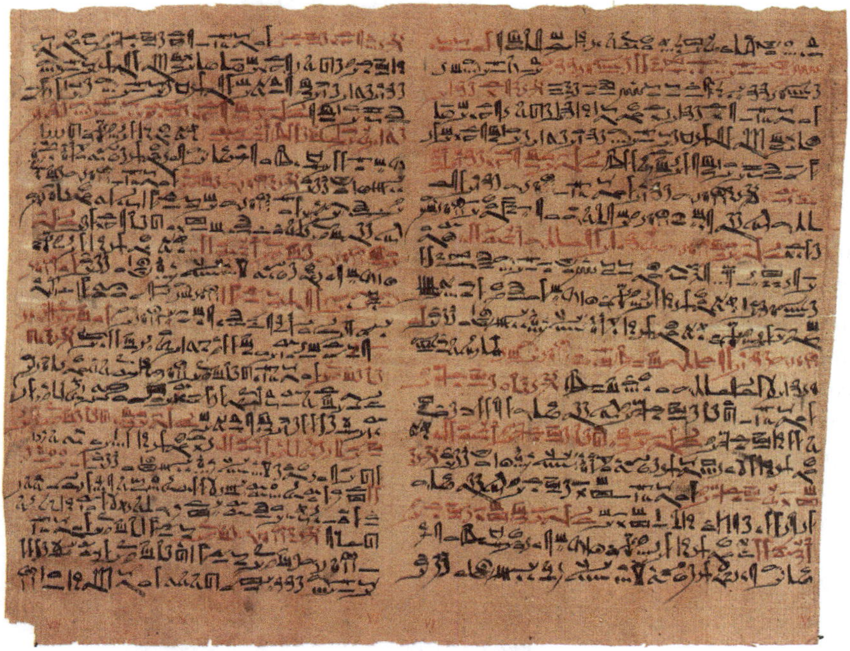

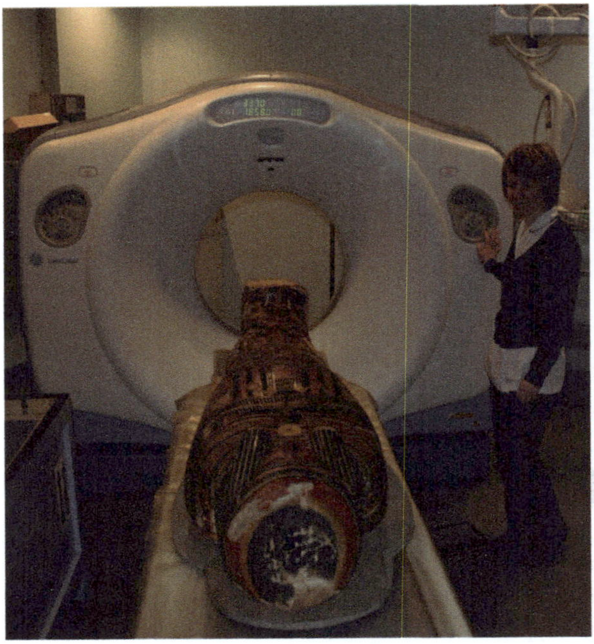

Plate 6. Three-dimensional CT (computer tomography) scanning of a mummy within a coffin at Manchester Royal Infirmary (courtesy of the KNH Centre, The University of Manchester).

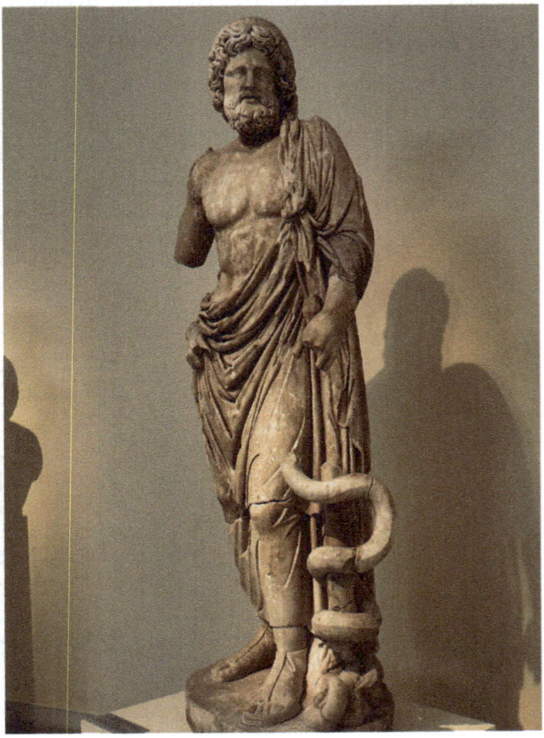

Plate 7. Statue of Asclepius. The god leans on a staff, around which his sacred animal, the snake, is coiled. Found in the Sanctuary of Asclepius at Epidaurus. Pentelic marble. *c.* AD 160. National Archaeological Museum of Athens, Greece, 263 (Wikipedia, Public Domain. Photographer G. E. Koronaios).

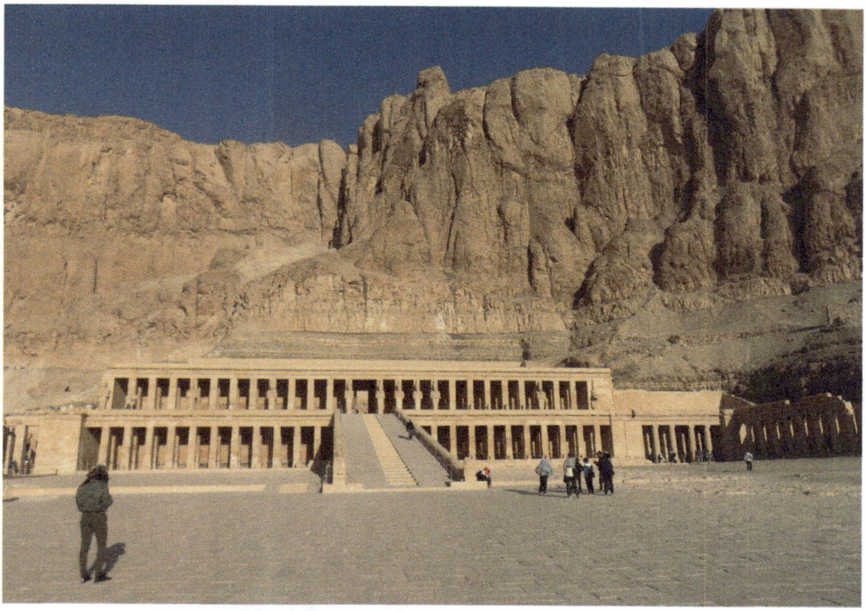

Plate 8. 18th Dynasty mortuary temple of Hatshepsut at Deir el-Bahri. Located on the west bank of the Nile opposite Karnak. In the Graeco-Roman Period this had accommodation for the healing cult of Imhotep and Amenhotep, son of Hapu (courtesy of K. N. White).

Plate 9. Temple of Kom Ombo situated on the Nile between Aswan and Edfu. The temple is dedicated equally to Sobek (the crocodile god) and to Haroeris or 'Horus the Elder', with the main features of the standard temple duplicated. Built during the Ptolemaic Period (although on the site of an older temple) with some later additions during the Roman Period (courtesy of R. David).

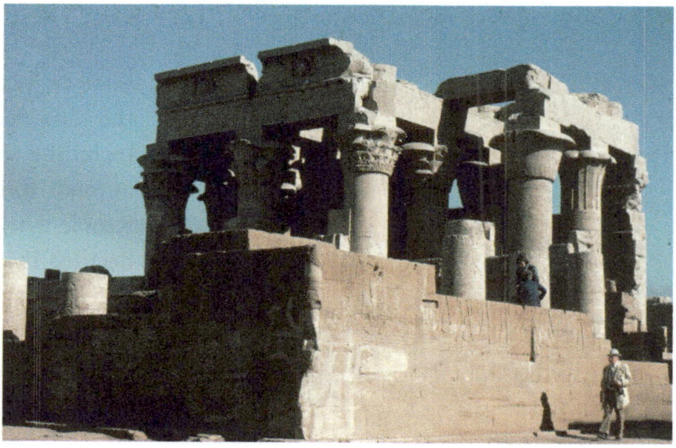

Plate 10. Statuette of the goddess Taweret, a deity associated with protection of mother and child during pregnancy and childbirth. Discovered in the Qena area, Upper Egypt. Ptolemaic Period. Faience. Metropolitan Museum of Art, New York, 26.7.1193 (courtesy of The Metropolitan Museum of Art. Purchase, Edward S. Harkness Gift, 1926).

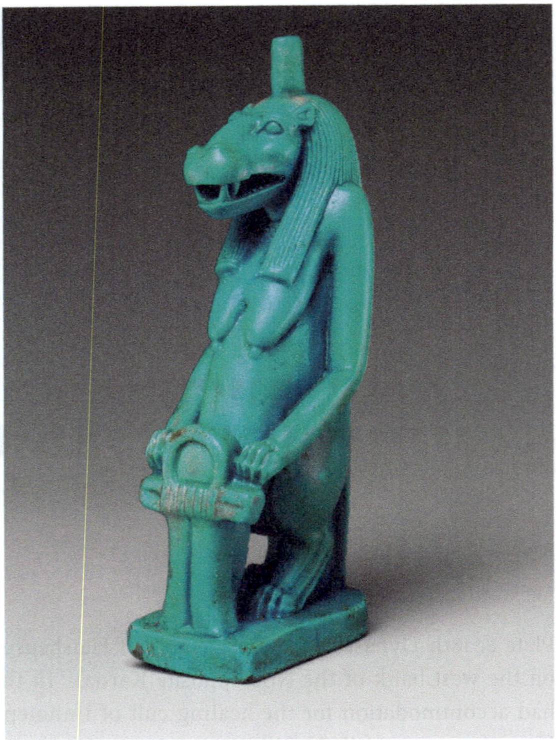

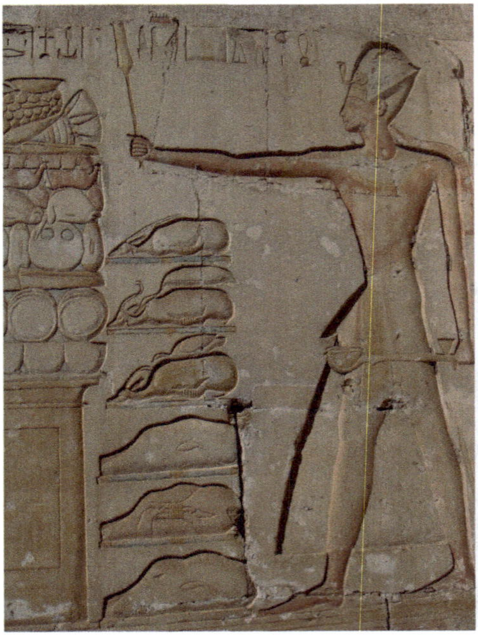

Plate 11. Wall relief showing the king dedicating offerings including sacrificial trussed animals to be presented to temple deities. Priests who decided if animals were fit for sacrifice may also have played a role as veterinary specialists. 19th Dynasty. Temple of Ramesses II, Abydos (courtesy of K. N. White).

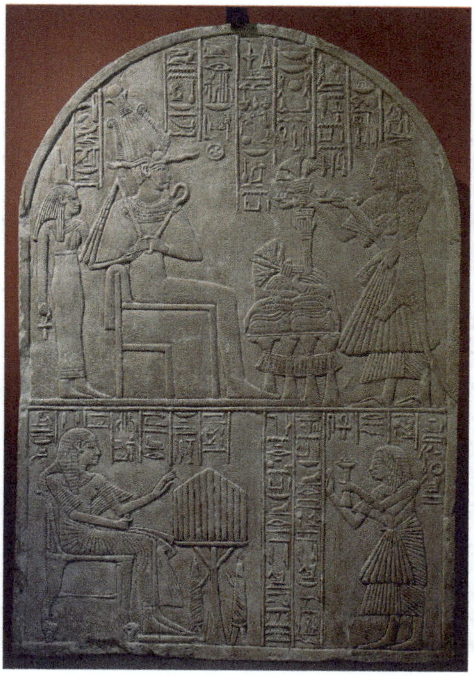

Plate 12. Stela of the physician Iuny. Upper register: Osiris and Isis; lower register: Iuny's son Khaemwaset, also a physician, presents him with gifts. Limestone, New Kingdom. Louvre, C89 (Wikimedia, Public Domain. Photographer: Jastrow).

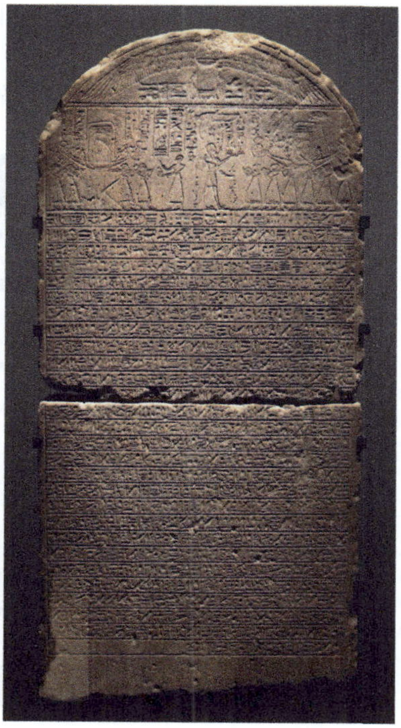

Plate 13. Bentresh Stela. Describes the story of Bentresh, daughter of the prince of Bakhtan, who fell ill and was cured by a healing statue. Discovered near the Khonsu temple of Ramesses III at Karnak. Dated to the Late or Ptolemaic Period. Black sandstone. Louvre, C 284 (Wikipedia, Public Domain. Photographer: Rama).

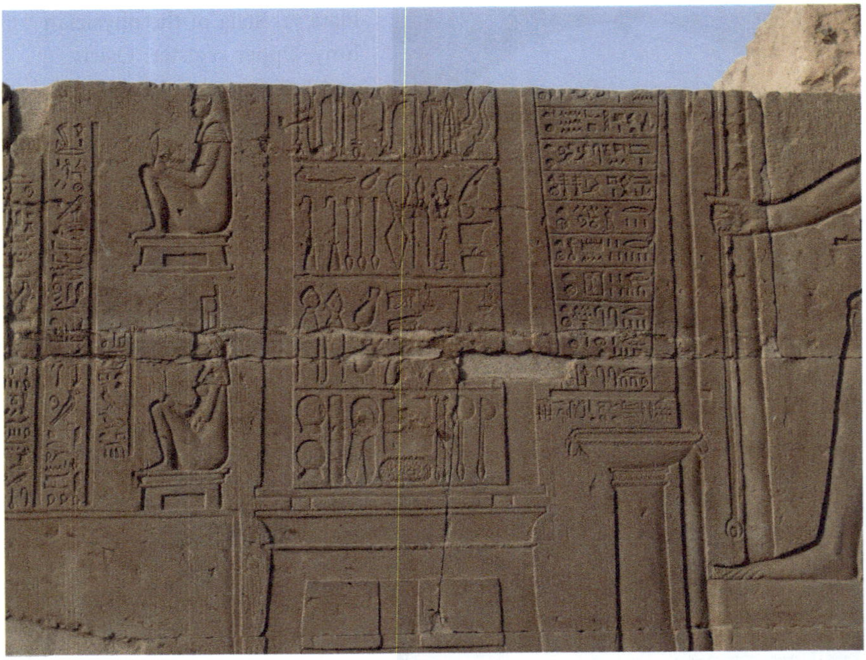

Plate 14. A scene carved on the north-western corner of the inner aspect of the outer enclosure wall of the Graeco-Roman temple at Kom Ombo. The relief depicts a series of implements often considered to represent surgical instruments (Wikipedia, Public Domain. Photographer: Ad Meskens).

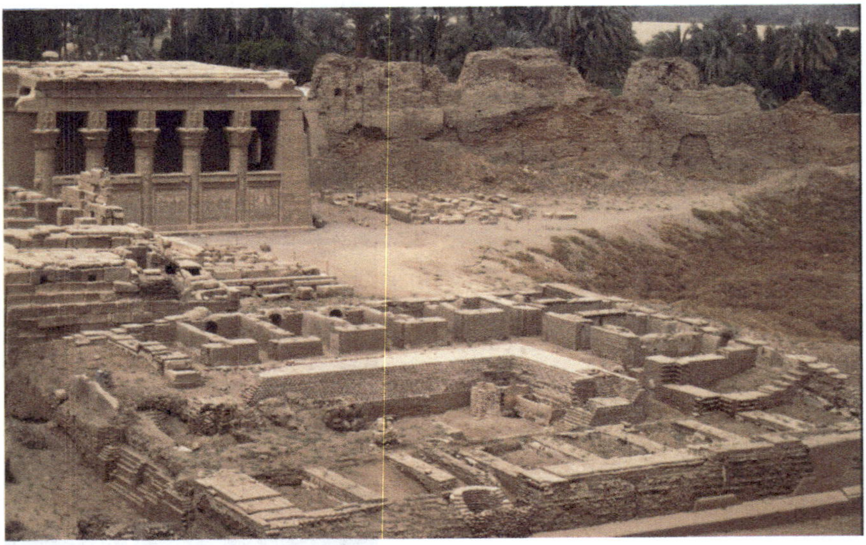

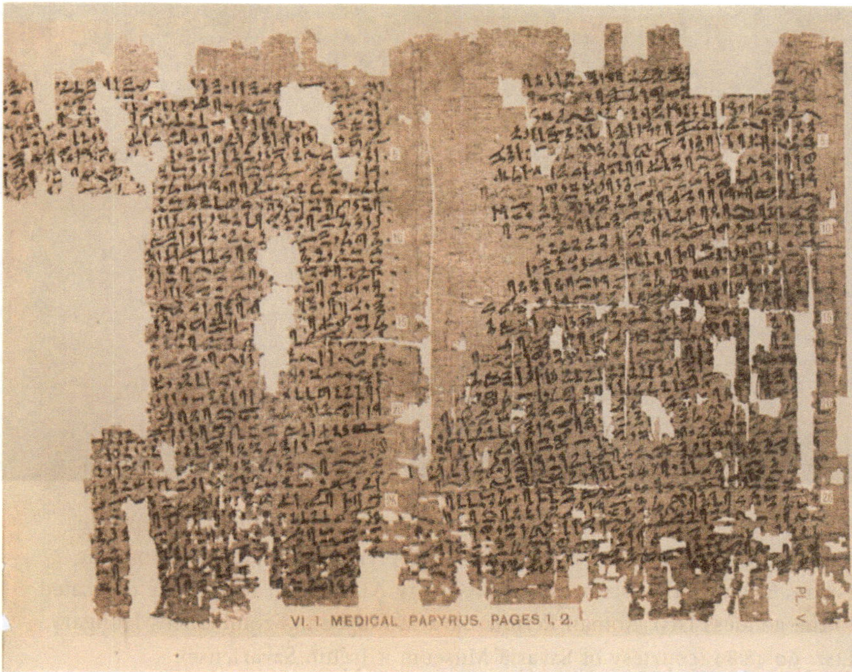

Plate 16. Pages 1 and 2 of the Kahun Papyrus, which is the earliest known manuscript on gynaecology in the world. It includes thirty-four cases dealing with women's health, including gynaecological diseases, fertility, pregnancy and contraception. It is dated to about 1800 BC and was found at Kahun by Flinders Petrie. Now housed at University College, London, UC 32057 (Wikimedia Commons, Public Domain).

Plate 15 (opposite). The mudbrick sanatorium (foreground) at the Temple of Hathor, Dendara. This building incorporates a series of cubicles where the patients were bathed with sacred water. Late Period/Graeco-Roman Period (courtesy of R. David).

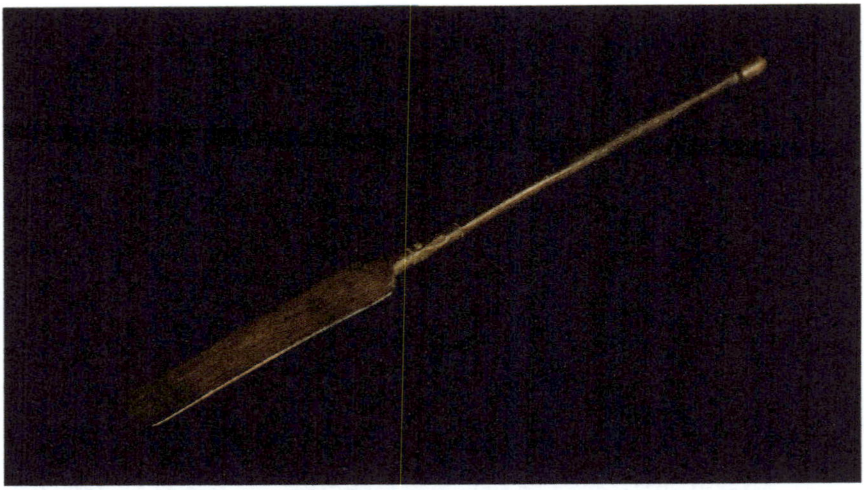

Plate 17. Bronze spatula possibly used as a medical instrument to separate the edges of a wound or for mixing and applying medicaments. From the Iseum, Savaria (The Iseum is a 2nd century AD Roman temple site dedicated to the goddess Isis). Roman Period. Savaria Museum, Szombathely, Hungary, Ltsz: 60:48:89 (courtesy of Savaria Museum – Iseum Savariense).

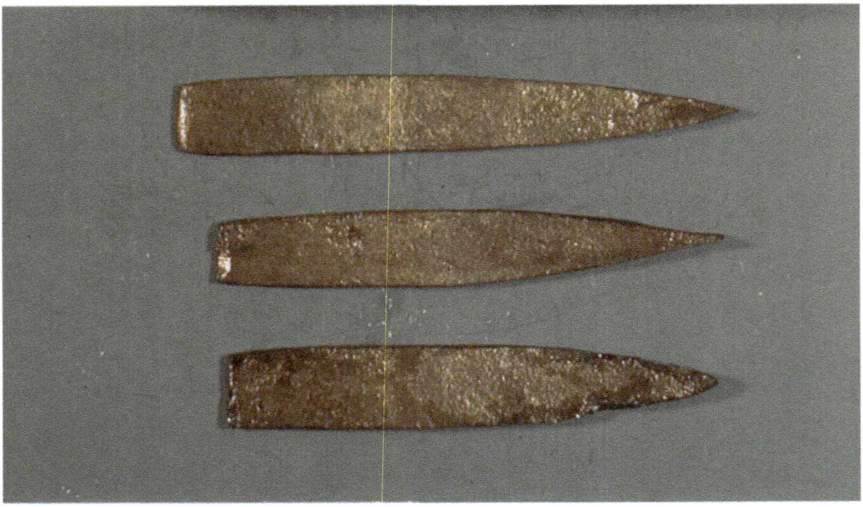

Plate 18. Three copper graves ('pointed knife'). Excavated by Petrie at Kahun and designated as foundation deposits. 12th Dynasty. Petrie Museum of Egyptian Archaeology, UC16134 (courtesy of the Petrie Museum of Egyptian and Sudanese Archaeology).

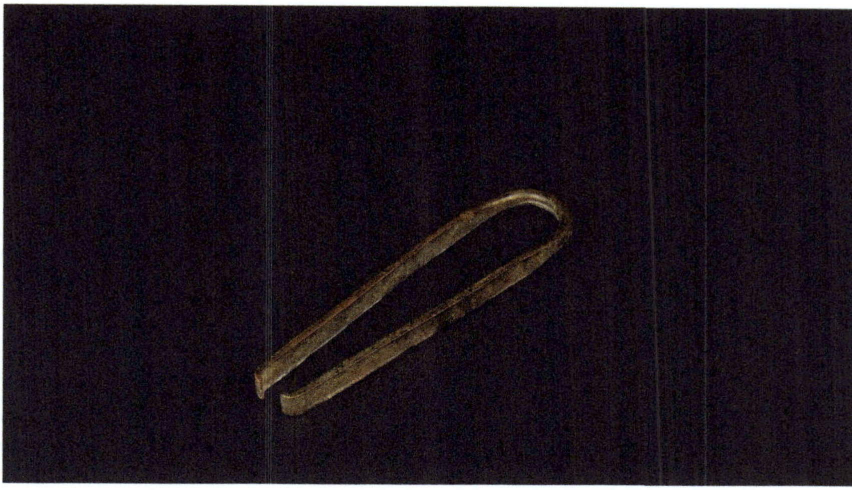

Plate 19. Bronze forceps with wide jaws used perhaps as a medical instrument, an embalming tool or a cosmetic implement. 17/18th Dynasty. From the Iseum, Savaria. Roman Period. Savaria Museum, Szombathely, Hungary Ltsz: 60:48:88 (courtesy of Savaria Museum – Iseum Savariense).

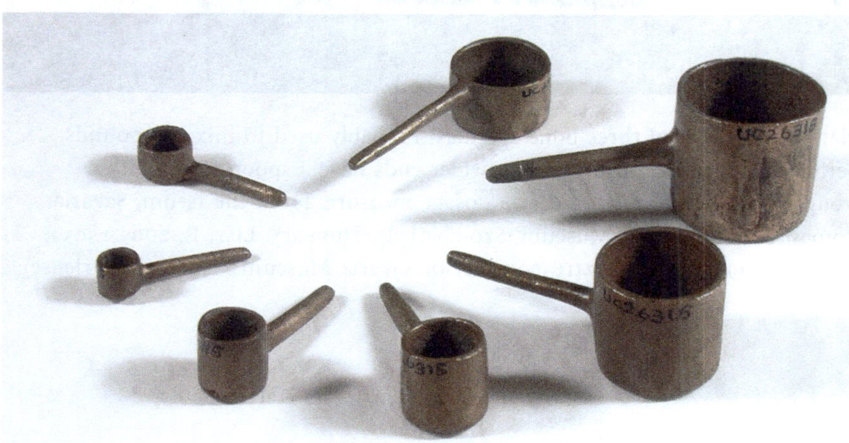

Plate 20. Seven cylindrical bronze measures with handles. Largest = 1/2 deben, H. 19mm; D. 20mm. Smallest 1/128 deben, H. 5mm; D. 5mm. Found at Kom Ombo by Petrie. 18th Dynasty. Petrie Museum of Egyptian Archaeology, UC26315 (courtesy of the Petrie Museum of Egyptian and Sudanese Archaeology).

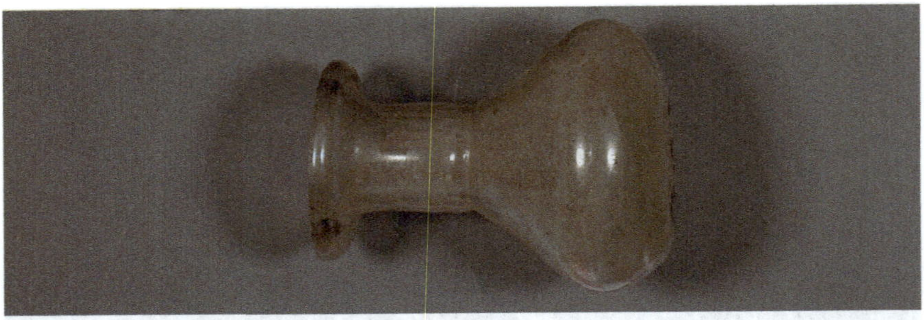

Plate 21. Glass flask with a conical body, heavy brim and flattened base. Perhaps used to store pharamaceutical preparations or cosmetics. Dated about AD 100–300. Petrie Museum of Egyptian Archaeology, UC22009 (courtesy of the Petrie Museum of Egyptian and Sudanese Archaeology).

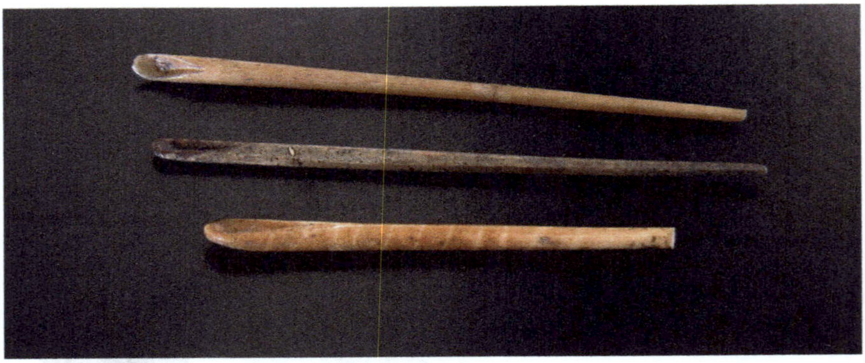

Plate 22. A group of three bone spatulas. Probably used to mix compounds, perhaps for medical purposes. The wider ends have a spoon shape with a trough-like cut probably used as a dosage measure. From the Iseum, Savaria. Roman Period. Savaria Museum, Szombathely, Hungary. Ltsz: R. 2009.2.5050; R. 2009.2.5198; R. 2009.2.7413 (courtesy of Savaria Museum – Iseum Savariense).

Plate 24 (opposite). Prosthetic device found attached to the right foot of a female mummy retrieved in parts from the burial chamber of a looted shaft tomb in Theban Tomb No. 95, Sheikh ʻAbd el-Qurna/Western Thebes. Third Intermediate Period/Late Period. Now housed in the National Museum of Egyptian Civilization, Cairo JE100016a (courtesy of the University of Basel, Project Life Histories of Theban Tombs. Photographer: Matjaž Kačičnik).

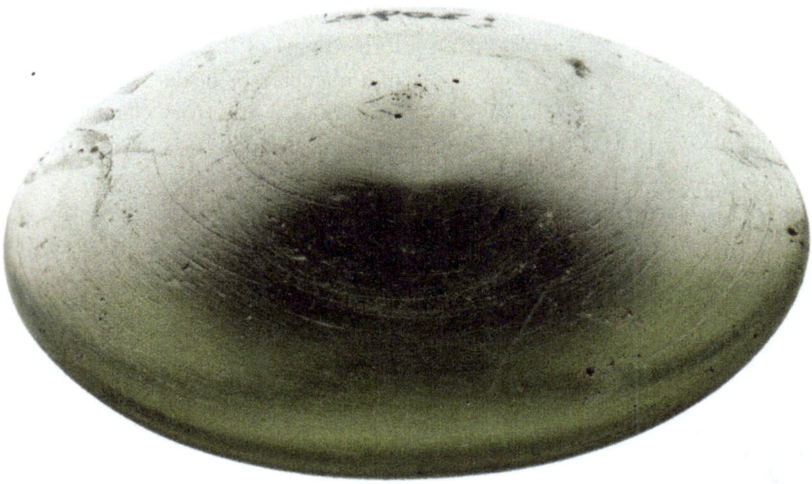

Plate 23. Glass convex lens, perhaps for magnification in reading documents or performing complex tasks such as medical procedures. Discovered at Hawara by Petrie in the 1880s. Roman, dating to the 1st century AD. Manchester Museum, 2090 (courtesy of The Manchester Museum, The University of Manchester).

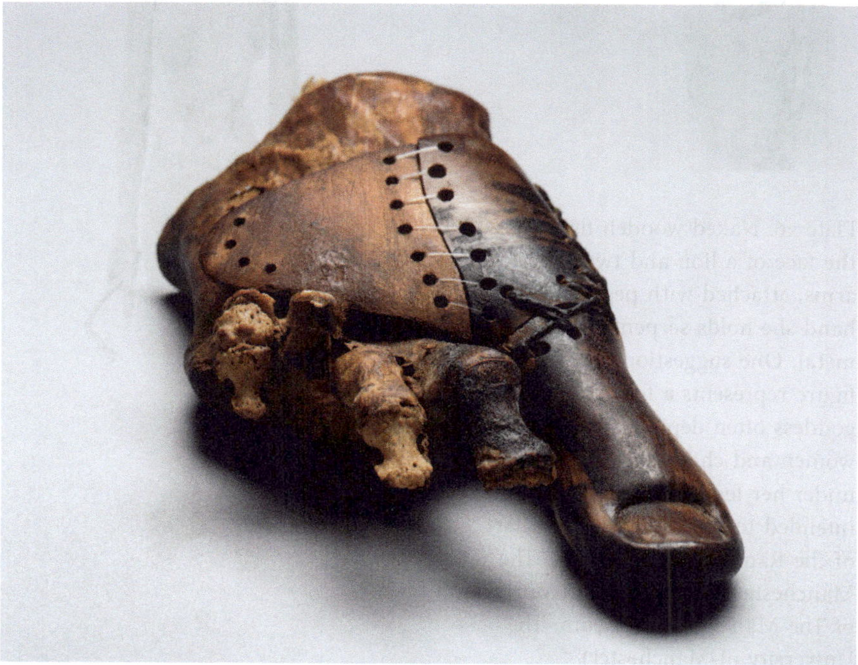

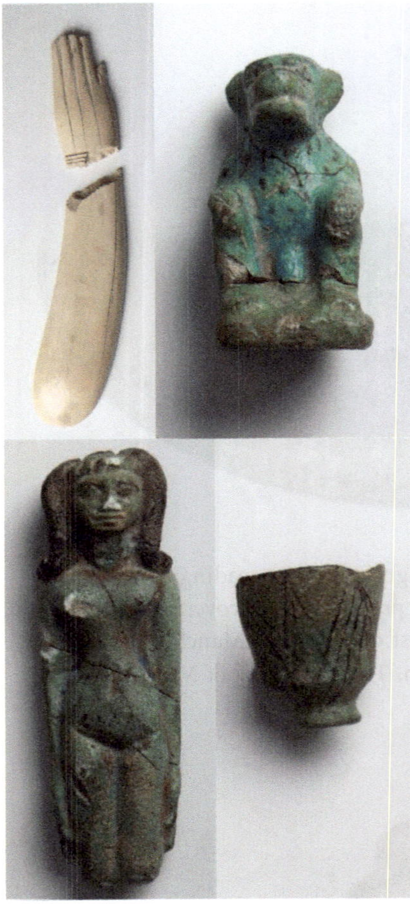

Plate 25. Items from the 'Ramesseum collection'. These artefacts may have formed part of the ritual equipment of a magician or healer. Clockwise from the left are: ivory clapper, 1796A; squatting baboon, 1835; miniature blue faience shaped cup, 1791; female fertility figurine, 1789. The Manchester Museum (courtesy of The Manchester Museum, The University of Manchester).

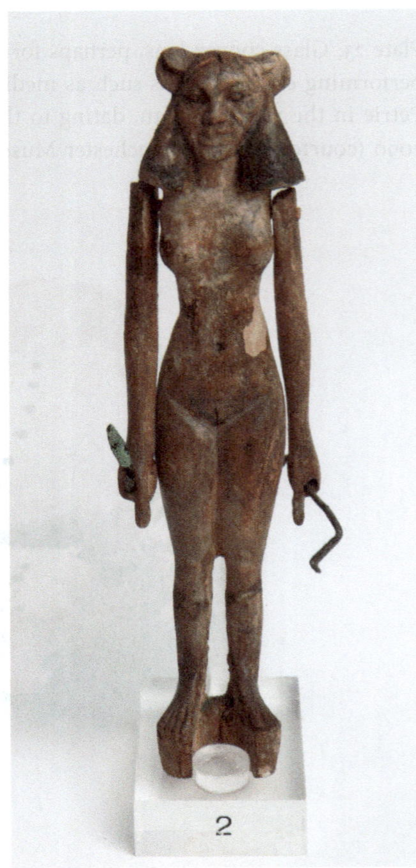

Plate 26. Naked wooden figurine with the face of a lion and two movable arms, attached with pegs. In each hand she holds serpents made of metal. One suggestion is that the figure represents a female Bes, a goddess often depicted as protecting women and children. Pieces of wood under her feet suggest that she was intended to stand on a plinth. Part of the Ramesseum collection. The Manchester Museum, 1790 (courtesy of The Manchester Museum, The University of Manchester).

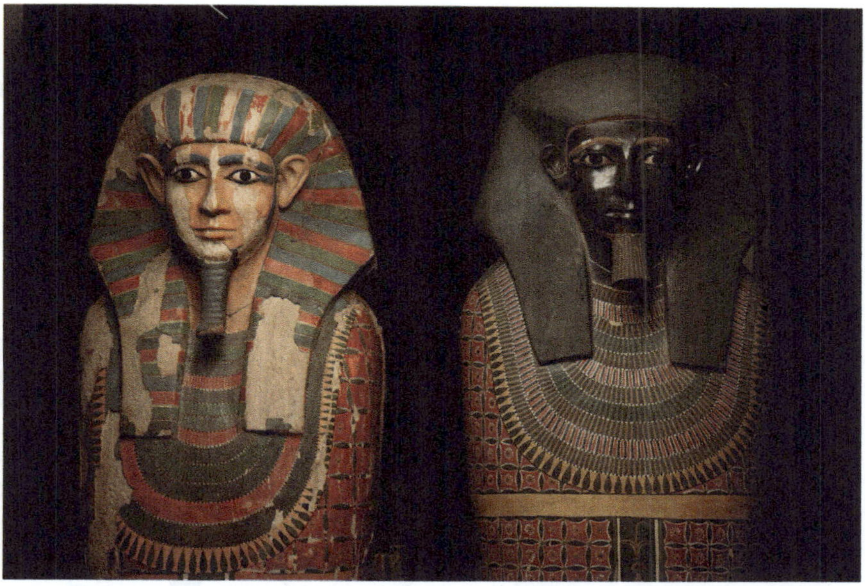

Plate 27. Painted wooden coffins of the Two Brothers, Nakht-ankh (left) and Khnum-Nakht. Studies on these mummies showed that the brothers suffered from several diseases, including sand pneumoconiosis and parasitic infestations. 12th Dynasty. From the Tomb of Two Brothers, Rifeh, now in The Manchester Museum, 4739, 4740 (courtesy of The Manchester Museum, The University of Manchester).

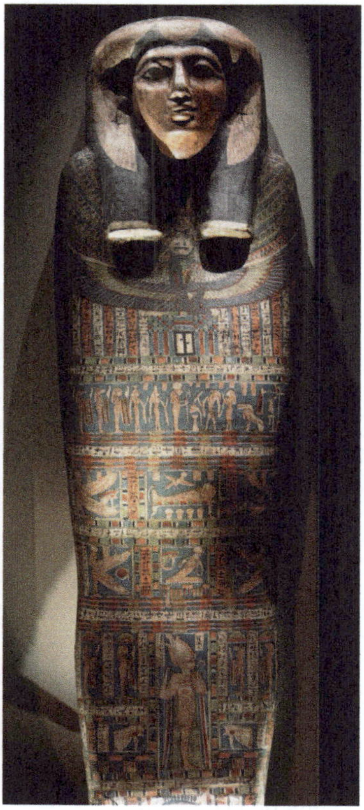

Plate 28. Painted wooden coffin of Asru, a Chantress in the Temple of Amun at Karnak. Scientific studies of the mummy indicate that she suffered from a range of parasitic and other diseases. Her estimated age at death, between fifty and sixty years, exceeded the normal lifespan. Late Period. Probably from Thebes, now in The Manchester Museum, 1777 (courtesy of The Manchester Museum, The University of Manchester).

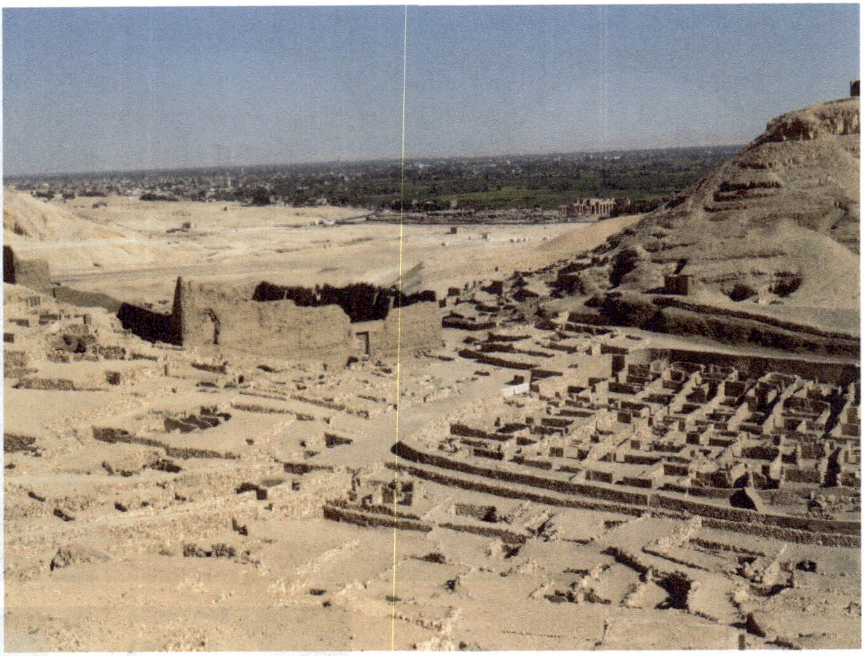

Plate 29. View of mudbrick houses in the Royal Workers' town at Deir el-Medina. New Kingdom. Living in close proximity to neighbours would have encouraged the spread of disease (courtesy of K. N. White).

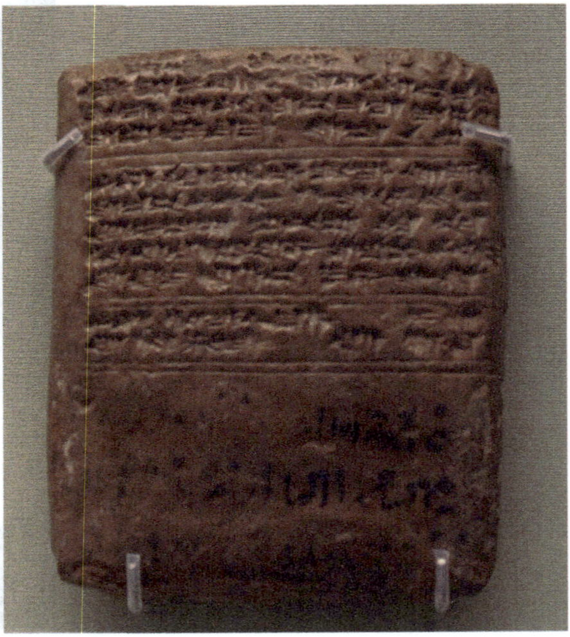

Plate 30. Amarna letter EA 23 (reverse). A communication from Tushratta of Mitanni to Amenhotep III of Egypt, about the possibility of the statue of goddess Ishtar of Nineveh being sent to Egypt. 18th Dynasty. Clay. British Museum (Wikipedia, Public Domain. Photographer: Zunkir).

Plate 31. Granite statue of Sekhmet, goddess of medicine, one of many erected during the reign of Amenhotep III (18th Dynasty), possibly as a response to plague in Egypt. Precinct of Mut, Temple of Karnak (courtesy of K. N. White).

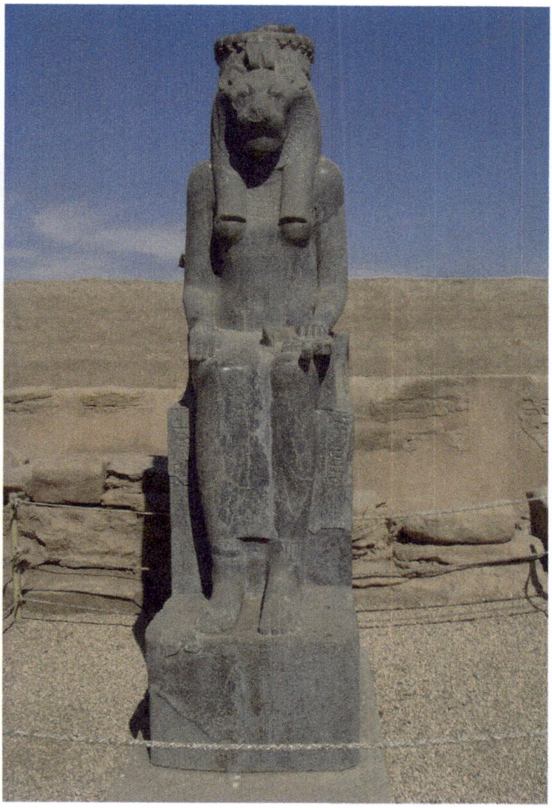

Plate 32. A histological skin specimen showing what is considered to be haemorrhagic smallpox in a child mummy (E: individual blood cells; M: a heavy deposit of melanin in the basal layer) (courtesy of KNH Centre for Biomedical Egyptology, The University of Manchester).

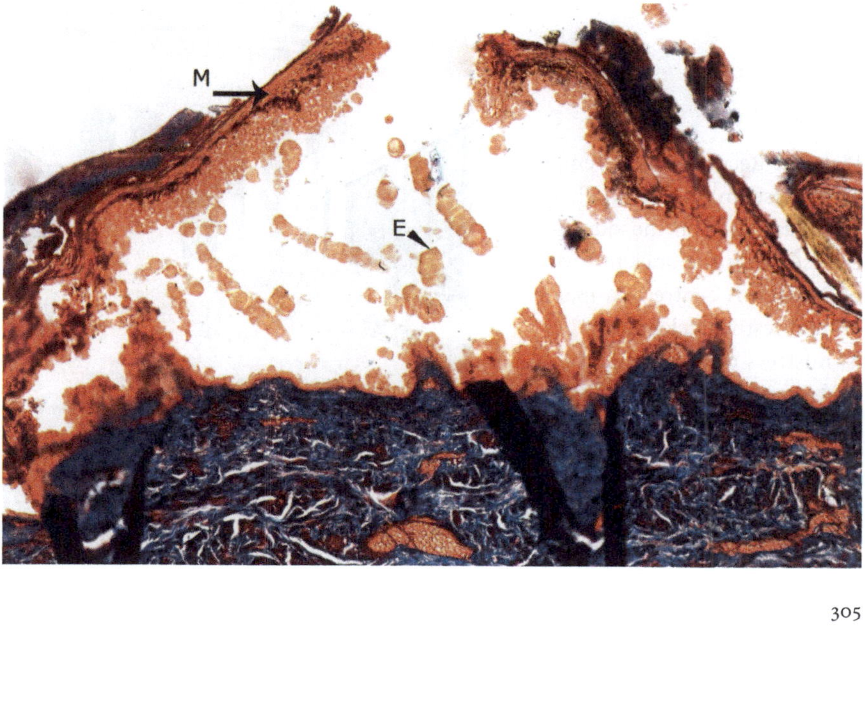

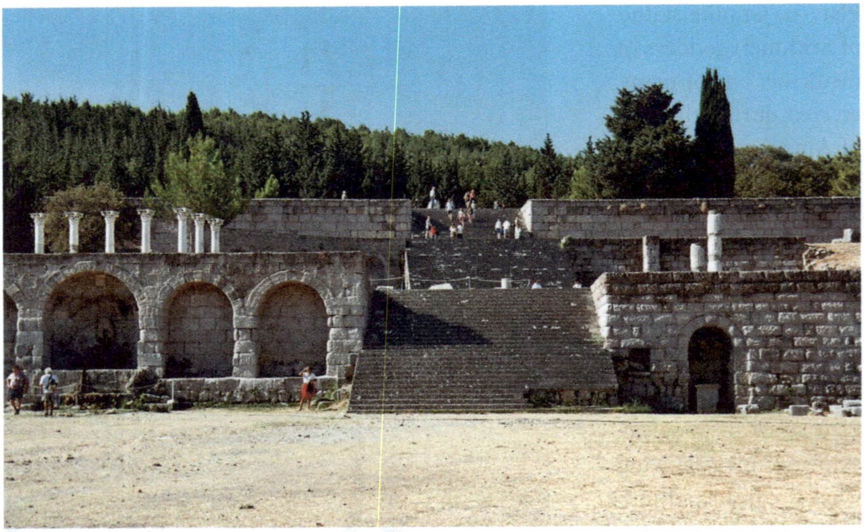

Plate 33. Panoramic view from the Asculapion on the island of Kos. This cult-centre for the Greek god of medicine, Asclepius, incorporated a main sanctuary and a self-contained area for healing procedures including incubation. Similar treatments were offered at the Temple of Hathor at Denderah. 4th century BC to 4th century AD (Wikipedia, Public Domain. Photographer: Briantist).

Plate 34. Reconstructed Temple of Isis (Iseum) at Szombothely, Hungary, built on the site of the Iseum in the ancient town of Savaria. A centre of a major annual festival celebrating Isis as mistress of the seas and protectress of rulers and peoples of the Roman Empire. Surgical instruments found at the site indicate that it was a sanctuary for medical treatment (courtesy of K. N. White).

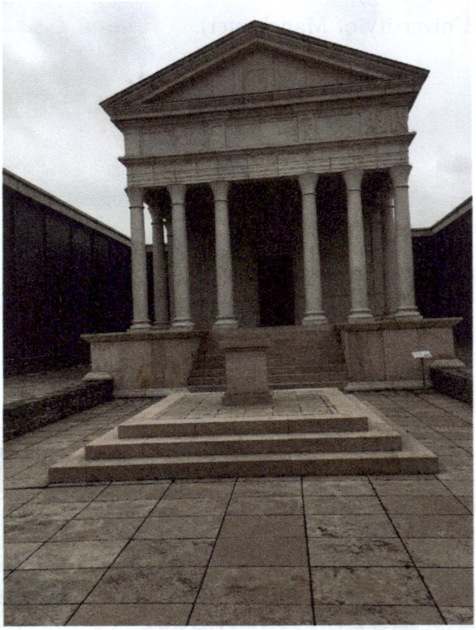

Printed and bound by CPI Group (UK) Ltd, Croydon, CR0 4YY
13/09/2026
14961100-0001